D1345256

Practical MR Imaging in the Head and Neck

Guest Editor

LAURIE A. LOEVNER, MD

MAGNETIC RESONANCE IMAGING CLINICS OF NORTH AMERICA

www.mri.theclinics.com

Consulting Editors
VIVIAN S. LEE, MD, PhD, MBA
LYNNE STEINBACH, MD
SURESH K. MUKHERJI, MD, FACR

August 2012 • Volume 20 • Number 3

SAUNDERS an imprint of ELSEVIER, Inc.

W.B. SAUNDERS COMPANY
A Division of Elsevier Inc.

1600 John F. Kennedy Boulevard • Suite 1800 • Philadelphia, Pennsylvania 19103-2899

http://www.theclinics.com

MRI CLINICS OF NORTH AMERICA Volume 20, Number 3
August 2012 ISSN 1064-9689, ISBN 13: 978-1-4557-4699-6

Editor: Sarah Barth
Developmental Editor: Donald Mumford

Magnetic Resonance Imaging Clinics of North America (ISSN 1064-9689) is published quarterly by Elsevier Inc., 360 Park Avenue South, New York, NY 10010-1710. Months of issue are February, May, August, and November. Business and Editorial Offices: 1600 John F. Kennedy Blvd., Ste. 1800, Philadelphia, PA 19103-2899. Customer Service Office: 3251 Riverport Lane, Maryland Heights, MO 63043. Periodicals postage paid at New York, NY and additional mailing offices. Subscription prices are $337.00 per year (domestic individuals), $541.00 per year (domestic institutions), $172.00 per year (domestic students/residents), $376.00 per year (Canadian individuals), $678.00 per year (Canadian institutions), $488.00 per year (international individuals), $678.00 per year (international institutions), and $249.00 per year (international and Canadian students/residents). International air speed delivery is included in all *Clinics* subscription prices. All prices are subject to change without notice. **POSTMASTER:** Send address changes to *Magnetic Resonance Imaging Clinics*, Elsevier Health Sciences Division, Subscription Customer Service, 3251 Riverport Lane, Maryland Heights, MO 63043. Customer Service (orders, claims, online, change of address): Elsevier Health Sciences Division, Subscription Customer Service, 3251 Riverport Lane, Maryland Heights, MO 63043. Tel:1-800-654-2452 (U.S. and Canada); 314-447-8871 (outside U.S. and Canada). Fax: 314-447-8029. E-mail: journalscustomerservice-usa@elsevier.com (for print support); journalsonlinesupport-usa@elsevier.com (for online support).

Reprints. For copies of 100 or more of articles in this publication, please contact the Commercial Reprints Department, Elsevier Inc., 360 Park Avenue South, New York, NY 10010-1710. Tel.: 212-633-3812; Fax: 212-462-1935; E-mail: reprints@elsevier.com.

Magnetic Resonance Imaging Clinics of North America is covered in the *RSNA Index of Imaging Literature, MEDLINE/PubMed (Index Medicus),* and *EMBASE/Excerpta Medica.*

Printed in the United States of America.

GOAL STATEMENT

The goal of *Magnetic Resonance Imaging Clinics of North America* is to keep practicing physicians up to date with current clinical practice by providing timely articles reviewing the state of the art in patient care.

ACCREDITATION

The *Magnetic Resonance Imaging Clinics of North America* is planned and implemented in accordance with the Essential Areas and Policies of the Accreditation Council for Continuing Medical Education (ACCME) through the joint sponsorship of the University of Virginia School of Medicine and Elsevier. The University of Virginia School of Medicine is accredited by the ACCME to provide continuing medical education for physicians.

The University of Virginia School of Medicine designates this enduring material activity for a maximum of 15 *AMA PRA Category 1 Credit*(s)™ for each issue, 60 credits per year. Physicians should claim only the credit commensurate with the extent of their participation in the activity.

The American Medical Association has determined that physicians not licensed in the US who participate in this CME enduring material activity are eligible for a maximum of **15** *AMA PRA Category 1 Credit*(s)™ for each issue, 60 credits per year.

Credit can be earned by reading the text material, taking the CME examination online at http://www.theclinics.com/home/cme, and completing the evaluation. After taking the test, you will be required to review any and all incorrect answers. Following completion of the test and evaluation, your credit will be awarded and you may print your certificate.

FACULTY DISCLOSURE/CONFLICT OF INTEREST

The University of Virginia School of Medicine, as an ACCME accredited provider, endorses and strives to comply with the Accreditation Council for Continuing Medical Education (ACCME) Standards of Commercial Support, Commonwealth of Virginia statutes, University of Virginia policies and procedures, and associated federal and private regulations and guidelines on the need for disclosure and monitoring of proprietary and financial interests that may affect the scientific integrity and balance of content delivered in continuing medical education activities under our auspices.

The University of Virginia School of Medicine requires that all CME activities accredited through this institution be developed independently and be scientifically rigorous, balanced and objective in the presentation/discussion of its content, theories and practices.

All authors/editors participating in an accredited CME activity are expected to disclose to the readers relevant financial relationships with commercial entities occurring within the past 12 months (such as grants or research support, employee, consultant, stock holder, member of speakers bureau, etc.). The University of Virginia School of Medicine will employ appropriate mechanisms to resolve potential conflicts of interest to maintain the standards of fair and balanced education to the reader. Questions about specific strategies can be directed to the Office of Continuing Medical Education, University of Virginia School of Medicine, Charlottesville, Virginia.

The faculty and staff of the University of Virginia Office of Continuing Medical Education have no financial affiliations to disclose.

The authors/editors listed below have identified no professional or financial affiliations for themselves or their spouse/partner:
Ashley Aiken, MD; Sarah Barth, (Acquisitions Editor); Douglas C. Bigelow, MD; Larissa T. Bilaniuk, MD; Gary Bouloux, MD, DDS; Mary Beth Cunnane, MD; Eduard de Lange, MD (Test Author); Kevin Emerick, MD; Lindell R. Gentry, MD; Christine M. Glastonbury, MBBS; Mari Hagiwara, MD; Michael J. Hartman, MD; Ellen Hoeffner, MD; Ken Kazahaya, MD; Robert Kersten, MD; Stephen F. Kralik, MD; Kim O. Learned, MD; Vivian S. Lee, MD, PhD, MBA (Consulting Editor); Kelly M. Malloy, MD; David M. Mirsky, MD, MBA; Suyash Mohan, MD, PDCC; Gul Moonis, MD; Brian L. Schmidt, MD, DDS, PhD; Karuna V. Shekdar, MD; and Richard H. Wiggins, MD III.

The authors/editors listed below identified the following professional or financial affiliations for themselves or their spouse/partner:
Brian M. Chin, MD, MBA authors and edits cases and chapters for Amirsys, Inc.
Hugh Curtin, MD is a consultant for WorldCare.
Christine M. Glastonbury, MBBS is a consultant and is on the Advisory Board for AMIRSYS, INC.
Patricia Hudgins, MD is a consultant, is on the Advisory Board, and is a stockholder for AMIRSYS, Inc.
Laurie A. Loevner, MD (Guest Editor) owns stock in GE.
Suresh Mukherji, MD (Consulting Editor) is a consultant for Philips Medical Systems.
Annette Nusbaum, MD is on the Advisory Board for Giffen Solutions, Inc.
Richard R. Orlandi, MD is a consultant for Entellus and Medtronic.
Lynne Steinbach, MD (Consulting Editor) is a consultant for Pfizer, Inc.

Disclosure of Discussion of non-FDA approved uses for pharmaceutical products and/or medical devices:
The University of Virginia School of Medicine, as an ACCME provider, requires that all faculty presenters identify and disclose any "off label" uses for pharmaceutical and medical device products. The University of Virginia School of Medicine recommends that each physician fully review all the available data on new products or procedures prior to instituting them with patients.

TO ENROLL

To enroll in the Magnetic Resonance Imaging Clinics of North America Continuing Medical Education program, call customer service at 1-800-654-2452 or visit us online at www.theclinics.com/home/cme. The CME program is available to subscribers for an additional fee of $196.00.

Contributors

CONSULTING EDITORS

VIVIAN S. LEE, MD, PhD, MBA
Professor of Radiology, Physiology, and
Neurosciences; Vice-Dean for Science; Senior
Vice-President and Chief Scientific Officer,
New York University Langone Medical Center,
New York, New York

LYNNE STEINBACH, MD
Professor of Clinical Radiology and
Orthopaedic Surgery, University of California
San Francisco, San Francisco, California

SURESH K. MUKHERJI, MD, FACR
Professor and Chief of Neuroradiology and
Head and Neck Radiology; Professor of
Radiology, Otolaryngology–Head Neck
Surgery, Radiation Oncology, Periodontics and
Oral Medicine, University of Michigan Health
System, Ann Arbor, Michigan

GUEST EDITOR

LAURIE A. LOEVNER, MD
Professor of Radiology, Otorhinolaryngology:
Head & Neck Surgery, and Neurosurgery,
Director of Head and Neck Imaging,
Department of Radiology, Division of
Neuroradiology, University of Pennsylvania
School of Medicine, Philadelphia, Pennsylvania

AUTHORS

ASHLEY AIKEN, MD
Assistant Professor, Neuroradiology Division,
Department of Radiology and Imaging
Sciences, Emory University School of
Medicine, Atlanta, Georgia

DOUGLAS C. BIGELOW, MD
Associate Professor of Otorhinolaryngology:
Head and Neck Surgery, University of
Pennsylvania School of Medicine, Philadelphia,
Pennsylvania

LARISSA T. BILANIUK, MD
Professor of Radiology, Assistant Chair,
Division of Neuroradiology, Department
of Radiology, The Children's Hospital of
Philadelphia, Perelman School of Medicine at
the University of Pennsylvania, Philadelphia,
Pennsylvania

GARY BOULOUX, MD, DDS
Chief of Service for Oral and Maxillofacial
Surgery, Division of Surgery, Assistant
Professor, Department of Oral Surgery,
Emory University School of Medicine; Director
of Clinical Research, Grady Memorial Hospital,
Atlanta, Georgia

BRIAN M. CHIN, MD, MBA
Department of Radiology, University of Utah,
Salt Lake City, Utah

MARY BETH CUNNANE, MD
Department of Radiology, Massachusetts Eye
and Ear Infirmary, Boston, Massachusetts

HUGH CURTIN, MD
Department of Radiology, Massachusetts Eye
and Ear Infirmary, Boston, Massachusetts

KEVIN EMERICK, MD
Department of Otorhinolaryngology,
Massachusetts Eye and Ear Infirmary, Boston,
Massachusetts

LINDELL R. GENTRY, MD
Professor of Radiology, Department of
Radiology, University of Wisconsin Hospital,
Madison, Wisconsin

CHRISTINE M. GLASTONBURY, MBBS
Professor of Radiology, University of California
San Francisco, San Francisco, California

MARI HAGIWARA, MD
Assistant Professor, Department of Radiology,
New York University School of Medicine,
New York, New York

MICHAEL J. HARTMAN, MD
Assistant Professor of Radiology, Department
of Radiology, University of Wisconsin Hospital,
Madison, Wisconsin

ELLEN HOEFFNER, MD
Clinical Associate Professor, Neuroradiology,
Department of Radiology, University of
Michigan Health System, Ann Arbor, Michigan

PATRICIA HUDGINS, MD
Professor, Neuroradiology Division,
Department of Radiology and Imaging
Sciences, Emory University School of
Medicine, Atlanta, Georgia

KEN KAZAHAYA, MD, MBA, FACS
Associate Director, Division of Pediatric
Otolaryngology, The Children's Hospital of
Philadelphia, Associate Professor of Clinical
Otorhinolaryngology/Head and Neck Surgery,
Perelman School of Medicine at the University
of Pennsylvania, Philadelphia, Pennsylvania

ROBERT KERSTEN, MD
Professor of Clinical Ophthalmology,
Ophthalmic Plastic and Reconstructive
Surgery, University of California,
San Francisco, San Francisco, California

STEPHEN F. KRALIK, MD
Assistant Professor of Radiology, Department
of Radiology, Riley Hospital for Children,
Indiana University School of Medicine,
Indianapolis, Indiana

KIM O. LEARNED, MD
Assistant Professor, Neuroradiology Division,
Department of Radiology, University of
Pennsylvania Health System, University of
Pennsylvania Perelman School of Medicine,
Hospital of the University of Pennsylvania,
Philadelphia, Pennsylvania

LAURIE A. LOEVNER, MD
Professor of Radiology, Otorhinolaryngology:
Head & Neck Surgery, and Neurosurgery,
Director of Head and Neck Imaging,
Department of Radiology, Division of
Neuroradiology, University of Pennsylvania
School of Medicine, Philadelphia, Pennsylvania

KELLY M. MALLOY, MD
Assistant Professor, Department of
Otorhinolaryngology–Head and Neck Surgery,
Hospital of the University of Pennsylvania,
University of Pennsylvania Perelman School
of Medicine, Philadelphia, Pennsylvania

DAVID M. MIRSKY, MD
Clinical Instructor, Division of Neuroradiology,
Department of Radiology, The Children's
Hospital of Philadelphia, Perelman School of
Medicine at the University of Pennsylvania,
Philadelphia, Pennsylvania

SUYASH MOHAN, MD, PDCC
Assistant Professor of Radiology, Division of
Neuroradiology, Department of Radiology,
University of Pennsylvania School of Medicine,
Philadelphia

GUL MOONIS, MD
Department of Radiology, Massachusetts Eye
and Ear Infirmary; Department of Radiology,
Beth Israel Deaconess Medical Center,
Boston, Massachusetts

ANNETTE NUSBAUM, MD
Assistant Professor, Department of Radiology,
New York University School of Medicine,
New York, New York

RICHARD R. ORLANDI, MD
Department of Otolaryngology, Head and Neck
Surgery, University of Utah, Salt Lake City, Utah

BRIAN L. SCHMIDT, DDS, MD, PhD
Professor, Department of Oral & Maxillofacial
Surgery, Director, Bluestone Center for Clinical
Research, New York University College of
Dentistry, New York, New York

KARUNA V. SHEKDAR, MD
Assistant Professor of Radiology, Division of
Neuroradiology, Department of Radiology, The
Children's Hospital of Philadelphia, Perelman
School of Medicine at the University of
Pennsylvania, Philadelphia, Pennsylvania

RICHARD H. WIGGINS III, MD
Department of Radiology; Department
of Otolaryngology, Head and Neck
Surgery; and Department of BioMedical
Informatics, University of Utah,
Salt Lake City, Utah

Contents

> MR imaging allows detailed evaluation of temporomandibular (TMJ) anatomy be-
> cause of its inherent tissue contrast and high resolution. Joint biomechanics can
> be assessed through imaging patients in the closed and open jaw positions. Despite
> the accuracy of MR imaging in detecting disc position, results must be interpreted
> together with clinical findings, because an anteriorly displaced disc can be seen in
> up to one-third of asymptomatic patients, and a normal disc position can be seen
> in up to one-quarter of symptomatic patients. Interpretation of MR imaging requires
> knowledge of the normal anatomy and an understanding of normal and abnormal
> biomechanics.

> A wide range of orbital disorders, including an orbital mass, infection, inflammation,
> systemic disease, or intracranial lesions, may be encountered with imaging. Evalu-
> ation of orbital disorders requires the combination of accurate and relevant clinical
> information with an understanding of anatomy and pathologic processes. An imag-
> ing approach to an orbital differential diagnosis includes assessment for alteration of
> a normal orbital structure, a lesion that does not belong in the orbit, or alteration of
> the orbit from bone or periorbital disorders. This approach, combined with key
> elements of clinical history, leads to a narrower differential diagnosis and improved
> patient care.

> Perineural tumor spread (PNS) is a mode of neoplastic spread whereby tumor cells
> use neural conduits to escape the borders of a primary tumor. MRI is generally
> favored over CT for evaluating PNS, and findings include obliteration of fat within
> skull base foramina, enlargement and enhancement of the involved nerves, and
> enlargement and destruction of the bony foramina. Careful examination of the entire
> course of the nerve allows detection of skip lesions. Recognition of the complete
> extent of PNS is crucial for correct treatment because it facilitates both surgical
> and radiotherapy targeting of entire extent of disease.

> Although uncommon, sinonasal malignancies and aggressive inflammatory pro-
> cesses are entities every radiologist will encounter during the evaluation of routine
> sinus imaging studies. A high index of suspicion is necessary for prompt diagnosis.
> It is important to consider aggressive inflammatory disease in all patients having

routine sinus computed tomography because any delay in diagnosis can adversely affect the patients' care. Magnetic resonance (MR) will often provide a better assessment of the lesion extent, allowing for better surgical treatment. MR is crucial for the accurate assessment of neoplastic lesions. A proficient understanding of the complex anatomy of the region is essential.

MR Assessment of Oral Cavity Carcinomas

Mari Hagiwara, Annette Nusbaum, and Brian L. Schmidt

Approximately half of head and neck carcinomas arise from the oral cavity. Imaging plays an essential role in the preoperative evaluation of oral cavity carcinomas. MR imaging is particularly advantageous in the evaluation of the oral cavity, with better depiction of the anatomy in this region and reduction of dental artifacts compared with CT. MR is also the preferred imaging modality for the evaluation of bone marrow invasion and perineural tumor spread, which are findings critical for treatment planning. Advanced MR imaging techniques may potentially better delineate true tumor extent, determine lymph node metastases, and predict treatment response.

Myocutaneous Flaps and Other Vascularized Grafts in Head and Neck Reconstruction for Cancer Treatment

Kim O. Learned, Kelly M. Malloy, and Laurie A. Loevner

This article addresses the clinical evaluation and some of the more common flaps and grafts used to reconstruct the surgical bed after excision of primary head and neck cancers and nodal metastases. This focused summary is intended to enhance the reader's understanding and improve the interpretation of posttreatment MR imaging. A practical approach to MR imaging evaluation of the postoperative reconstructed neck is presented. Readers of this article will become familiar with the normal appearances of commonly used flaps, recognize common complications, be able to delineate residual and recurrent neoplasm, and learn to avoid interpretative pitfalls.

Evaluation of the Sellar and Parasellar Regions

Brian M. Chin, Richard R. Orlandi, and Richard H. Wiggins III

The article reviews the anatomy and imaging evaluation of the sellar and parasellar regions. Both common and uncommon sellar and suprasellar masses are reviewed, focusing on a systematic approach to analysis and when appropriate, differential creation.

Applications of Magnetic Resonance Imaging in Adult Temporal Bone Disorders

Suyash Mohan, Ellen Hoeffner, Douglas C. Bigelow, and Laurie A. Loevner

Magnetic resonance (MR) imaging has new applications in the assessment of temporal bone disorders. This article summarizes current MR imaging applications in evaluating adult temporal bone lesions according to their location, beginning from the most common indication, vestibular schwannoma. Inner ear lesions, petrous lesions, and middle ear lesions are discussed, including the role of diffusion-weighted imaging in cholesteatomas, external ear lesions, and a few systemic conditions. Although this article emphasizes the role of MR imaging, the diagnostic value of computed tomography scan associated with MR imaging is also stressed. The main indications of temporal bone MR imaging are summarized.

Evaluation of neck lesions in the pediatric population can be a diagnostic challenge, for which magnetic resonance (MR) imaging is extremely valuable. This article provides an overview of the value and utility of MR imaging in the evaluation of pediatric neck lesions, addressing what the referring clinician requires from the radiologist. Concise descriptions and illustrations of MR imaging findings of commonly encountered pathologic entities in the pediatric neck, including abnormalities of the branchial apparatus, thyroglossal duct anomalies, and neoplastic processes, are given. An approach to establishing a differential diagnosis is provided, and critical points of information are summarized.

Abnormalities of the fetal head and neck may be seen in isolation or in association with central nervous system abnormalities, chromosomal abnormalities, and syndromes. Magnetic resonance imaging (MRI) plays an important role in detecting associated abnormalities of the brain as well as in evaluating for airway obstruction that may impact prenatal management and delivery planning. This article provides an overview of the common indications for MRI of the fetal head and neck, including abnormalities of the fetal skull and face, masses of the face and neck, and fetal goiter.

MAGNETIC RESONANCE IMAGING CLINICS OF NORTH AMERICA

FORTHCOMING ISSUES

Contrast Agents
Juan E. Gutierrez, MD, and
Marco Essig, MD, *Guest Editors*

MR Imaging of Hip Disorders
Miriam Bredella, MD, *Guest Editor*

Modern Imaging Evaluation of the Brain, Body, and Spine
Lara Brandão, MD, *Guest Editor*

RECENT ISSUES

May 2012
MRI of the Shoulder
Jenny Bencardino, MD, *Guest Editor*

February 2012
MRI of the Newborn, Part 2
Claudia M. Hillenbrand, PhD, and
Thierry A.G.M. Huisman, MD, *Guest Editors*

November 2011
MRI of the Newborn, Part 1
Thierry A.G.M. Huisman, MD, and
Claudia M. Hillenbrand, PhD, *Guest Editors*

RELATED INTEREST

PET Clinics, October 2012
Head and Neck PET Imaging
Min Yao, MD, PhD, and Peter F. Faulhaber, MD, *Guest Editors*

Preface

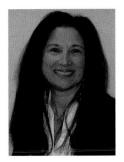

Laurie A. Loevner, MD
Guest Editor

It was a pleasure to synthesize and edit this issue of *Magnetic Resonance Imaging Clinics*, which focuses on state-of-the-art timely applications of MRI in evaluating pathology affecting the neck. It is titled "Practical MR Imaging in the Head and Neck," which accurately reflects its contents thanks to the significant contributions of so many talented authors and coauthors. This issue illustrates the knowledge and dedicated efforts of many of our young investigators and clinicians. Every article's "leading author" is an assistant professor, and each was closely paired with some of our most nationally and internationally recognized head and neck neuroradiologists known for their expertise in selected areas as coauthors. Every article also includes valuable input and coauthorship from our clinical colleagues, subspecialists in related disciplines. I have tried to focus this edition on anatomic locations and disease processes in the neck and skull base that MR imaging in particular provides in the way of valuable diagnostic information. In addition, emerging technologies such as fetal MRI in head and neck pathology are addressed. The authors in this issue cover the continent from east to west with stops in the mid-sections too and the issue reflects the outstanding work from many wonderful academic institutions. This issue is multidisciplinary, reflecting the essential teamwork required to adequately diagnose and treat diseases of the head and neck.

The opening article addresses one of the hidden, overlooked areas of the skull base, the TMJ. Dr Aiken and her coauthors provide an organized approach to evaluating pathology and radiologic mimics affecting these joints. The MRI illustrations of pathology are wonderful, and the wording is carefully chosen to provide a clear and succinct lesson you won't forget. Next, the orbits and optic pathways are covered, with attention to detail and the literature, by Drs Kralik and Glastonbury. The orbit article is well organized, providing a simplified algorithm for evaluating orbital pathology and the cranial nerves related to eye function, and it is illustrated by well-chosen MR images. In the third article, patterns of peineural spread in head and neck cancers are covered with great expertise and beautiful MR images by the combined efforts of its energetic first author Dr Moonis, and her colleagues Drs Cunnane and Curtin. Innervation never looked so easy.

The middle of this issue begins with a comprehensive, magnificently illustrated article by Drs Hartman and Gentry on aggressive inflammatory and neoplastic processes affecting the paranasal sinuses and nasal cavity illustrating the roles of MR and CT imaging in evaluating the ventral skull base. It is followed by another comprehensive, beautifully illustrated article by Dr Hagiwara and her colleagues on the assessment of oral cavity carcinoma with an emphasis on assessing disease extent and issues affecting resectability. The middle of the issue continues to build momentum with what I feel is one of the most succinct, well-organized, well-illustrated, practical articles on assessing myocutaneous flaps and other grafts in head and neck reconstruction following cancer surgery. Its leading author is my colleague, Dr Learned, with whom it is a pleasure to work with. She makes it look easy and interesting, reviewing surgical approaches, graft selection, and imaging evaluation.

The final articles of this issue are equally interesting and informative, addressing the central

Magn Reson Imaging Clin N Am 20 (2012) xiii–xiv
http://dx.doi.org/10.1016/j.mric.2012.07.001
1064-9689/12/$ – see front matter © 2012 Published by Elsevier Inc.

and posterior skull base, and finishing strong with two articles addressing head and neck MRI in the pediatric population. The sella and parasellar regions are covered with clarity and thoughtful attention to detail and anatomy of the sella and its surrounding areas by Dr Chin and coauthors. The images and illustrations are outstanding; they are worth a thousand words. Applications of MR imaging in temporal bone pathology are covered with clarity, depth, and organization by my wonderful colleague, Dr Mohan, and coauthors, who did a great job breaking the temporal bone down into its parts and exquisitely illustrating the role of MRI in assessing temporal bone pathology through well-chosen images that accurately reflect the content of this article. The last two articles in the issue focus on the MRI evaluation of children with head and neck masses, and the emerging technology of fetal MR imaging, respectively. They were mentored by Dr Bilaniuk, one of our greats in pediatric head and neck radiology. Dr Shedkar and colleagues provide a rational, comprehensive approach for evaluating children with neck masses, with patient safety also at the forefront. The article is beautifully illustrated with thoughtfully selected images and makes the pediatric neck look easy. The book closes with a final article on state-of-the-art MR imaging of children in utero. It is first-authored by Dr Mirsky, a rising

star of pediatric neuroradiology, and whom I had the pleasure and honor of working with during his fellowship at PENN and CHOP. He did a wonderful job introducing the technology and demonstrating the advantages of this emerging technology through well-selected, wonderful images. It was the perfect way to close this book.

Throughout this issue, neuroradiologists and a spectrum of subspecialized clinicians work together to provide a rational, interesting, thorough approach in the evaluation and multidisciplinary care of patients with head and neck pathology. I hope that you will find the pages that follow as informative and educational as I believe them to be. A special thank-you to all of the trainees—our fellows, residents, and medical students—who enlighten our careers through their inquisitive nature and keep us on our toes! I hope you enjoy reading this issue.

Laurie A. Loevner, MD
Department of Radiology
Division of Neuroradiology
University of Pennsylvania School of Medicine
3400 Spruce Street
Philadelphia, PA 19104, USA

E-mail address:
laurieloevner@aol.com

MR Imaging of the Temporomandibular Joint

Ashley Aiken, MD[a],[*], Gary Bouloux, MD, DDS[b,c,d],
Patricia Hudgins, MD[a]

KEYWORDS

- TMJ • Temporomandibular joint • Internal derangement • Articular disc • Osteoarthritis • MRI
- Synovial joint • Anterior displacement

KEY POINTS

- Internal derangement of the temporomandibular joint (TMJ) is very common.
- MR imaging is the preferred study for evaluating the TMJ.
- Key TMJ features to evaluate include disc position, disc morphology, condylar translation, presence of a joint effusion, and superimposed osteoarthritis.
- Disc position can be classified as normal, anteriorly displaced with recapture, and anteriorly displaced without recapture.
- MR imaging is also useful to exclude other diagnoses that may mimic internal derangement, including infection and inflammatory arthritis.

INTRODUCTION

Up to 20% to 30% of the population experiences pain related to the temporomandibular joint (TMJ), and 3% to 7% seek treatment.[1–3] TMJ disorder or dysfunction (TMD) is an umbrella term that encompasses several clinical entities that affect the TMJ, muscles of mastication, or both.[4] Internal derangement of the disc and joint mechanics is the most common of these various clinical diagnoses. Internal derangement of the TMJ is defined as an abnormal positional and functional relationship between the disc and articulating surfaces.[5] Common clinical symptoms include pain and joint sounds (clicking or crepitus), but joint sounds are nonspecific as they are found in up to 35.8% of asymptomatic persons under 18 years of age.[6] However, the clinical evaluation can be unreliable as many symptoms of internal derangement overlap with myofascial pain dysfunction, which is often a stress-related psychophysiologic disorder.[4,7,8] Therefore, MR imaging has become part of the standard evaluation of TMD. Less common entities affecting the TMJ include infection, trauma, neoplasm, and inflammatory arthritis.

MR imaging allows detailed evaluation of TMJ anatomy because of its inherent tissue contrast and high resolution using surface coils. MR also allows assessment of joint biomechanics through imaging patients in the closed and open jaw positions. Furthermore, a dynamic study can be obtained with cine MR imaging as the patient opens and closes the jaw.[4,9–11] Despite the sensitivity and specificity of MR imaging in detecting disc position, results must be interpreted together with clinical findings, because an anteriorly displaced disc can be seen in up to 34% of asymptomatic patients, and a normal disc position can be seen

[a] Department of Radiology and Imaging Sciences, Neuroradiology Division, Emory University School of Medicine, 1364 Clifton Road, Atlanta, GA 30322, USA; [b] Department of Oral Surgery, Emory University School of Medicine, 1364 Clifton Road, Atlanta, GA 30322, USA; [c] Division of Oral and Maxillofacial Surgery, Department of Surgery, Emory University School of Medicine, 1364 Clifton Road, Atlanta, GA 30322, USA; [d] Grady Memorial Hospital, The Emory Clinic 'B', 1364 Clifton Road, Atlanta, GA 30322, USA
* Corresponding author.
E-mail address: ashley.aiken@emoryhealthcare.org

Magn Reson Imaging Clin N Am 20 (2012) 397–412
http://dx.doi.org/10.1016/j.mric.2012.05.002
1064-9689/12/$ – see front matter © 2012 Elsevier Inc. All rights reserved.

in up to 23% of symptomatic patients.[12–15] Interpretation of MR imaging of the TMJ requires knowledge of the normal anatomy and an understanding of normal and abnormal biomechanics.

NORMAL ANATOMY

The TMJ is an unusual synovial joint in that the articular surfaces are covered with fibrocartilage rather than hyaline cartilage.[16] The articular capsule is attached to the edges of the glenoid fossa, including the articular tubercle, and to the neck of the mandible. The fibrocartilaginous articular disc, or meniscus, lies within the articular capsule between the mandibular condyle and glenoid fossa, dividing the synovial cavity into superior and inferior synovial compartments (**Fig. 1**). The lateral pterygoid muscle inserts anteriorly on the mandibular condyle at the pterygoid fovea and the anterior band of the disc.[17] The articular disc, or meniscus, is a biconcave avascular connective tissue structure composed of three segments: anterior band, intermediate zone, and posterior band.

The anterior and posterior bands are triangular in shape and connected by the thin intermediate zone. The anterior band is attached to the joint capsule, condylar head, and superior belly of the lateral pterygoid muscle, whereas the posterior band attaches to the bilaminar zone or retrodiscal tissue, which is a rich neurovascular tissue. The bilaminar zone, also known as the *posterior ligament*, provides stability to the disc by attaching the posterior band of the disc to the mandibular condyle and the temporal bone (see **Fig. 1**).[4]

MR Imaging

On sagittal MR imaging, the normal disc appears as a biconcave structure with homogenous low signal on T1- and T2-weighted imaging. Rarely, bright signal can be seen within the intermediate zone on T2-weighted imaging, resembling a centrally hydrated disc.[18–21] The fibrofatty bilaminar zone, or retrodiscal tissue, has a higher signal intensity than muscle on proton density and T1-weighted sequences. More fibers of the posterior attachment with intermediate signal intensity are seen extending from the superior aspect of the posterior band of the disc to attach to the temporal bone, and another band originates from the inferior aspect of the posterior band and attaches to the condylar neck (**Fig. 2**).

NORMAL BIOMECHANICS

The TMJ is primarily a hinge and glide articulation, but also allows side-to-side motion. The muscles of mastication are responsible for the opening and closing of the jaw. The temporalis, medial pterygoid, and masseter muscles facilitate jaw closure. The lateral pterygoid contributes to jaw opening. In a normal joint in the closed mouth position, the disc is positioned between the condylar head inferiorly, the glenoid fossa superiorly, and the articular eminence anteriorly. The disc is often sigmoid-shaped and lies in the anterior half of the joint space (see **Fig. 2C**). In the closed mouth position, the junction of the posterior band and bilaminar zone should lie immediately above the condylar head near the 12 o'clock position (**Fig. 3**). The junction of the posterior band and bilaminar zone should

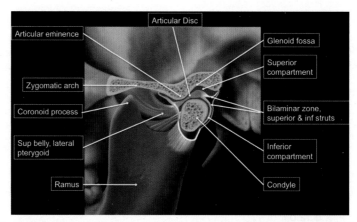

Fig. 1. Normal anatomy of the TMJ. Lateral graphic image shows the relationship of the condylar head to the glenoid fossa of the skull base. The normal bowtie-shaped disc is located between the condylar head and glenoid fossa, separating the joint space into superior and inferior compartments (*shaded yellow-green*). The articular disc has thicker anterior and posterior bands and a thinner intermediate zone. The lateral pterygoid insertion attaches to the anterior band. The posterior band attachments are called the *bilaminar zone*. The superior strut of the bilaminar zone attaches to the posterior mandibular fossa and the inferior strut attaches to the mandibular condyle.

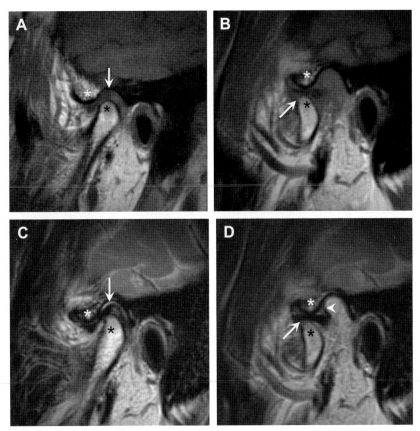

Fig. 2. Normal MR image of the TMJ. (*A*) Sagittal T1-weighted image in the closed mouth position shows the biconcave disc with posterior margin at 12 o'clock (*arrow*). The disc is hypointense on T1, but often the margins of the disc are not as well defined as on the T2-weighted image. Also note the normal position and T1-hyperintense marrow signal of the mandibular condyle (*black asterisk*) and articular eminence (*white asterisk*). (*B*) Sagittal T1-weighted image in the open mouth position shows adequate opening and normal anterior translation of the disc (*arrow*) and mandibular condyle (*black asterisk*) to a position under the articular eminence (*white asterisk*). (*C*) Sagittal T2-weighted image in the closed mouth position shows the biconcave disc with posterior margin at 12 o'clock (*arrow*) and the normal appearance of the articular eminence (*white asterisk*) and condyle (*black asterisk*). (*D*) Sagittal T2-weighted image in the open mouth position shows adequate opening and normal anterior translation of the disc (*arrow*) and mandibular condyle (*black asterisk*) to a position under the articular eminence (*white asterisk*). The posterior attachment (bilaminar zone) is also better appreciated (*arrowhead*).

fall within 10° of vertical to be within the 95th percentile of normal.[13,22,23] However, controversy exists over this definition of normal versus abnormal, because this definition results in anterior displacement in a large number of asymptomatic volunteers (33%).[15] Rammelsberg and colleagues[24] suggested that a disc should be considered anteriorly displaced beyond 30° from the vertical. At Emory, the term *partial anterior displacement* is used to describe discs that do not fall within 10° from the 12 o'clock position, but rather lie around the 10 to 11 o'clock position.

During jaw opening, two motions occur at the TMJ. First, rotation occurs around a horizontal axis through the condylar heads. The second motion is anterior translation of the condyle and

disc to a position beneath the articular eminence. The disc slides into a position between the condylar head and articular eminence and takes on a more "bow tie" appearance (see **Fig. 2D**; **Fig. 4**). The loose tissue of the bilaminar zone allows a remarkable range of motion of the disc. In the open mouth position, the disc rotates posteriorly on the condyle and the entire complex moves anteriorly.

On coronal images, the medial and lateral borders of the disc are aligned with the condylar head and do not bulge medially or laterally.

MR IMAGING PROTOCOL

MR imaging is the standard imaging choice for evaluating the TMJ for internal derangement.[20]

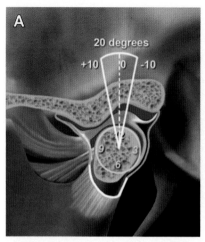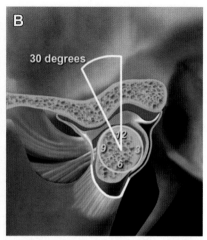

Fig. 3. Normal range of position of the disc in the closed mouth position. (*A*) The junction of the posterior band and bilaminar zone should fall within 10° of vertical to be within the 95th percentile of normal. (*B*) Because the first definition may result in up to 30% false-positives, Rammelsberg and colleagues[24] suggested that a disc should be considered anteriorly displaced beyond 30° from the vertical.

The authors' TMJ imaging is performed with a standard noncontrast protocol that includes static and cine imaging in open and closed mouth positions (**Table 1**). Dual-surface coils are used to provide excellent detail of the joint with a small field of view and high signal-to-noise ratio.

Coronal and axial T1-weighted images are routinely obtained to exclude other pathologies in the masticator space and to evaluate the contour and marrow signal of the mandibular condyles. Additionally, the coronal images are needed to identify lateral or medial disc displacement. The

oblique or parasagittal images are corrected sagittal images (approximately 30° from the true sagittal) that are scanned in a plane perpendicular to the horizontal long axis of the mandibular condyle. The authors do not routinely use intravenous contrast for TMJ imaging, although early reports suggested that gadolinium-enhanced T1-weighted images with fat saturation may improve detection of disruption or injury to the posterior disc attachment.[25] Dynamic information can be

Fig. 4. Normal translation of the mandibular condyle and position of the disc in the open and closed mouth. As the mouth opens, the condyle moves anteriorly to a position just below the articular eminence. Similarly, the disc moves anteriorly to a position between the articular eminence and the mandibular condyle in the open mouth.

Table 1
TMJ protocol: without contrast

#	Sequence	Plane	Comment
1	T1: TR 500, TE min, 3 mm, 0.5 skip	COR	Closed mouth
2	T1: TR 500, TE min, 2 mm, 0 skip	AX	Closed mouth
3	T2 & PD, TR 3500, TE min & 85	Left SAG OBL	Closed mouth
4	T2 & PD, TR 3500, TE min & 85	Right SAG OBL	Closed mouth
5	T2 & PD, TR 3500, TE min & 85	LEFT SAG OBL	Open mouth
6	T2 & PD, TR 3500, TE min & 85	Right SAG OBL	Open mouth
7	T2, TR 1180, TE 64, cine	Left SAG OBL	Dynamic
8	T2, TR 1180, TE 64, cine	Right SAG OBL	Dynamic

Abbreviations: AX, axial; COR, coronal; Min, minimum; OBL, oblique; PD, proton density; SAG, sagittal; T1, T1-weighted; T2, T2-weighted; TE, echo time; TR, repetition time.

obtained with MR imaging by acquiring static images with spin echo techniques at progressive increments from closed to open position and then displaying the images sequentially in a back-and-forth closed cine loop.[4,26] Other authors have also described using a balanced steady-state free procession sequence at 3T for dynamic MR imaging of the TMJ.[11]

Although MR is the preferred imaging study for internal derangement of the TMJ, CT may be complementary to MR for evaluating inflammatory arthritis, infection, or tumors. CT may also be complementary in the setting of coexistent internal derangement and osteoarthritis (**Box 1**).

INTERNAL DERANGEMENT

The most common abnormality of the TMJ is internal derangement, which is an abnormal relationship of the disc with respect to the mandibular condyle, articular eminence, and glenoid fossa. The incidence of symptomatic internal derangement peaks in the second to fourth decade of life, with a female-to-male ratio of 3:1.[27] Patients most often present with jaw pain on biting and opening, clicking and locking when opening or closing, and decreased maximum incisal opening. Headaches and myofascial pain may occur secondarily or be unrelated to the internal derangement. Internal derangement is considered an acquired, progressive degenerative process.[28] Wilkes[29] classified various stages of internal derangement, progressing from an early stage with only reciprocal clicking and no pain, to a late stage characterized by pain, restriction of motion, and grinding symptoms. In the earliest stages, only mild anterior displacement of a morphologically normal disc is present in the closed mouth position, whereas the late stage is characterized by anterior displacement without recapture of a thinned disc with perforation and arthritic changes (**Box 2**). It is important to

---

Box 1
Pathology and primary imaging modalities

- Internal derangement: MR is the primary imaging modality
- Osteoarthritis (often complication of internal derangement): MR and CT may be complimentary
- Infection: MR and CT may be complementary
- Tumor: MR and CT may be complementary
- Inflammatory arthritis: MR and CT may be complementary
- Trauma: CT is the primary imaging modality

Box 2
Wilkes staging criteria for internal derangement of the TMJ

I. Early stage

Clinical: no significant mechanical symptoms, other than reciprocal clicking

Radiologic: slight anterior displacement, but good anatomic contour of disc

Surgical: normal anatomic form and slight anterior displacement

II. Early/intermediate stage

Clinical: occasional joint tenderness and temporal headaches, increase in intensity of clicking sounds, and beginning transient subluxations or joint locking

Radiologic: slight anterior displacement and thickening of posterior edge of disc

Surgical: anterior displacement, early anatomic deformity (slight thickening of posterior edge)

III. Intermediate stage

Clinical: multiple episodes of pain, joint tenderness, temporal headaches, major mechanical symptoms—sustained locking, restriction of motion, and pain with function

Radiologic: anterior displacement with significant anatomic deformity (moderate to marked thickening of posterior edge)

Surgical: marked anatomic deformity with displacement, variable adhesions (anterior, lateral, and posterior recesses)

IV. Intermediate/late stage

Clinical: chronic episodic pain, headaches, restriction of motion, undulating course

Radiologic: increase in severity over intermediate stage with early to

moderate degenerative remodeling of the mandibular condyle and glenoid fossa

Surgical: degenerative remodeling changes of both bearing surfaces, osteophytic projections, multiple adhesions, but no perforation of disc or attachment

V. Late stage

Clinical: crepitus grinding symptoms, chronic episodic pain, restriction of motion

Radiologic: anterior displacement, disc perforation with gross anatomic deformity of disc, severe degenerative arthritic changes

Surgical: perforation of posterior disc attachments, erosions of bearing surfaces with sclerosis and flattening of the condyle, osteophytic projections, subcortical cysts

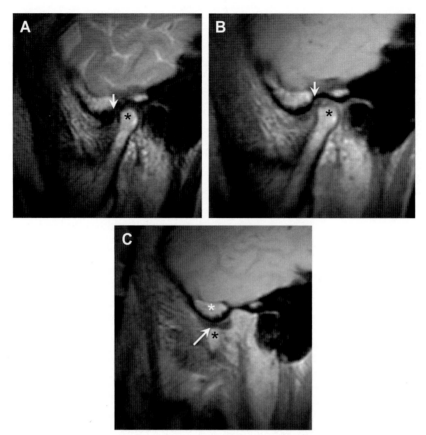

Fig. 5. Partial anterior displacement with recapture. (*A*) Sagittal T2-weighted image in the closed mouth position shows anterior displacement of the disc (*arrow*) in front of the condyle (*black asterisk*). Notice that on the T2-weighted image, the dark signal of the disc can often appear inseparable from the dark cortical signal of the articular eminence and condyle (*black asterisk*). In these cases, the proton density sequence may be helpful to more accurately assess the position of the disc. (*B*) Sagittal proton density–weighted image in the closed mouth position also shows anterior displacement of the disc (*arrow*) in front of the condyle (*black asterisk*). However, the proton density shows that the posterior margin of the disc in between 10 and 11 o'clock, and therefore partially displaced. (*C*) Sagittal proton density–weighted image in the open mouth position shows recapture of the disc (*white arrow*) between the mandibular condyle (*black asterisk*) and articular eminence (*white asterisk*).

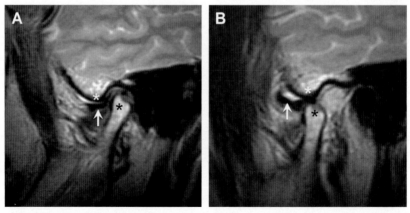

Fig. 6. Anterior displacement without recapture. (*A*) Sagittal T2-weighted image in the closed mouth position shows anterior displacement of the disc (*arrow*) in front of the condyle (*black asterisk*). The condylar eminence is also shown (*white asterisk*). (*B*) Sagittal T2-weighted image in the open mouth position shows adequate anterior translation of the condyle (*black asterisk*) beneath the eminence (*white asterisk*), and therefore adequate opening, but the disc (*arrow*) remains displaced anteriorly with no recapture.

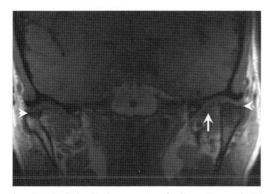

Fig. 7. Medial displacement of disc. Coronal T1-weighted image shows medial displacement of the left disc (*white arrow*). Notice the severe degenerative changes of the mandibular condyles (*arrowheads*) bilaterally with flattening, loss of joint space, and abnormally dark marrow signal on T1-weighted image (which could be edema or sclerosis).

understand the Wilkes staging system, because many TMJ surgeons use this system to classify and treat patients.

At Emory, the average age of patients undergoing MR imaging for symptoms of TMD with clinical suspicion of internal derangement is 42 years. An overwhelming percentage of patients are female (92%) and most proceed to arthroscopy (63%).

Disc displacement may be unidirectional or multidirectional. Most commonly, it is anterior and unidirectional. It may also be multidirectional in an anteromedial direction, or rarely in an anterolateral direction. Unidirectional transverse and posterior disc displacements are rare.[6,28]

Although Wilkes describes five stages or levels of severity, other authors simplify the categorization of internal derangement on imaging from least to most severe as follows[4]:

- Anterior disc displacement with recapture on mouth opening (**Fig. 5**)
- Anterior disc displacement without recapture on mouth opening (**Fig. 6**)
- Chronic anterior disc displacement with disc perforation or disruption of the posterior attachment of the disc to the bilaminar zone and features of degenerative joint disease (**Figs. 7–9**)

Complications of chronic internal derangement include osteoarthritis, bone marrow abnormalities, and avascular necrosis. It is well recognized that many cases of osteoarthritis are the result of internal derangement. Osteoarthritis is present in up to 20% of patients with internal derangement on initial presentation.[30–32] Osteoarthritis also becomes more common with longer duration of internal derangement. However, the presence of osteoarthritis does not necessarily impact the degree of pain and discomfort in patients with internal derangement. Furthermore, older patients with osteoarthritis of the TMJ may be completely asymptomatic.[4,33,34]

Conservative treatment of internal derangement includes soft diet, rest, heat, nonsteroidal antiinflammatory drugs, muscle relaxants, occlusal

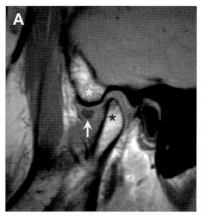

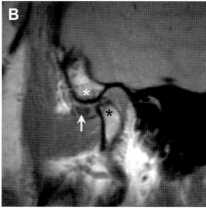

Fig. 8. Severe anterior displacement without recapture, perforation of posterior attachments, and restriction of motion. (*A*) Sagittal T1-weighted image in the closed mouth position shows far anterior displacement of the disc (*arrow*) in front of the condyle (*black asterisk*). Note the globular morphology of the disc and lack of visualization of the posterior attachment (bilaminar zone), which is disrupted. Also note the chiseled appearance of the condyle, suggesting degenerative arthritic changes. The articular eminence is also shown (*white asterisk*). (*B*) Sagittal T1-weighted image in the open mouth position shows suboptimal anterior translation of the condyle (*black asterisk*) in relation to the articular eminence (*white asterisk*) in this patient with restriction of motion. The disc (*arrow*) remains displaced anteriorly with no recapture.

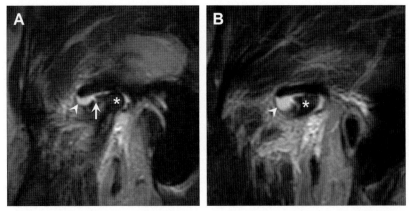

Fig. 9. Severe internal derangement with effusion and osteoarthritis. (*A*) Sagittal T2-weighted image in the closed mouth position shows a moderate effusion (*arrowhead*), flattening and irregularity of the mandibular condyle with abnormally dark marrow signal (*white asterisk*), and thinned disc with focal perforation (*arrow*). (*B*) Sagittal T2-weighted image in the closed mouth position slightly more lateral also shows the moderate effusion (*arrowhead*) and flattening and irregularity of the mandibular condyle with abnormally dark marrow signal (*white asterisk*).

Box 3
Six key features to evaluate on the TMJ MRI

1. Position of the disc
- Normal
- Anterior displacement

  Recapture- seen best on sagittals (**Fig. 5**)

  No recapture- seen best on sagittals (**Fig. 6**)
- Medial or lateral displacement seen best on coronal T1-weighted image (**Fig. 7**)

2. Morphology and signal of the disc
- Normal bow-tie appearance (**Fig. 2D**)
- Thin
- Globular (**Fig. 8**)
- Perforated: implies focal high signal on T2 weighted image (**Fig. 9**)

3. Condylar translation
- Normal/ adequate
- Limited (**Fig. 8**)
- None

4. Masticator space

The axial and coronal T1-weighted sequences will occasionally reveal other causes for TMJ discomfort within the masticator space, such as infection or osteochondroma (**Fig. 10**)

5. Joint Effusion
- No (or trace)
- Yes (**Fig. 9**)

6. Osteoarthritis: Morphology and signal of mandibular condyle
- Normal
- Flattened, irregular with or without erosions (**Fig. 7**)
- Abnormal low signal on T1 weighted sequences
- Osteophytyes (**Fig. 11**)

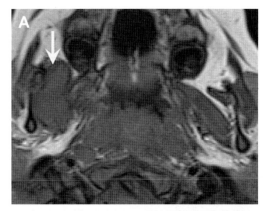

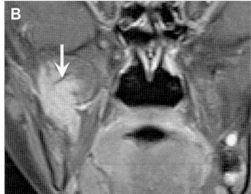

Fig. 10. Desmoid tumor or aggressive fibromatosis involving the masticator space in a 46-year-old woman with trismus, initially thought to be related to TMD. (*A*) Axial T1-weighted image shows an infiltrative isointense mass centered in the right masticator space (*white arrow*), involving the lateral pterygoid muscle and extending from the ramus to the pterygoid plates. (*B*) Coronal T1-weighted image post gadolinium shows intense enhancement of this mass (*white arrow*) and better shows its involvement of both medial and lateral pterygoid muscles.

splints, and physical therapy. Surgical intervention is reserved for patients with refractory pain. Disc plication and repositioning can be performed easily with open surgery (arthrotomy), although successful disc repositioning with advanced surgical arthroscopy is also possible. Disc repositioning is typically performed with either resorbable or nonresorbable sutures, or with the use of mini bone anchors placed in the head of the condyle. In patients with morphologically abnormal discs or discs that cannot be mobilized adequately, a simple discectomy with or without a disc replacement can be performed.

Considerable controversy exists with respect to the most ideal surgical treatment. Patients with Wilkes stage I, II, and early III internal derangement (see **Box 2**) are the most frequent group treated with disc plication. Patients with Wilkes late stage III internal derangement may be more problematic in terms of disc reposition, and patients in this category may be best treated with discectomy. When discectomy is completed, the decision to replace the disc is also controversial. The presence of degenerative joint disease (features of Wilkes stage IV and V internal derangement) often mandates some form of interposition grafting. Options for disc replacement include temporalis muscle, auricular cartilage, fat, dermis, and temporary silastic. Preoperative MR imaging is helpful in staging patients according to Wilkes criteria, allowing a better understanding of disc position and morphology (disease severity), which can be helpful in planning for disc repositioning or discectomy and the potential need for an interpositional graft. Severe degenerative joint disease seen on MR imaging may indicate a potential need for alloplastic total joint replacement.

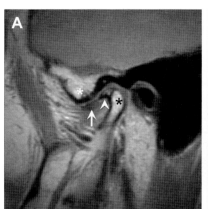

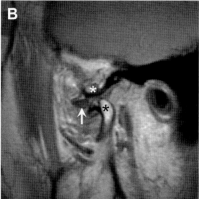

Fig. 11. Severe internal derangement with osteoarthritis. (*A*) Sagittal T1-weighted image in the closed mouth position shows an anteriorly displaced disc, immediately below the articular eminence (*white asterisk*). Also, note the osteophyte (*arrowhead*) along the anterior margin of the condyle (*black asterisk*). (*B*) Sagittal T1-weighted image in the open mouth position shows persistent anterior displacement without reduction (*arrow*).

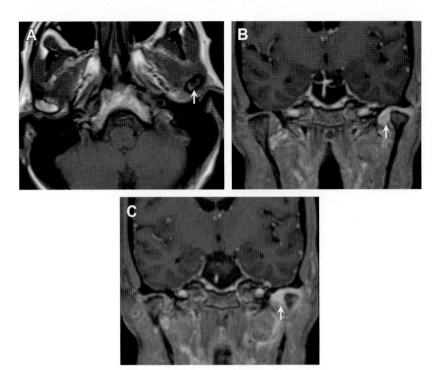

Fig. 12. Synovitis in a patient with rheumatoid arthritis. (*A*) Axial T1-weighted image shows abnormal low signal intensity in the left mandibular condyle (*arrow*). (*B, C*) Coronal magnetization-prepared rapid gradient-echo image post gadolinium shows synovial enhancement (*arrow*).

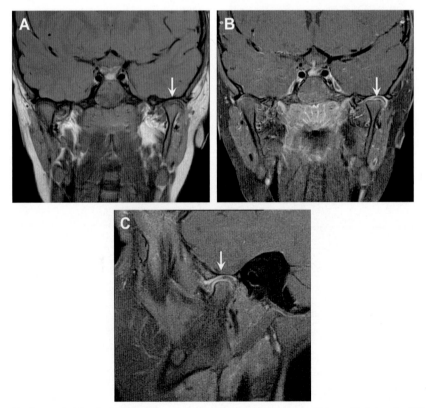

Fig. 13. Juvenile rheumatoid arthritis (JRA) in a 14-year-old boy with known JRA and joint pain. (*A*) Coronal T1-weighted image shows irregular flattening of the left mandibular condyle (*arrow*). (*B*) Coronal T1-weighted image post gadolinium shows synovial enhancement and increases the conspicuity of this abnormality (*arrow*). (*C*) Sagittal T1-weighted image post gadolinium also shows synovial enhancement (*arrow*).

Key MR Imaging Features of Internal Derangement and its Complications

There are six key imaging features or anatomic subsites to evaluate on every MRI of the TMJ (Box 3). These include the position of the disc, the morphology and signal of the disc, condylar translation, the adjacent masticator space, the presence of a joint effusion and signs of osteoarthritis.

Anterior disc displacement is the most common internal derangement of the TMJ. With anterior displacement, the posterior attachment (bilaminar zone) is stretched and may be thickened or redundant.[17] In general, if the disc position is normal in the closed mouth position, then the position is normal. If the disc is anteriorly displaced in the closed mouth position, the next step is to evaluate the position in the open mouth position to determine if there is recapture. The best sequences to

evaluate anterior disc displacement are the oblique sagittal PD or T2 weighted sequences. Often, a severely degenerated disc can be difficult to evaluate on the static images. In this scenario, the authors find the dynamic cine images very helpful to identify disc position.

Condylar translation refers to the anterior movement of the condyle during jaw opening. It is critical to determine whether there has been adequate jaw opening. If there is adequate opening, there is anterior translation of the condyle just below the articular eminence. The cause of limited or no normal condylar translation may be pathologic such as a stuck disc or restriction of motion or it could be patient cooperation. Stuck or fixed disc may result from intracapsular adhesions. MR does not directly visualize the adhesions, but the fixed position of the disc is suggestive.[35–37] Occasionally, the condyle and

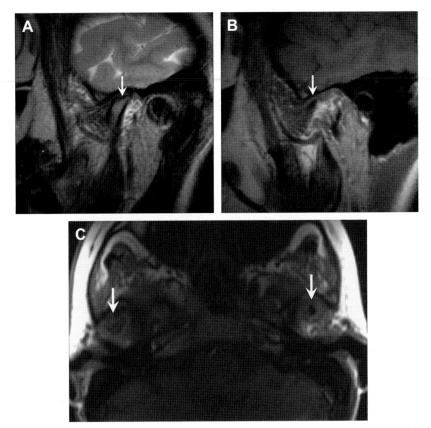

Fig. 14. Idiopathic condylar resorption in a 17-year-old girl with severe bilateral TMJ pain and dysfunction. (A) Sagittal T2-weighted image in the closed mouth position on the right shows nearly complete resorption of the normal condyle. Note the chiseled, pointed appearance (arrow). (B) Sagittal T1-weighted image in the closed mouth position on the left shows complete resorption of the left mandibular condyle. The glenoid fossa is essentially empty when scanning through all sagittal images. The only remnant of the condyle is seen just posterior to the eminence (arrow). (C) Axial T1-weighted image shows the markedly abnormal morphology and signal of the bilateral mandibular condyles (arrows). The left has been resorbed to an even greater extent. Note that the axial T1-weighted images are also obtained with the dual surface coil so that the deeper structures are not as well visualized.

disc may move anterior to the articular eminence during maximum incisal opening.

A small amount of effusion can be seen in normal joints, but moderate to large effusions are only seen in abnormal joints. It has been suggested that the presence of an effusion may reflect synovitis, but a statistical significance has not been shown.[38]

Osteoarthritis in the TMJ, like other synovial joints, manifests in narrowing of the joint space, articular erosion, eburnation and osteophytosis.

MR IMAGING OF OTHER TMJ ARTHROPATHIES

A wide range of inflammatory arthropathies can also involve the TMJ, including rheumatoid arthritis, gout, calcium pyrophosphate dihydrate crystal deposition disease, pigmented villonodular synovitis (PVNS), and infection.

Rheumatoid arthritis is characterized by both soft tissue and bone involvement. Contrast-enhanced MR imaging is most sensitive to evaluate both the soft tissue abnormalities of synovial proliferation (**Fig. 12**) and bone abnormalities, such as joint space narrowing, articular erosion, and flattening of the condylar head.[37] However, synovial enhancement is not specific for inflammatory arthritis; it (along with retrodiscal soft tissue enhancement) has been reported in patients with internal derangement and osteoarthritis.[25] Contrast-enhanced MR imaging is particularly important for evaluating TMJ involvement in children with juvenile arthritis (**Fig. 13**), because a delay in diagnosis could compromise normal facial growth.[39] Other inflammatory arthropathies, such as psoriatic arthritis, ankylosing spondylitis, and systemic lupus erythematosus, can also affect the TMJ and might be radiographically indistinguishable from rheumatoid arthritis.

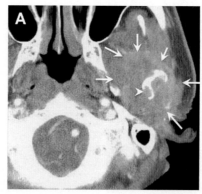

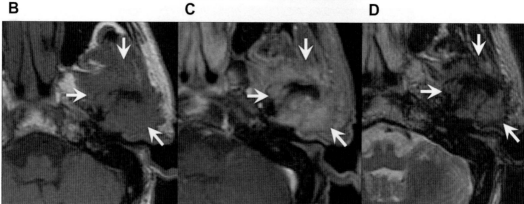

Fig. 15. PVNS in a 70-year-old male who had an enlarging left preauricular mass for 1 year. The patient presented with increasing pain on jaw opening. (*A*) Axial contrast-enhanced CT shows an enhancing soft tissue mass surrounding the left TMJ (*arrows*) with erosions of the mandibular condyle (*arrowhead*). Note the absence of calcified loose bodies. (*B*) Axial T1-weighted image shows an isointense to mildly hypointense mass surrounding the left TMJ (*white arrows*), with involvement of the left mandibular condyle. (*C*) Axial T1-weighted image post gadolinium shows intense enhancement of this mass (*white arrows*). (*D*) Axial T2-weighted image shows the characteristic low T2 signal intensity secondary to hemosiderin deposition (*white arrows*). The absence of calcified loose bodies on the CT favors PVNS on imaging. (*Courtesy of* Dr Brian Bast of UCSF Oral and Maxillofacial Surgery.)

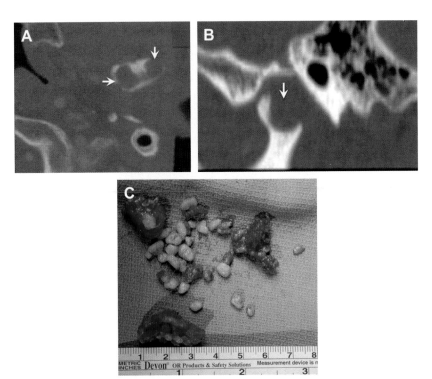

Fig. 16. Synovial chondromatosis in a 47-year-old man with progressive pain on the left with jaw opening. (*A, B*) Axial and coronal CT show abnormal widening of the left TMJ with erosions of the mandibular condyle (*arrows*). However, no calcified loose bodies were seen. The differential considerations included PVNS and synovial chondromatosis. (*C*) At surgery, multiple loose bodies were identified and chondrometaplasia was confirmed histologically.

Idiopathic condylar resorption, also known as "cheerleaders syndrome," is a poorly understood disease process that specifically affects the TMJ, usually in teenage girls participating in sports activities. Although the pathogenesis is unknown, theories exist of estrogen hormone mediation leading to an exaggerated response after minor trauma, orthodontics, or orthognathic surgery.[40] Although many of the inflammatory arthritides (described earlier) may also cause condylar resorption, idiopathic condylar resorption is a separate disease entity characterized by loss of vertical height of the condyle leading to deformity, TMJ dysfunction, and pain. Expected findings on MR imaging include striking decreased condylar size and volume, anterior disc displacement, and thick retrodiscal soft tissue (**Fig. 14**). The best results are achieved with early detection and surgical management.[40]

Other synovial processes, which more commonly occur in large joints, such as PVNS and synovial osteochondromatosis, are also rarely seen involving the TMJ. PVNS is a tumefactive synovial disease of uncertain origin characterized by abnormal proliferation of the synovium. On MR imaging, characteristic areas of low signal intensity on T1- and T2-weighted images are caused by hemosiderin deposition (**Fig. 15**).[41]

Synovial osteochondromatosis is another benign tumor-like disorder that can involve the TMJ. It is thought to be secondary to synovial metaplasia, leading to multiple loose bodies in the joint (**Fig. 16**). If the loose bodies do not calcify, synovial osteochondromatosis can mimic PVNS on CT and

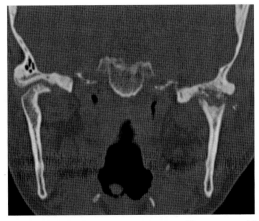

Fig. 17. Septic arthritis in a 43-year-old woman with intense left TMJ pain for 2 weeks and progressive tenderness and swelling. Arthroscopic diagnosis and culture grew streptococcus. Coronal CT shows destruction and erosion of the glenoid fossa and mandibular condyle.

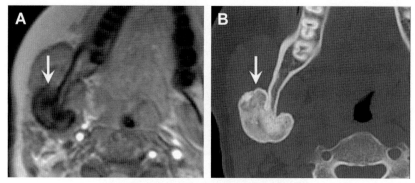

Fig. 18. Osteochondroma in a 19-year-old man with right TMJ pain mimicking internal derangement. (*A*) Axial T1-weighted image shows a hypointense, pedunculated mass involving the mandibular ramus and condyle (*arrow*). (*B*) Axial CT confirmed characteristic features of an osteochondroma, including continuity with the parent mandibular bone, continuous medullary bone, and uninterrupted cortex.

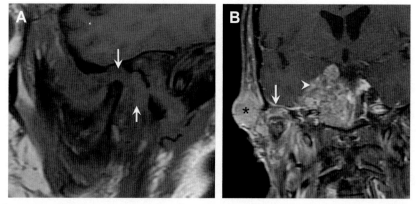

Fig. 19. Contiguous spread from parotid acinic cell carcinoma. (*A*) Sagittal T1-weighted image shows abnormal T1-isointense soft tissue surrounding the left mandibular condyle and extending into the TMJ (*white arrows*). (*B*) Coronal T1-weighted image, post gadolinium shows a parotid mass (*asterisk*) invading the TMJ (*arrow*). Also note the bulky intracranial extension (*arrowhead*).

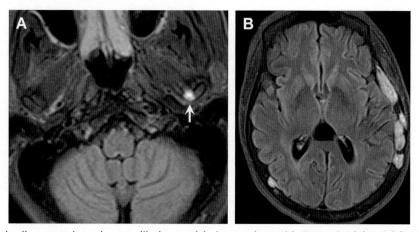

Fig. 20. Renal cell metastasis to the mandibular condyle in a patient with TMJ pain. (*A*) Axial fluid attenuated inversion recovery (FLAIR) MR image shows focal abnormal signal in the left mandibular condyle (*arrow*). (*B*) Axial FLAIR MR image shows multiple additional calvarial metastases.

MR imaging. In most cases (70%) the loose bodies calcify and CT can be helpful to distinguish between the two entities when there is overlap of MR imaging features, because PVNS virtually never calcifies.

Infectious arthritis of the TMJ is rare. Like septic arthritis anywhere, inoculation can be direct or hematogenous and the clinical course can be rapid. Early recognition is key because aggressive joint destruction can occur, leading to ankylosis and fibrosis of the TMJ (**Fig. 17**).[42]

MR IMAGING OF TMJ NEOPLASMS

Osteochondroma is the most common benign tumor that involves the TMJ (**Fig. 18**).[4] Other benign tumors and tumor-like conditions, including osteoma, giant cell tumor, nonossifying fibroma, and aneurysmal bone cysts, are seen rarely. Most malignant neoplasms affecting the TMJ are the sequela of direct spread from a bone primary, such as osteosarcoma or a primary parotid tumor (**Fig. 19**). Metastases from primary sites such as the breast, lung, and kidney are more common to the body of the mandible than to the TMJ (**Fig. 20**).

REFERENCES

1. Poveda Roda R, Bagan JV, Diaz Fernandez JM, et al. Review of temporomandibular joint pathology. Part I: classification, epidemiology and risk factors. Med Oral Patol Oral Cir Bucal 2007;12(4):E292–8.

2. Guralnick W, Kaban LB, Merrill RG. Temporomandibular-joint afflictions. N Engl J Med 1978;299(3):123–9.

3. Solberg WK, Woo MW, Houston JB. Prevalence of mandibular dysfunction in young adults. J Am Dent Assoc 1979;98(1):25–34.

4. Rao VM, Bacelar MT. MR imaging of the temporomandibular joint. Neuroimaging Clin N Am 2004;14(4):761–75.

5. Sommer OJ, Aigner F, Rudisch A, et al. Cross-sectional and functional imaging of the temporomandibular joint: radiology, pathology, and basic biomechanics of the jaw. Radiographics 2003;23(6):e14.

6. Nebbe B, Major PW. Prevalence of TMJ disc displacement in a pre-orthodontic adolescent sample. Angle Orthod 2000;70(6):454–63.

7. Larheim TA. Role of magnetic resonance imaging in the clinical diagnosis of the temporomandibular joint. Cells Tissues Organs 2005;180(1):6–21.

8. Marguelles-Bonnet RE, Carpentier P, Yung JP, et al. Clinical diagnosis compared with findings of magnetic resonance imaging in 242 patients with internal derangement of the TMJ. J Orofac Pain 1995;9(3):244–53.

9. Brooks SL, Westesson PL. Temporomandibular joint: value of coronal MR images. Radiology 1993;188(2):317–21.

10. Katzberg RW, Bessette RW, Tallents RH, et al. Normal and abnormal temporomandibular joint: MR imaging with surface coil. Radiology 1986;158(1):183–9.

11. Yen P, Katzberg RW, Buonocore MH, et-al. Dynamic MR imaging of the temporomandibular joint using a balanced steady-state free precession sequence at 3T. AJNR Am J Neuroradiol, in press.

12. Kaplan PA, Tu HK, Williams SM, et al. The normal temporomandibular joint: MR and arthrographic correlation. Radiology 1987;165(1):177–8.

13. Drace JE, Enzmann DR. Defining the normal temporomandibular joint: closed-, partially open-, and open-mouth MR imaging of asymptomatic subjects. Radiology 1990;177(1):67–71.

14. Westesson PL, Eriksson L, Kurita K. Reliability of a negative clinical temporomandibular joint examination: prevalence of disc displacement in asymptomatic temporomandibular joints. Oral Surg Oral Med Oral Pathol 1989;68(5):551–4.

15. Katzberg RW, Westesson PL, Tallents RH, et al. Anatomic disorders of the temporomandibular joint disc in asymptomatic subjects. J Oral Maxillofac Surg 1996;54(2):147–53 [discussion: 153–5].

16. Hollinshead H. Anatomy for surgeons: the head and neck. 3rd edition. Philadelphia: Lippincott; 1982.

17. Schellhas KP, Wilkes CH, Fritts HM, et al. Temporomandibular joint: MR imaging of internal derangements and postoperative changes. AJR Am J Roentgenol 1988;150(2):381–9.

18. Katzberg RW. Temporomandibular joint imaging. Radiology 1989;170(2):297–307.

19. Murphy W, Kaplan P. Temporomandibular joint. In: Resnick D, editor. Diagnosis of bone and joint disorders. Philadelphia: Saunders; 1995. p. 1699–754.

20. Helms CA, Kaplan P. Diagnostic imaging of the temporomandibular joint: recommendations for use of the various techniques. AJR Am J Roentgenol 1990;154(2):319–22.

21. Schwaighofer BW, Tanaka TT, Klein MV, et al. MR imaging of the temporomandibular joint: a cadaver study of the value of coronal images. AJR Am J Roentgenol 1990;154(6):1245–9.

22. Tomas X, Pomes J, Berenguer J, et al. MR imaging of temporomandibular joint dysfunction: a pictorial review. Radiographics 2006;26(3):765–81.

23. Harms SE, Wilk RM. Magnetic resonance imaging of the temporomandibular joint. Radiographics 1987;7(3):521–42.

24. Rammelsberg P, Pospiech PR, Jager L, et al. Variability of disc position in asymptomatic volunteers and patients with internal derangements of the TMJ. Oral Surg Oral Med Oral Pathol Oral Radiol Endod 1997;83(3):393–9.

25. Suenaga S, Abeyama K, Noikura T. Gadolinium-enhanced MR imaging of temporomandibular disorders: improved lesion detection of the posterior disc attachment on T1-weighted images obtained with fat suppression. AJR Am J Roentgenol 1998;171(2):511–7.

26. Bell KA, Miller KD, Jones JP. Cine magnetic resonance imaging of the temporomandibular joint. Cranio 1992;10(4):313–7.

27. Isberg A, Hagglund M, Paesani D. The effect of age and gender on the onset of symptomatic temporomandibular joint disc displacement. Oral Surg Oral Med Oral Pathol Oral Radiol Endod 1998;85(3):252–7.

28. Larheim TA, Westesson P, Sano T. Temporomandibular joint disc displacement: comparison in asymptomatic volunteers and patients. Radiology 2001;218(2):428–32.

29. Wilkes CH. Internal derangements of the temporomandibular joint. Pathological variations. Arch Otolaryngol Head Neck Surg 1989;115(4):469–77.

30. Katzberg RW, Keith DA, Guralnick WC, et al. Internal derangements and arthritis of the temporomandibular joint. Radiology 1983;146(1):107–12.

31. Westesson PL, Rohlin M. Internal derangement related to osteoarthrosis in temporomandibular joint autopsy specimens. Oral Surg Oral Med Oral Pathol 1984;57(1):17–22.

32. Toller PA. Osteoarthrosis of the mandibular condyle. Br Dent J 1973;134(6):223–31.

33. Sano T, Westesson PL, Larheim TA, et al. The association of temporomandibular joint pain with abnormal bone marrow in the mandibular condyle. J Oral Maxillofac Surg 2000;58(3):254–7 [discussion: 258–9].

34. Sano T. Recent developments in understanding temporomandibular joint disorders. Part 1: bone marrow abnormalities of the mandibular condyle. Dentomaxillofac Radiol 2000;29(1):7–10.

35. Rao VM, Vinitski S. High resolution spin-echo imaging of the temporomandibular joint. Magn Reson Imaging 1993;11(5):621–4.

36. Rao VM, Liem MD, Farole A, et al. Elusive "stuck" disc in the temporomandibular joint: diagnosis with MR imaging. Radiology 1993;189(3):823–7.

37. Suenaga S, Ogura T, Matsuda T, et al. Severity of synovium and bone marrow abnormalities of the temporomandibular joint in early rheumatoid arthritis: role of gadolinium-enhanced fat-suppressed T1-weighted spin echo MRI. J Comput Assist Tomogr 2000;24(3):461–5.

38. Segami N, Nishimura M, Kaneyama K, et al. Does joint effusion on T2 magnetic resonance images reflect synovitis? Comparison of arthroscopic findings in internal derangements of the temporomandibular joint. Oral Surg Oral Med Oral Pathol Oral Radiol Endod 2001;92(3):341–5.

39. Kuseler A, Pedersen TK, Herlin T, et al. Contrast enhanced magnetic resonance imaging as a method to diagnose early inflammatory changes in the temporomandibular joint in children with juvenile chronic arthritis. J Rheumatol 1998;25(7):1406–12.

40. Wolford LM. Idiopathic condylar resorption of the temporomandibular joint in teenage girls (cheerleaders syndrome). Proc (Bayl Univ Med Cent) 2001;14(3):246–52.

41. Bemporad JA, Chaloupka JC, Putman CM, et al. Pigmented villonodular synovitis of the temporomandibular joint: diagnostic imaging and endovascular therapeutic embolization of a rare head and neck tumor. AJNR Am J Neuroradiol 1999;20(1):159–62.

42. Hekkenberg RJ, Piedade L, Mock D, et al. Septic arthritis of the temporomandibular joint. Otolaryngol Head Neck Surg 1999;120(5):780–2.

Evaluation of Orbital Disorders and Cranial Nerve Innervation of the Extraocular Muscles

Stephen F. Kralik, MD[a],*, Robert Kersten, MD[b],
Christine M. Glastonbury, MBBS[c]

KEYWORDS

- Orbit • Cranial nerves • Magnetic resonance imaging • Differential diagnosis • Imaging approach

KEY POINTS

- Critical clinical information required for evaluating orbital disorders includes age of the patient, primary sign/symptom, acuity, and presence of pain.
- Differentiation of orbital pseudotumor from lymphoma or sarcoid isolated to the orbit remains challenging because of a variety of overlapping orbital imaging patterns.
- Orbital infection requires critical evaluation of extent relative to the orbital septum and intracranial extension.
- An acute third nerve palsy with pupillary involvement must be evaluated for an aneurysm with computed tomography angiography or magnetic resonance angiography as initial imaging.

INTRODUCTION

Evaluation of the visual pathways covers the gamut from orbital masses to intracranial lesions to systemic disease. Orbital masses may affect any part of the orbit from the globe to the muscles to the orbital fat or lacrimal gland. Intracranial disease may manifest with visual symptoms such as diplopia from cranial neuropathies or brainstem injury, or with visual field defects from disorders affecting the optic pathway from the optic nerves to the occipital lobes. Systemic diseases may manifest in the lacrimal glands (such as sarcoidosis or lymphoma), in the extraocular muscles (thyroid ophthalmopathy), or with orbital masses or infiltrating disease (such as Wegener granulomatosis or metastases).

For the radiologist to best protocol, perform, and interpret an imaging study, it is helpful to have a clear understanding of the visual pathways and orbital disease. Integration of clinical history and imaging findings is essential to generate an accurate differential diagnosis. This article presents a review of orbital disorders and intracranial disease manifesting with visual symptoms, reviews cranial nerve innervation of the extraocular muscles, and shares our method for evaluating orbital lesions. It begins with a review of the imaging techniques and protocols, followed by a 3-step process for establishing a differential diagnosis.

IMAGING TECHNIQUES

Nonenhanced computed tomography (CT) is the imaging modality of choice for orbital trauma and foreign bodies, and has a complimentary role with magnetic resonance (MR) imaging for complete evaluation of lesions of the bony orbit.

[a] Department of Radiology and Imaging Sciences, Indiana University School of Medicine, 702 Barnhill Drive, Room 1053, Indianapolis, IN 46202, USA; [b] Ophthalmic Plastic and Reconstructive Surgery, University of California San Francisco, 505 Parnassus Avenue, San Francisco, CA 94143, USA; [c] Department of Radiology and Biomedical Imaging, University of California San Francisco, 505 Parnassus Avenue, San Francisco, CA 94143, USA
* Corresponding author.
E-mail address: steve.kralik@gmail.com

Magn Reson Imaging Clin N Am 20 (2012) 413–434
doi:10.1016/j.mric.2012.05.005
1064-9689/12/$ – see front matter Published by Elsevier Inc.

Contrast-enhanced CT is the modality of choice in the initial evaluation of acute infection affecting the orbits, which is most commonly of sinus origin. Contrast-enhanced CT also has a role for those patients who have contraindications to MR imaging. Slice thickness is less than or equal to 2 mm, and coronal and sagittal reformats should be routinely obtained, preferably with slice overlap to minimize distortion. For all infections and most inflammatory disease, it is important to include the entire paranasal sinuses with orbital imaging because of the close association of sinus and orbital disorders.

MR is the preferred modality for evaluation of orbital soft tissues including muscles, lacrimal gland, orbital fat, and the globe, as well as the intracranial structures. High-resolution MR imaging can be performed in a standard head coil at 1.5 T or 3T (**Box 1**). T2-weighted (T2W) fast spin echo (FSE) sequences (with or without fat saturation) best evaluate the optic nerve, although saturation of both water and fat is more sensitive for detection of subtle optic nerve signal abnormality.[1] Chemical-selective fat saturation techniques are important with postcontrast imaging to differentiate disorders from the normal orbital fat, which is intrinsically hyperintense on T1-weighted (T1W) imaging. Additional brain imaging may reveal associated findings related to systemic diseases, such as demyelinating plaques in association with optic neuropathy.

RADIOLOGICAL AND CLINICAL EVALUATION OF ORBITAL DISORDERS

The evaluation of orbital disorders begins with obtaining an accurate clinical history, demographic factors such as patient age, and any additional information such as prior trauma and known systemic disease. The integration of imaging findings with clinical signs and symptoms is essential.

When evaluating an orbital lesion it is important to accurately identify the components of the orbit that are involved, such as the extraocular muscles (muscle cone) and the intraconal and extraconal spaces. It is paramount to distinguish preseptal (periorbital) from postseptal (orbital) involvement. However, this spatial approach is not always helpful in generating a differential diagnosis. We find that a more useful approach is to categorize orbital lesions into 1 of 3 groups: alteration of a normal orbital structure, lesion that does not belong in the orbit, or alteration of the orbit from bone or periorbital disorders.

When there is a known contributing history such as neurofibromatosis, Graves disease, or sarcoidosis, imaging is often not used to make a diagnosis but to evaluate the extent of disease in the orbit and intracranial structures.

ALTERATION OF A NORMAL ORBITAL STRUCTURE

Imaging assessment for proptosis can be performed by drawing a line between the right and left zygomatic borders (interzygomatic line) at the level of the lens in primary gaze, followed by drawing a perpendicular line to the apex of the cornea (Hertel index) or from the interzygomatic line to the posterior globe margin. The normal mean distance from the interzygomatic line to the posterior margin of the globe is 9.4 mm (2 standard deviation range 5.9–12.8 mm) or approximately one-third of the globe posterior to the interzygomatic line, whereas a Hertel index greater than 22 mm is abnormal (**Fig. 1**).[2,3]

Orbital disorders may result in enlargement or, less commonly, decrease in size of a normal structure (**Table 1**).[4] Often, the change in size or volume of a structure is evident by observation alone, but, for more subtle disorders, reference values may be helpful for confirming change in size of structures (**Table 2**).[5–10]

Enlargement of the Optic Nerve or Nerve Sheath

The primary differential for an enlarged optic nerve is a glioma or optic neuritis. These may be differentiated clinically by the more rapid onset of vision loss and pain with optic neuritis compared with the slowly progressive visual loss with an optic glioma. Optic nerve gliomas associated with childhood sporadic gliomas and neurofibromatosis type 1 (NF-1) are of low-grade disorders (World Health Organization [WHO] grade I or II), whereas

---

Box 1
MR imaging orbital protocol

Routine

- Axial, coronal, and/or sagittal T1-weighted; slice thickness 3 to 4 mm, field of view (FOV) 16 cm, matrix 256 × 192 to 256
- Coronal T2-weighted FSE with fat saturation; slice thickness 3 to 4 mm, FOV 16 cm, matrix 256 × 256
- Axial and coronal T1-weighted contrast enhanced fat suppressed; slice thickness 3 to 4 mm, FOV 16 to 18 cm, matrix 256 × 192 to 256

Additional sequences

- Three-dimensional T2-weighted FSE; slice thickness 1 mm, matrix 256 × 256
- Diffusion weighted

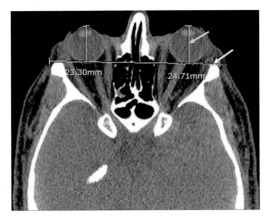

Fig. 1. Measurement of proptosis. Axial CT shows the interzygomatic line (*white arrow*) and Hertel index (*yellow arrow*). A Hertel index value greater than 22 mm is abnormal, as is seen here.

the uncommon adult optic nerve gliomas are frequently anaplastic astrocytomas (WHO III) or glioblastomas (WHO IV). An optic glioma may be seen in 10% to 30% of NF-1, although only about half of the patients develop related signs or symptoms.[11,12] Optic nerve gliomas show 2 growth patterns and corresponding MR patterns: (1) intraneural glial proliferation seen as fusiform nerve enlargement with variable increased T2W hyperintensity and contrast enhancement, or (2) extraneural extension with growth into the adjacent subarachnoid space (perineural arachnoidal gliomatosis) (**Fig. 2**), which shows T2W hyperintensity with mild to moderate enhancement in the sheath surrounding a normal-appearing optic nerve (pseudo–cerebrospinal fluid [CSF] sign).[13] This is more common in NF-1. When a glioma is identified, the optic nerve, chiasm, optic tracts, and

Table 1
Differential diagnosis: enlargement of a normal orbital structure

Structure	Common	Uncommon	Rare

Optic nerve	Multiple sclerosis
	Optic nerve glioma
		Infection: viral
		  (VZV, HIV, CMV), syphilis
		Granulomatous:
		  sarcoidosis
		NMO
			Neuritis: Lyme disease,
			  tuberculosis,
			  radiotherapy
			Ganglioglioma
			Medulloepithelioma
			Hemangioblastoma
			Erdheim-Chester disease

Optic nerve sheath	Meningioma	Orbital pseudotumor
		Carcinomatosis
		Lymphoma
			Granulomatosis with
			  polyangiitis (Wegener
			  disease)
			Giant cell arteritis
			Hemangiopericytoma

Extraocular muscle(s)	Thyroid orbitopathy Orbital pseudotumor	Carotid-cavernous fistula Metastatic disease Sarcoidosis Lymphoma Cellulitis	Rhabdomyosarcoma Trauma System lupus erythematosus

Superior ophthalmic vein(s)	Carotid-cavernous fistula
	Cavernous sinus
	  thrombosis
	Venous varix
		Dural arteriovenous fistula
		Cavernous sinus mass
		  (meningioma,
		  schwannoma,
		  hemangioma)
		Increased intracranial
		  pressure
		Thyroid orbitopathy
			—

Lacrimal gland	Dacryoadenitis
	Sarcoidosis
	Lymphoma
	Orbital pseudotumor
	Pleomorphic adenoma
		Adenoid cystic carcinoma
		Sjögren disease
		Granulomatosis with
		  polyangiitis (Wegener
		  disease)
			—

Abbreviations: CMV, cytomegalovirus; HIV, human immunodeficiency virus; NMO, neuromyelitis optica; VZV, varicella-zoster virus.
  Data from Miller NR. Primary tumors of the optic nerve and its sheath. Eye 2004;18:1026–37.

Table 2
Normal anatomic sizes of orbital structures

Structure	Measurement (mm)
Superior rectus muscle	3.1–5.6
Inferior rectus muscle	3.7–6.0
Medial rectus muscle	3.2–4.9
Lateral rectus muscle	2.6–4.8
Superior oblique	2.4–4.1
Optic nerve (nerve sheath)[a]	Average diameter 5 mm posterior to the globe, 3.23 (5.72) Average diameter 10 mm posterior to the globe, 2.94 (4.53) Average diameter 15 mm posterior to the globe, 2.67 (3.98)
Superior ophthalmic vein	Diameter 1.5–3
Lacrimal gland	Axial AP axis length: average 14.5/14.7 (L/R) (10%–90% range 10.3/10.9–18.3/18.3) Coronal CC axis length: average 16.9/17.7 (L/R) (10%–90% range 12.8/ 13.9–20.8/21.8)

Published normative values of extraocular muscles vary slightly based on CT versus MR imaging measurement technique, differences in windowing when obtaining CT measurements, patient ethnicity, or small but statistically significant difference in size of the extraocular muscles in men and women.[5,9,10]

Abbreviations: AP, anterior to posterior; CC, cranial to caudal; L, left; R, right.

[a] Optic nerve decreases in diameter as distance increases posteriorly from the globe, which causes discrepancies in published optic nerve diameters or areas.[6]

Data from Refs.[5–10]

radiations must be carefully assessed. Compared with NF-1–associated optic gliomas, sporadic optic gliomas more frequently involve the chiasm and hypothalamus (rather than the optic nerve), extend beyond the optic pathways, show cystic areas, and are more likely to enlarge over time.[14]

Inflammation of the optic nerve, optic neuritis, is most often associated with multiple sclerosis. MR imaging shows variably increased T2W signal intensity and a mildly enlarged enhancing optic nerve in up to 90% to 95% of patients (**Fig. 3**). Imaging of the brain aids in assessing the risk for development of multiple sclerosis because there is correlation between the number of white matter lesions identified on baseline imaging and an increasing risk of multiple sclerosis.[15] A diagnosis other than multiple sclerosis should be considered when there is progressive visual worsening for more than 2 weeks or lack of improvement after 8 weeks.[15] Recognition of other causes, including sarcoidosis, neuromyelitis optica (NMO), lupus, viral infections (such as varicella-zoster), or as a complication of prior radiotherapy, are important in the management and prognosis of optic neuritis.

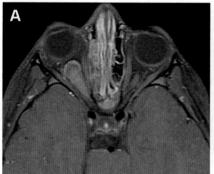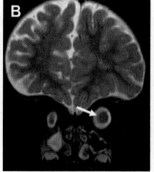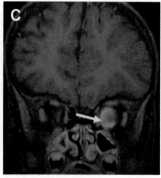

Fig. 2. Optic nerve glioma appearances. (*A*) A 5-year-old child with NF-1 with mild right proptosis and poor vision. Axial enhanced fat-suppressed T1W MR shows fusiform enlargement and mild enhancement of the right optic nerve. (*B, C*) A 3-year-old with NF-1 with a left optic nerve glioma. Coronal T2W MR (*B*) shows fusiform enlargement of the optic nerve (*arrow*), whereas coronal enhanced fat-suppressed T1W MR (*C*) shows perineural sheath enhancement (*arrow*) consistent with perineural arachnoid gliomatosis.

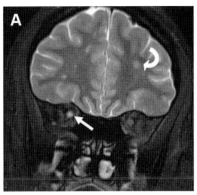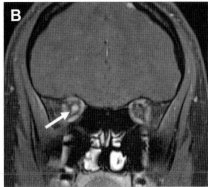

Fig. 3. Optic neuritis from multiple sclerosis. A 15-year-old patient presented with acute onset of right eye pain and blurred vision. (*A*) Coronal fat-suppressed T2W MR shows abnormal right optic nerve hyperintensity (*white arrow*) as well as the presence of intracranial white matter lesions (*curved arrow*) related to demyelination. (*B*) Coronal enhanced fat-suppressed T1W MR shows abnormal enhancement of the right optic nerve (*white arrow*).

When an enlarged optic nerve sheath is encountered, there is a key distinction to make: is the nerve sheath enlarged from dural ectasia, such as can be seen with NF-1, or is there a thickened, abnormally enhancing nerve sheath caused by perineuritis, an optic nerve sheath meningioma (**Fig. 4**), or carcinomatosis. The clinical history often differentiates perineuritis from a meningioma. An optic nerve sheath meningioma presents with gradually progressive, painless vision loss.[16] They are more frequent in women (80%), with an average age at presentation of 40 years. Presentation in childhood can be seen in patients with neurofibromatosis type 2 (NF-2).[16] Optic nerve meningiomas are unilateral in 95% of patients.[16] Optic perineuritis is an uncommon inflammation of the nerve sheath that may represent a manifestation of idiopathic orbital inflammation (orbital pseudotumor), sarcoidosis, syphilis, or granulomatosis with polyangiitis (previously called Wegener syndrome). Perineuritis typically presents similarly to optic neuritis, with acute onset of eye pain and/or vision loss. MR imaging shows abnormal nerve sheath thickening and enhancement rather than enhancement of the optic nerve itself (the tram-track sign). Distinction of optic perineuritis from optic neuritis is important because patients with optic perineuritis show a dramatic response to steroids, do not have a risk of developing multiple sclerosis, and have a good prognosis, because most (80%) return to baseline vision.[17]

In addition, a thickened, enhancing optic nerve sheath may be associated with leukemic or carcinomatous infiltration of the meninges, as well as granulomatosis processes such as sarcoid.

Decreased Size of the Optic Nerve

Decreased size of the optic nerve is seen with optic nerve hypoplasia (congenital) or atrophy (acquired).

The role of imaging with optic nerve hypoplasia is to identify associated congenital intracranial abnormalities such as septo-optic dysplasia. The diagnosis of septo-optic dysplasia requires both ophthalmologic examination and neuroimaging because the diagnosis of optic nerve hypoplasia is only made in 50% of these patients with neuroimaging.[11] Common intracranial findings seen in septo-optic dysplasia include cortical malformations (schizencephaly, gray matter heterotopia, partial absence of the septum), white matter hypoplasia, pituitary abnormalities (absent gland, ectopic posterior gland, small or absent infundibulum), or hypogenesis of the corpus callosum. Identification of intracranial findings assists in determining prognosis

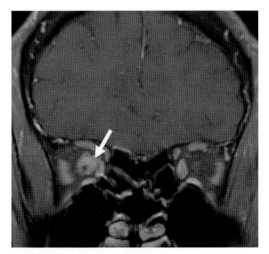

Fig. 4. Optic nerve meningioma. A 36-year-old patient presents with painless progressive right eye vision loss. Coronal enhanced fat-suppressed T1W MR shows a homogeneously enhancing mass arising from the right optic nerve sheath (*white arrow*) surrounding the hypointense optic nerve, consistent with a meningioma.

because those with hemispheric or pituitary anomalies carry a worse prognosis. Many other causes of optic atrophy (metabolic, vascular, and nutritional) have no specific imaging findings. In such cases, the optic nerve head shows pallor on funduscopy, but the cross-sectional diameter of the nerve on imaging is normal. Imaging may still be useful to exclude orbital disorders compressing the optic nerve. Optic nerve atrophy may also be evident on imaging in patients with prior history of optic neuritis.

Enlargement of Extraocular Muscles

Diffuse enlargement of the extraocular muscles may occur with thyroid orbitopathy, the myositic form of pseudotumor, granulomatous disease, tumor (lymphoma, metastatic disease), or carotid-cavernous fistula (CCF) in which increased venous pressure results in engorgement of the extraocular muscles.

Thyroid orbitopathy, also known as thyroid ophthalmopathy, or Graves ophthalmopathy, is the most common cause of exophthalmos in adults (80% of bilateral, 15%–28% of unilateral).[18] It is a complex disease process with both antigen-specific and antigen-independent pathways that seem to target orbital fibroblasts.[19] Presentation occurs in the third to fifth decades and women are affected 7 to 8 times more often than men. Patients are usually hyperthyroid (80%–90%) but may be hypothyroid or euthyroid (10%–20%).[20] Disease may occur before, after, or simultaneously with hyperthyroidism. Nearly all patients with thyroid orbitopathy have the presence of thyrotropin receptor antibodies.[21]

The role of imaging includes differentiation of thyroid orbitopathy from other causes of proptosis, evaluation for acute or chronic stages of disease to guide treatment, and to evaluate for optic neuropathy from stretching of the optic nerve (which is thinned at the orbital apex and prechiasmatic segment) or orbital apex compression by concentric enlargement of the extraocular muscles. Although patients may clinically have unilateral eye findings, bilateral orbital involvement is found in up to 75% of cases.[2] Imaging findings include proptosis, increase in orbital fat, enlargement of the extraocular muscles with sparing of the myotendinous junction, and fat deposition in the extraocular muscles, as is seen in the chronic state of the disease (**Fig. 5**). MR imaging is more sensitive than CT in distinguishing active inflammatory changes (muscle edema) from chronic/fibrotic changes (fat deposition in the muscle).[2] Findings that should raise suspicion for an alternative cause include associated orbital inflammation, rapid progression of symptoms, enlarged superior ophthalmic vein and cavernous sinus, involvement of myotendinous junction, or isolated involvement of the lateral rectus muscle.

Idiopathic orbital inflammation, orbital pseudotumor, is a benign nongranulomatous inflammatory disease without a defined pathogenesis that more commonly presents as unilateral rather than bilateral disease (except in children). Presentation is typically acute over hours to days, with inflammatory symptoms including pain, swelling, erythema, chemosis, optic neuropathy, and extraocular muscle dysmotility. Orbital pseudotumor includes any combination of lacrimal gland enlargement, extraocular muscle enlargement with involvement of the myotendinous junction, optic nerve sheath thickening and enhancement (perineuritis), replacement of orbital fat with ill-defined inflammation or a well-defined focal mass, and uveoscleral thickening (**Fig. 6**). MR imaging shows variable T2W signal intensity that may be hypointense, particularly with infiltrative sclerosing form, which

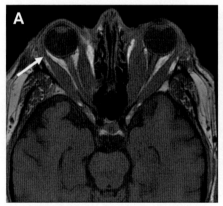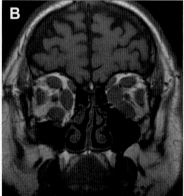

Fig. 5. Thyroid orbitopathy. A 58-year-old patient with Graves disease and proptosis. (*A*) Axial T1W and (*B*) coronal T1W MR images show proptosis and bilateral enlargement of the extraocular muscles with sparing of the myotendinous junction (*arrow*).

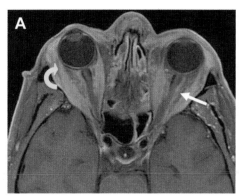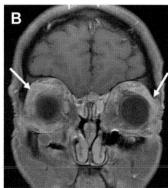

Fig. 6. Idiopathic orbital inflammation. A 58-year-old patient with afebrile acute onset of bilateral eye pain and proptosis. (*A*) Axial enhanced fat-suppressed T1W MR image shows bilateral abnormal enhancement of the orbital fat, left optic nerve sheath enhancement (*white arrow*) consistent with perineuritis, and enlarged extraocular muscles with involvement of the myotendinous junction (*curved arrow*). (*B*) Coronal enhanced fat-suppressed T1W MR shows bilateral enlarged homogeneously enhancing lacrimal glands (*arrows*). Biopsy reveled nongranulomatous inflammatory infiltrate consistent with pseudotumor.

shows significant homogeneous enhancement in areas of involvement.[22] Inflammation may extend to the orbital apex or cavernous sinus resulting in Tolosa-Hunt syndrome, also known as painful ophthalmoplegia because of inflammatory dysfunction of cranial nerves 3, 4, V1 and 6 as they traverse the superior orbital fissure. Orbital pseudotumor is a diagnosis of exclusion, and histology reveals nongranulomatous inflammatory cell infiltrates. Recently, in a small series comparing orbital pseudotumor with orbital lymphoma, diffusion-weighted imaging (DWI) with an apparent diffusion coefficient (ADC) threshold of 1.0×10^{-3} mm^2/s and ADC$_{lesion}$/ADC$_{normal\ frontal\ lobe\ white\ matter}$ ratio of 1.2 suggested a 100% sensitivity and specificity in differentiation between pseudotumor and lymphoma.[23] Orbital pseudotumor responds to steroids and immunosuppressive therapy; however, incomplete resolution or recurrence may be seen in 25% to 52% of cases.[24] Sclerosing orbital inflammation is a related disorder characterized by dense desmoplastic fibrosis containing a scant inflammatory cellular response. It is usually refractory to steroids, antiinflammatory medications and radiation.

Decreased Size of Extraocular Muscles

Decrease in size of extraocular muscles is uncommon and may be congenital or acquired. Knowledge and evaluation of the cranial nerve innervation is necessary (**Table 3**). Congenital causes include fibrosis syndromes and may present with decreased eye motility or abnormal eye position. When evaluating for congenital causes of strabismus, thin-section images are necessary to detect subtle volume loss or fibrosis of an extraocular muscle or,

rarely, the presence of an accessory muscle or fibrous band. Sporadic congenital absence of extraocular muscles (usually the inferior rectus) has rarely been reported. Thin-section T2W images are also necessary for detection of associated absence or hypoplasia of cranial nerves, particularly cranial nerves 3 and 6. Acquired causes of extraocular muscle atrophy presenting with abnormal eye motility are rare and may be caused by a myopathy from denervation, prior inflammation, linear scleroderma, myasthenia gravis, or a mitochondrial disease.[25] Chronic progressive external ophthalmoplegia, a mitochondrial cytopathy, may present at any age with blepharoptosis followed by slowly progressive, symmetric, painless loss of extraocular muscle function. Imaging shows decreased size of extraocular muscles and/or intrinsic T1W hyperintensity within the extraocular muscles (**Fig. 7**).[26] Extraocular muscle atrophy caused by denervation requires imaging from the globe to the brainstem and is described later.

Enlargement of Superior Ophthalmic Veins

Enlargement of the superior ophthalmic vein(s) may occur with a CCF, venous varix, cavernous sinus mass or thrombosis, or increase of intracranial pressure.

A CCF is caused by an abnormal communication between the cavernous segment of the internal carotid artery with the cavernous sinus itself, and is classified as direct or indirect. Direct CCF may occur as a result of trauma, surgery, rupture of an aneurysm, arterial dissection, or fibromuscular dysplasia.[27] An indirect CCF results from communication of small dural branches of the external carotid or internal carotid artery with

Table 3
Cranial nerve anatomy and clinical functions

Nerve	Course	Innervation	Clinical Signs
Oculomotor CN3	Nuclei: paramedian midbrain posterior to red nuclei Edinger-Westphal (PS) nuclei are dorsal Exits brain: interpeduncular cistern Cistern: between SCA and PCA Cavernous sinus: superior lateral wall of the sinus Exits skull: superior orbital fissure	Superior, medial, and inferior rectus and inferior oblique levator palpebrae superiorus PS: sphincter pupillae and ciliary	Isolated CN3: Ptosis, downward and abducted globe, absent accommodation, pupillary dilatation CN3 palsy with pupil involvement must exclude aneurysm With other CN: CN3 palsy + CN4 + CN6 must evaluate cavernous sinus or superior orbital fissure
Trochlear CN4	Nuclei: midbrain below CN3 Exits brain: dorsally below inferior colliculi after crossing in superior medullary velum Cistern: ambient; between PCA and SCA inferolateral to CN3 Cavernous sinus: in lateral wall below CN3 Exits skull: superior orbital fissure	Superior oblique	Isolated CN4: Outward rotation of globe (extorsion) ± head tilt away from affected side Isolated CN4 palsy uncommon, often trauma With other CN: CN4 palsy + CN3 + CN6 must evaluate cavernous sinus or superior orbital fissure
Abducens CN6	Nuclei: dorsal pons deep to facial colliculus Exits brain: prepontine cistern at pontomedullary junction Cistern: prepontine to Dorello canal Cavernous sinus: within sinus inferolateral to internal carotid artery Exits skull: superior orbital fissure	Lateral rectus	Isolated CN6: Inability to deviate eye laterally Isolated CN6 palsy is most common extraocular muscle palsy With other CN: CN6 + CN3 + CN4 suggests cavernous sinus or superior orbital fissure CN6 + CN5 suggests petrous apex lesion CN6 + CN7 suggests pontine lesion

Abbreviations: CN, cranial nerve; PCA, posterior cerebral artery; PS, parasympathetic, SCA, superior cerebellar artery.

the cavernous sinus. Risk factors for development of an indirect CCF include pregnancy, surgery, sinusitis, or prior cavernous sinus thrombosis.[27] MR imaging or CT imaging findings of a CCF include an enlargement of the superior ophthalmic vein and ipsilateral cavernous sinus, enlargement of extraocular muscles from venous congestion, edematous orbital fat, and proptosis (**Fig. 8**). Catheter angiography provides both dynamic display of early filling of the cavernous sinus with carotid artery injection as well as the opportunity to repair the fistula by transvenous or transarterial routes.

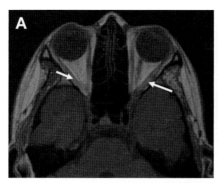
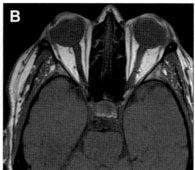

Fig. 7. Chronic progressive external ophthalmoplegia. Patient 1: a 25-year-old patient with horizontal diplopia, bilateral weakness of adduction (left > right). (*A*) Axial T1W MR image shows atrophy of the bilateral lateral rectus muscles with fatty infiltration (*white arrows*), and enophthalmos. Patient 2: a 45-year-old patient with chronic progressive external ophthalmoplegia. (*B*) Axial T1W MR image shows diffuse bilateral extraocular muscle atrophy.

A venous varix should be differentiated from an enlarged superior ophthalmic vein. Although a venous varix is uncommon, it is the most common cause of spontaneous orbital hemorrhage and presents with rapidly developing proptosis.[28,29] Other patients may present with intermittent (usually with Valsalva) or reversible proptosis or sustained proptosis if there is thrombosis of the varix.[30] A venous varix can be diagnosed with contrast-enhanced CT imaging performed before and with Valsalva maneuver, which shows enlargement of the intensely enhancing varix on Valsalva (**Fig. 9**).

Cavernous sinus thrombosis may lead to enlarged superior ophthalmic vein(s) caused by increased intracranial venous pressure. Most often, thrombosis is a complication of sinusitis, (most frequently sphenoid). Most patients present with headaches, and there may be associated orbital pain, vision loss, and/or ophthalmoplegia. Contrast-enhanced CT or MR imaging shows a convex lateral margin of the cavernous sinus with a filling defect or complete lack of enhancement. If orbital MR imaging is used to assess for cavernous sinus thrombosis, it is important to obtain unenhanced T1W images to distinguish suppressed fat from nonenhancing clot. Early diagnosis and treatment are critical to reduce morbidity and mortality.

Enlargement of Lacrimal Glands

In most cases, enlargement of the lacrimal gland(s) is caused by an inflammatory or lymphoproliferative process. On imaging, the gland typically appears diffusely enlarged, and retains its configuration contouring around the superolateral perimeter of the globe, with homogeneous enhancement. Inflammatory lesions include pseudotumor (the lacrimal gland is the most common site of orbital pseudotumor), sarcoidosis, granulomatosis with polyangiitis (Wegener), and Sjögren disease. Lymphomatous involvement of the lacrimal gland has a similar imaging appearance and is the most common site of orbital lymphoma, accounting for 50% of orbital lymphomas. It is bilateral in 20% of cases. A minority of lacrimal gland lesions represent epithelial tumors, although older pathology series have reported near-equal incidences of inflammatory/lymphoproliferative masses and epithelial tumors.[31] In general, lacrimal gland tumors are usually unilateral, present with chronic symptoms, and display heterogeneity on MR imaging with a focal enlargement (a mass) arising within the gland.

Sarcoidosis can involve any portion of the orbit; however, the most common site on imaging is within the lacrimal glands, which may occur in up to 50% to 60% of cases.[32] Between 20% and 25% of patients with systemic sarcoidosis have orbital involvement.[33,34] Sarcoidosis isolated to the orbit without systemic involvement is uncommon and patients most often present with a diffusely enlarged lacrimal gland.[33] Involved lacrimal gland(s) show homogeneous enhancement, whereas involved extraocular muscles may show hypointensity on T2W imaging.[35] Histology shows noncaseating granulomas. Differentiation from orbital pseudotumor or lymphoma remains challenging, particularly in the setting of disease limited to the lacrimal gland without additional systemic or intracranial findings.

A primary lacrimal gland tumor should be suspected if imaging findings show a unilateral enlarged lacrimal gland with a focal heterogeneous mass. One-half of lesions are malignant (mucoepidermoid, adenocarcinoma, adenoid cystic, squamous cell carcinoma) and the other 50% are pleomorphic adenomas (benign mixed

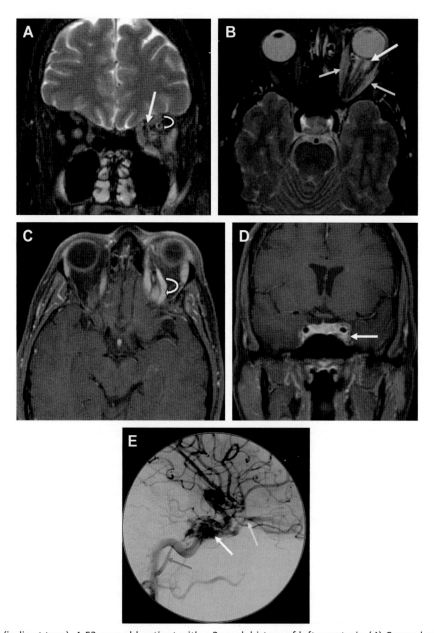

Fig. 8. CCF (indirect type). A 52-year-old patient with a 3-week history of left proptosis. (*A*) Coronal and (*B*) axial fat-suppressed T2W MR images show hyperintense edema in the intraconal space (*white arrow*), enlarged superior ophthalmic vein (*curved arrow*), and edematous and enlarged extraocular muscles (*yellow arrows*). (*C*) Axial and (*D*) coronal enhanced fat-suppressed T1W MR images show an enlarged superior ophthalmic vein (*curved arrow*) and an enlarged left cavernous sinus (*white arrow*). (*E*) Digitally subtracted cerebral angiogram lateral projection image shows abnormal early filling of the cavernous sinus (*white arrow*), superior ophthalmic vein (*yellow arrow*), and the inferior petrosal sinus (*red arrow*) consistent with an indirect CCF.

tumors).[36] Tumors arise more frequently from the orbital lobe of the lacrimal gland rather than the palpebral lobe, and therefore posterior rather than anterior extension is more common.[31] MR imaging is the modality of choice for differentiation of an epithelial tumor from an inflammatory or lymphoproliferative process, characterizing extent

of tumor involvement including assessment of perineural spread of malignancies. Pleomorphic adenoma is the most common benign epithelial tumor of the lacrimal gland and presents as a slowly enlarging, painless mass. Pain, diplopia, and/or rapid growth are not common and should suggest potential uncommon malignant

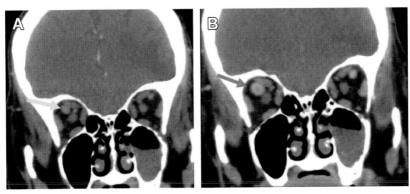

Fig. 9. Venous varix. A 75-year-old patient with an incidentally detected enlarged structure on noncontrast head CT. (*A, B*) Coronal reformat contrast-enhanced CT performed at rest (*A*) and with Valsalva (*B*) shows the characteristic dilatation of a venous varix with Valsalva (*arrows*).

transformation.[31] Adenoid cystic carcinoma is the most common malignant epithelial neoplasm of the lacrimal gland and often presents as a painful, firm mass with little proptosis. These tumors are not encapsulated and, on imaging, frequently show poorly defined margins, infiltration into the bone, and propensity for posterior extension and perineural invasion (**Fig. 10**).

LESIONS THAT DO NOT BELONG IN THE ORBIT

The most common disorders that result in lesions not normally in the orbit are foreign bodies, congenital malformations, infectious/inflammatory processes, and tumors. The patient's age, history, and acuity of symptoms are the most helpful clinical features when differentiating these lesions. Most pediatric lesions are infectious or benign, although aggressive tumors such as rhabdomyosarcoma may occur.

Orbital infection should be clinically apparent; however, adequate clinical assessment is limited because of the presence of edema. As such, imaging is essential to assess the extent of infection and associated complications. Most orbital cellulitis is secondary to sinusitis. Other causes of orbital infections include retained foreign body or penetrating injury. The imaging evaluation of orbital infection and treatment revolves around the orbital septum. The orbital septum is a thin sheet of fibrous tissue located beneath the orbicularis oculi muscle, which is continuous with the periosteum, which is loosely attached to bone, creating a potential space except at sites of firm attachment (sutures, fissures and foramina). Small defects in the orbital septum occur where vessels and nerves penetrate it. Preseptal soft tissue drains through superficial venous structures, whereas postseptal tissue drains by deep venous structures (superior and inferior ophthalmic veins,

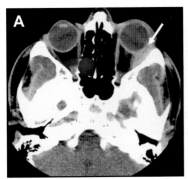
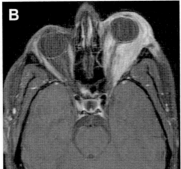
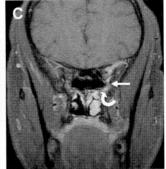

Fig. 10. Lacrimal gland adenoid cystic carcinoma in a 27-year-old man. (*A*) Axial enhanced CT shows asymmetric heterogeneous enlargement of the left lacrimal gland (*arrow*). There is mild proptosis, and no bone involvement. (*B*) Axial enhanced fat-suppressed T1W MR image performed 11 months later for eye pain shows marked proptosis and enhancing tissue in all compartments of the left orbit extending to the orbital apex, as well in the periorbital region. The cavernous sinus is normal. (*C*) Coronal enhanced fat-suppressed T1W MR image extending from the apex to the pterygopalatine fossa (*curved arrow*) via the inferior orbital fissure (*arrow*).

infraorbital vein, deep facial vein) toward the cavernous sinus, putting the patient at risk for cavernous sinus thrombosis.

Orbital infection is the most common complication of sinusitis, and is the most common cause of unilateral proptosis in a child (in adults, pseudotumor and thyroid ophthalmopathy are the most common causes of proptosis). Preseptal infection generally occurs in the pediatric population with periorbital swelling, erythema, and tenderness without impaired extraocular muscle movement or proptosis. Sinus-related orbital infection may occur by direct extension through congenital or acquired bone deficiencies, or indirectly through valveless draining veins. Imaging of orbital infections is initially performed with contrast-enhanced CT, and images are evaluated for extent of involvement (preseptal, postseptal, intracranial) and complicating features (orbital abscess, osteomyelitis, venous/cavernous sinus thrombosis, meningitis, subdural empyema, epidural abscess) (**Fig. 11**). Abscesses are present in one-half of all cases of orbital cellulitis caused by sinusitis, and usually develop in the subperiosteal space adjacent to the involved sinus.

Infantile hemangiomas are the most common benign tumors of infancy. They appear shortly after birth, undergo a proliferative phase around the age of 6 to 12 months, follow by involution over 5 to 7 years, and are replaced by fibrofatty tissue.[29] Infantile hemangiomas may be transpatial, although there is a predilection for involvement of the superior orbit. MR imaging shows a mildly hyperintense mass on T2W images with small linear flow voids, and intense homogeneous contrast enhancement indicating high-flow vascular tumor (**Fig. 12**). The role of imaging includes characterization of the mass and identifying its extent. Although these are benign tumors, their growth in the developing orbit of a child poses the potential for unique complications such as astigmatism, strabismus, and amblyopia. Rarer complications of orbital hemangiomas include hemorrhage or optic nerve compression. Treatment options include observation, steroids, interferon, laser therapy, and/or surgical excision. More recently, propranolol, either systemically or topically, has shown some success in the treatment of infantile hemangiomas.

Venous malformations are slow-flow vascular malformations that are soft and compressible,

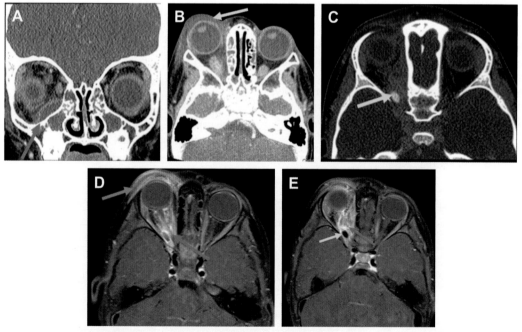

Fig. 11. Orbital cellulitis. Patient 1: a 13-month-old baby with sickle cell anemia presented with acute right proptosis, fever, and preseptal swelling. (*A*) Coronal reformat contrast- enhanced CT shows a subperiosteal abscess (*red arrow*) in the extraconal inferior right orbit associated with acute sinusitis. (*B*) Axial contrast-enhanced CT shows preseptal soft tissue thickening (*yellow arrow*) consistent with cellulitis, and right proptosis. Patient 2: a 2-year-old child with right eye pain and swelling following orbital trauma from a pencil 2 weeks earlier. (*C*) Axial contrast-enhanced CT shows a radiodense foreign body (*yellow arrow*) in the postseptal orbit and surrounding intraconal inflammation consistent with postseptal cellulitis. Inflammation extends to the superior orbital fissure. (*D, E*) Axial enhanced fat-suppressed T1W MR images show preseptal (*green arrow*) and postseptal intraconal (*red arrow*) enhancing tissue consistent with cellulitis, and a foreign body (*yellow arrow*).

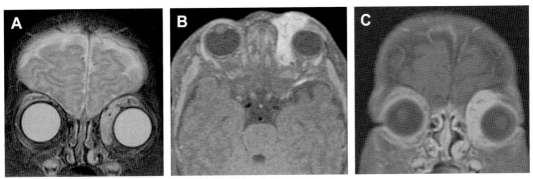

Fig. 12. Infantile hemangioma in an 8-week-old baby with left proptosis. (*A*) Coronal fat-suppressed T2W MR image shows a homogeneous T2W hyperintense mass involving all compartments of the orbit with small linear hypointense flow voids. (*B*) Axial and coronal (*C*) enhanced fat-suppressed T1W MR images show a homogeneously enhancing trans-spatial orbital mass involving the preseptal and postseptal orbit.

and represent the most common vascular malformation of the head and neck. Venous malformations of the orbit have been called cavernous hemangiomas, although these represent vascular malformations rather than tumors. These lesions may be found anywhere in the orbit, but are most commonly intraconal. They grow slowly as the patient grows and are either detected incidentally or, if there is painless proptosis, by imaging. An association between development of abrupt proptosis and pregnancy or puberty has been described.[29] On MR imaging, venous malformations appear as demarcated, often lobular, T2 hyperintense (similar to CSF) masses that show progressive enhancement with contrast (**Fig. 13**). Phleboliths, present in 50% of lesions, are characteristic and are seen as focal rounded calcification

on CT, and T2W hypointensity on MR imaging. If there are symptomatic effects of the mass, these lesions can be surgically excised, otherwise orbital venous malformations are often observed, although they progressively enlarge in most patients.

Lymphatic or mixed venous and lymphatic malformations frequently present in the first decade of life with painless proptosis, but may present with rapidly developing proptosis caused by spontaneous hemorrhage simulating infection or malignancy. Unlike a venous malformation, the lymphatic malformation is noncompressible on physical examination. MR imaging shows a unilocular or multiseptated transpatial mass with T2 hyperintensity. There are no flow voids and there is only thin peripheral enhancement in the lymphatic

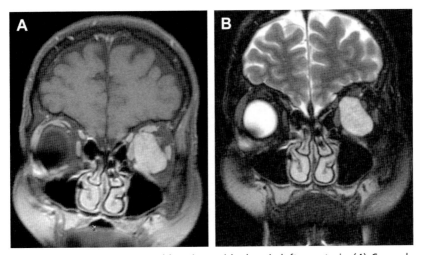

Fig. 13. Venous malformation in a 53-year-old patient with chronic left proptosis. (*A*) Coronal enhanced fat-suppressed T1W MR image shows a well-defined, avidly enhancing intraconal mass medial to the optic nerve and distinctly separate from it. (*B*) Coronal fat-suppressed T2W MR image shows that the demarcated mass is homogeneously hyperintense.

component, whereas the venous component shows larger areas of enhancement. Fluid-fluid levels are characteristic and result from propensity of these lesions to hemorrhage (**Fig. 14**).

Rhabdomyosarcoma is the most common soft tissue sarcoma in the pediatric population and the second most common head and neck malignancy. Rhabdomyosarcoma in the orbit often presents with rapidly progressive proptosis. Orbital rhabdomyosarcomas involve the orbit in 1 of 2 ways. Isolated intraorbital tumors arise in the soft tissues, usually in the superonasal orbit, and rarely invade bone. They occur most commonly in children in the first decade of life. Parameningeal rhabdomyosarcomas tend to develop in the paranasal sinuses and secondarily invade the orbit causing significant bone destruction. CT and MR imaging are important in evaluating extent of disease. Rhabdomyosarcomas most commonly are homogeneous and avidly enhance.[37,38] On occasion, these tumors may have similar appearance to an infantile hemangioma. The atypical age of the patient, unusual growth pattern, aggressive features, and low ADC signal intensity with diffusion imaging aid in the correct diagnosis (**Fig. 15**).[39] Orbital rhabdomyosarcoma is less likely to develop metastatic disease, which is typically by hematogenous spread to bone or lungs rather than to regional lymph nodes. There are 3 histologic types of rhabdomyosarcomas: embryonal (75%), alveolar (20%), and pleomorphic (5%).[40] The alveolar type is more common in older children and carries a worse prognosis than the embryonal type.

Other malignant neoplasms that may involve the orbit include lymphoma, leukemia, and metastatic disease. Lymphomas are the most common malignant orbital neoplasm in adults and have been increasing on an age-adjusted basis rapidly over the past several decades. Most are low-grade B-cell non-Hodgkin neoplasms with marginal zone B-cell lymphomas (MALT) representing more than 50% in most series. Most lymphomas occur in older adults and often have an indolent course. Up to 5% of systemic lymphoma may secondarily involve the orbit, but most orbital lymphomas develop a priori, and a significant number (25%–81%) may develop systemic disease.[41,42] Presenting symptoms most often are those of a painless orbital mass. Orbital lymphoma may develop anywhere in the orbit, but is particularly common in the eyelid, conjunctiva, and lacrimal gland. Approximately 50% develop in the lacrimal gland, which is more common than epithelial lacrimal gland tumors. MR of indolent orbital lymphoma shows a homogeneously enhancing orbital mass that conforms to the orbit and does not result in aggressive bony destruction (**Fig. 16**). Bilateral orbital involvement occurs in approximately 20% of cases and significantly increases the likelihood of subsequent systemic disease. ^{18}F-fluorodeoxyglucose (FDG) positron emission tomography (PET)/CT has a clear role for staging and monitoring systemic lymphoma; however, it has a less defined role for the surveillance of isolated orbital lymphoma. Orbital lymphoma shows increased uptake on ^{18}F-FDG PET/CT; however, orbital pseudotumor can also show increased uptake.[43] DWI has shown the potential ability to differentiate between orbital lymphoma and pseudotumor, although generalized differentiation of benign from malignant orbital disorders with diffusion imaging is likely confounded by the multiple different histologies.[23] DWI has its highest sensitivity and specificity when evaluating an infiltrative T2W hypointense orbital

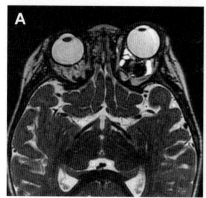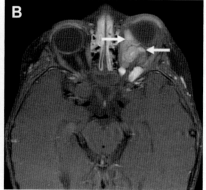

Fig. 14. Venolymphatic malformation in a 14-month-old baby with proptosis. (*A*) Axial fat-suppressed T2W image shows a multiloculated retrobulbar orbital mass. There are areas of T2W hyperintensity as well as areas of marked T2 hypointensity with fluid-fluid levels consistent with hemorrhage. (*B*) Axial enhanced fat-suppressed T1W MR image shows fluid-fluid levels (*arrows*) and serpiginous areas of enhancement.

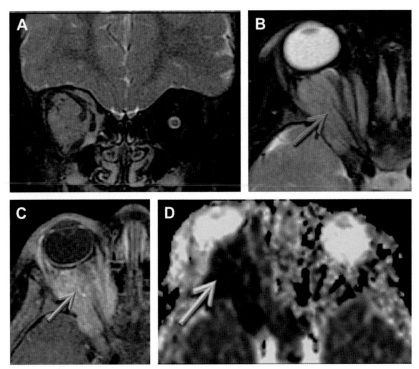

Fig. 15. Rhabdomyosarcoma in a 2-year-old child with 5-day history of progressive proptosis. (*A*) Coronal and axial (*B*) fat-suppressed T2W MR images show a postseptal intraconal and extraconal hyperintense orbital mass engulfing the extraocular muscles with probable small flow voids (*red arrow*). (*C*) Axial enhanced fat-suppressed T1W MR image shows solid homogeneous enhancement of the mass (*blue arrow*). (*D*) Axial ADC MR image shows marked hypointensity (*yellow arrow*) of the mass, consistent with restricted diffusion. The clinical history and restricted diffusion support rhabdomyosarcoma rather than infantile hemangioma. Pathology confirmed embryonal rhabdomyosarcoma.

because the disorders are likely to be hypocellular inflammatory lesions with fibrosis showing increased ADC versus aggressive hypercellular tumors with low ADC.[23] Aggressive higher grade orbital lymphomas (large B-cell lymphomas) occur infrequently but are more likely to exhibit bony invasion.

Retinoblastoma is the most common primary malignancy of childhood. The mean age of presentation is 18 months, and 95% present before 5

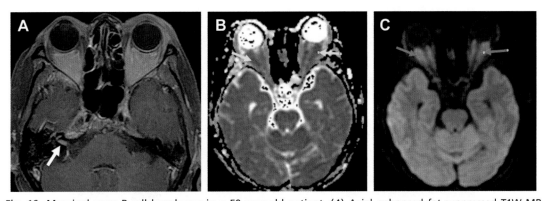

Fig. 16. Marginal zone B-cell lymphoma in a 59-year-old patient. (*A*) Axial enhanced fat-suppressed T1W MR image shows extensive infiltrating, enhancing masses replacing the retrobulbar fat and involving the extraocular muscles in bilateral orbits. Note intracranial involvement with enhancement in the Meckel cave bilaterally, and enhancing tumor in the right internal auditory canal (*arrow*). (*B*) Axial ADC shows low signal intensity of the tissue (*yellow arrows*), and (*C*) DWI shows hyperintensity (*red arrows*) favoring a neoplastic cause, in particular lymphoma, which was proved with biopsy.

years of age.[44] Leukocoria is the most common clinical sign but is not specific and the differential diagnosis, in addition to retinoblastoma, can include Coats disease, toxocariasis, retinopathy of prematurity, persistent hyperplastic primary vitreous, or drusen. The nonhereditary form occurs as unilateral disease in 70% of patients, whereas the bilateral hereditary form occurs in 30%.[45] CT imaging shows characteristic intraocular mass that may show characteristic calcification. Aside from showing an enhancing intraocular mass with restricted diffusion, MR is performed to evaluate for extraocular spread of malignancy, particularly into the postlaminar optic nerve or the orbit as well as for intracranial involvement of the disease that may involve the pineal gland (trilateral retinoblastoma) or, rarely, the pineal gland and suprasellar cistern (quadrilateral retinoblastoma) (**Fig. 17**). Other less common intraocular lesions are described in **Table 4**.[44–46]

ALTERATION OF THE ORBIT CAUSED BY BONE DISORDERS OR PERIORBITAL DISORDERS

Bone disorders or periorbital disorders may result in mass effect on orbital structures. A bone lesion may expand bone or extend from the bone into the orbital soft tissues. The age of the patient and acuity of symptoms aid in establishing a differential diagnosis. MR and CT are complementary in characterizing the bone lesion. CT assessment of a bone lesion includes evaluation of the margins (well defined with or without sclerosis, permeative, or moth eaten), periosteal reaction, and bone matrix. MR imaging is helpful for assessing soft tissue extension and the signal characteristics of the bone lesion such as the presence of fat, enhancement, or fluid-fluid levels. In children, bone lesions may be congenital (dermoid or epidermoid cysts), primary bone lesions (fibro-osseous lesions, Langerhans cell histiocytosis, Ewing sarcoma), or hematogenous metastatic disease (most commonly neuroblastoma). In older patients, fibro-osseous, metastatic disease or primary bone tumors (intraosseous hemangioma, chondrosarcoma, osteosarcoma) may be seen. Dermoid and epidermoid cysts are included in this article because of the commonly periorbital position and close association with the orbital bone. They are most frequently found near sutures (zygomaticofrontal and frontoethmoidal) and present as a painless, palpable mass. More than 80% are found in the superolateral orbit near the zygomaticofrontal suture.[47] Dermoid and epidermoid cysts slowly expand as their epithelial lining sloughs keratinaceous debris and adnexal secretions (in the case of dermoid cysts). On CT imaging, dermoid cysts are well-defined lesions that may show fat density because of their oily adnexal secretions, whereas epidermoid cysts are well defined but the sloughed keratin lining has a fluid density. The adjacent bone may show smooth long-standing pressure erosion. MR imaging of an epidermoid cyst shows T2W and fluid-attenuated inversion recovery hyperintensity, and high signal intensity on diffusion (low ADC signal indicating reduced diffusion), whereas a dermoid cyst shows T1W hyperintensity that loses signal intensity on fat saturation because of lipid material from sebaceous secretions (**Fig. 18**).

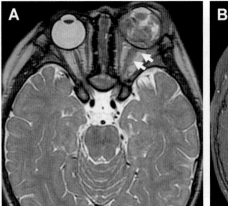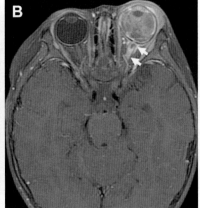

Fig. 17. Retinoblastoma. A 2-year-old child treated previously with chemotherapy for retinoblastoma. (*A*) Axial T2W MR image shows hypointense intraocular masses in an enlarged left globe with hazy periocular fat indicating infiltration of tumor. Note the enlarged left optic nerve sheath complex representing tumor infiltration (*arrows*). (*B*) Axial enhanced fat-suppressed T1W image shows extensive enhancement of the infiltrating tumor. Note enhancing tumor surrounding and involving the optic nerve and sheath (*small arrows*).

Table 4
Summary of intraocular lesions

Diagnosis	Clinical	Imaging
Coats disease	Retinal telangiectasia with exudative retinal detachment Unilateral 80%–90%, M > F; age 6–8 y (2/3 before age 10 y)	CT: hyperdense vitreous without calcification MR imaging: nonenhancing subretinal fluid
Toxocariasis	Unilateral endophthalmitis Eosinophilic granuloma caused by *Toxocara cani/ Toxocara cati* Older children	CT: hyperdense vitreous without calcification unless late stage of disease; possible retinal detachment MR imaging: enhancing retrolental or vitreous mass; thick enhancing intravitreal bands; enhancing intraocular abscess
Persistent primary hyperplastic vitreous	Full-term infant Cataract	Unilateral small globe Cone-shaped retrolental tissue Posterior hyaloid detachment No calcification unless late stages of disease in older children in the lens or in the detached retina
Retinopathy of prematurity	Premature infant with prior oxygen therapy Bilateral retinal fibrovascular tissue	Small globe Retinal detachment Calcification uncommon unless late in disease course (lens, choroid, retrolental tissue)
Choroidal osteoma	Young women Well-defined, rare, benign tumor (choristoma), involves the choroid near the optic disk	Calcification present
Choroidal hemangioma	Congenital vascular lesion Solitary form: middle aged or elderly adults Diffuse form: Sturge-Weber syndrome	MR imaging: T2W hyperintensity, intense enhancement
Retinal astrocytoma	Tuberous sclerosis or NF-1	May have calcification
Melanoma	Arises in the uvea	May show intrinsic T1 shortening from melanin
Metastatic disease	Usually breast or lung cancer	Uveal lesion

Abbreviations: F, female; M, male.
Data from Refs.[44–46]

Neither a dermoid or an epidermoid shows central enhancement, although a dermoid cyst may also show wall enhancement and/or have calcifications. Dermoid and epidermoid cysts are usually excised because, over time, they inevitably leak their secretions giving rise to a significant inflammatory reaction. A lesion that may mimic a dermoid or epidermoid cyst is a chronic hematic cyst (also known as a cholesterol granuloma). A chronic hematic cyst occurs when a subperiosteal hematoma imbibes fluid and progressively expands, leading to adjacent lytic bony changes. Patients are usually in the fourth or fifth decade of life with a clinical history of prior blunt trauma to the orbital rim and report progressive mass effect from a superolateral orbital lesion.[48] CT imaging shows

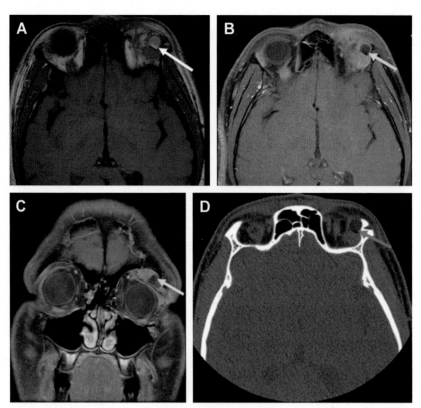

Fig. 18. Dermoid cyst with inflammation. Patient presented with acute left eye swelling. (*A*) Axial T1W MR image shows a focal mass in the left superolateral extraconal orbit with intrinsic T1 high signal (*arrow*) surrounded by the enlarged lacrimal gland. (*B*) Axial and (*C*) coronal enhanced fat-suppressed T1W MR images show lack of enhancement and loss of signal intensity in the lesion (*yellow arrow*) indicating the presence of fat/lipid products, with enhancing surrounding enlarged lacrimal gland. Note preseptal periorbital soft tissue enhancement consistent with inflammation. (*D*) Unenhanced CT confirms the presence of fat/lipid within the mass (*red arrow*). Pathology confirmed a dermoid cyst.

a lytic bone lesion, whereas MR imaging shows characteristic T1W and T2W hyperintensity. Curettage is curative.[48]

Langerhans cell histiocytosis (LCH) of the orbit most frequently involves the frontal bone.[47] LCH most commonly occurs in patients less than 4 years of age, and commonly presents with proptosis, pain, and periorbital swelling, as well as diabetes insipidus related to hypothalamic involvement.[47] On CT, LCH is well defined and lytic, often with an associated soft tissue mass (**Fig. 19**). MR imaging shows an enhancing mass with variable T2W signal intensity. Additional imaging of the body with skeletal survey radiographs or technetium 99m (Tc-99m) methylene diphosphonate skeletal scintigraphy are helpful for assessing systemic extent. Treatment includes local curettage of isolated monostotic lesions, systemic chemotherapy, or glucocorticoid therapy.[47]

Fibrous dysplasia is characterized by gradual replacement of medullary bone with fibrous tissue. Craniofacial involvement is seen in 10% to 27% of

monostotic fibrous dysplasia and 50% of polyostotic fibrous dysplasia, with the orbits affected in 20% to 39% of patients with craniofacial fibrous dysplasia.[47] Mass effect caused by the bone expansion may present with facial asymmetry, proptosis, extraocular muscle dysfunction, or decreased vision. CT imaging shows characteristic bone expansion with ground-glass appearance and relative sparing of the cortex (**Fig. 20**). MR imaging of fibrous dysplasia usually shows T1W hypointensity, variable T2W signal intensity, and solid enhancement that may lead to misinterpretation as neoplasm without CT imaging. Rare complications of fibrous dysplasia include malignant transformation in 1% of cases, which may present as new onset of pain, new soft tissue mass, or a new area of lytic destruction within the underlying fibrous lesion.

Primary malignant bone tumors of the orbit are uncommon but should be considered if a bone lesion shows rapid growth, aggressive features of the bone with osteoid matrix (osteosarcoma),

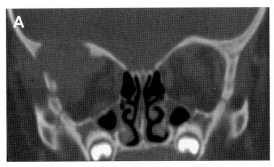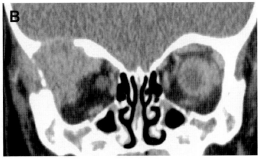

Fig. 19. LCH. An 11-month-old baby with progressive proptosis and extraocular dysmotility. (A, B) Unenhanced CT scans show a well-defined lytic bone lesion involving the right orbital roof and lateral wall with an associated extraosseous soft tissue mass. MR imaging (not shown) showed a solid enhancing mass.

cartilaginous matrix (chondrosarcoma), or an associated soft tissue mass in a pediatric patient (Ewing sarcoma). Other primary bone lesions such as an aneurysmal bone cyst (ABC), giant cell tumor, giant cell granuloma, or an intraosseous hemangioma are also uncommon. Presence of a lytic expansile bone lesion with internal fluid-fluid levels suggests an ABC, giant cell tumor, or a primary bone tumor with a secondary ABC. An ABC may result in spontaneous hemorrhage, resulting in rapidly progressive proptosis. Metastatic disease or myeloma involving the bony orbit is overwhelmingly accompanied by additional sites of disease in the bone, which aids in the diagnosis.

The paranasal sinuses all interface with the orbit. The bony orbit and the periorbita (periosteum) are the primary defense against paranasal sinus spread into the orbit. However, the bone is thin and perforated by small vessels and nerves, allowing a conduit of spread of sinus disease toward the orbit. The periorbita is the next barrier in limiting disease spread into the orbit. Mucoceles are caused by an obstruction of sinus drainage, resulting in accumulation of secretions. Over time, a mucocele results in sinus expansion and pressure erosion or dehiscence of the sinus wall. Although the periorbita remains intact, the rigidity of the bone is lost, allowing the mucocele to exert mass effect on orbital structures and resulting in decreasing vision, proptosis, and ocular dysmotility. However, if a sinus is obstructed and negative pressure develops within the sinus resulting in an atelectatic sinus, this may result in displacement of the bone toward the sinus and away from the orbital soft tissues causing enophthalmos, or may be mistaken for contralateral proptosis.[49]

OPTIC PATHWAYS AND CRANIAL NERVE INNERVATION OF THE EXTRAOCULAR MUSCLES

Compression of the intracranial optic nerve, optic chiasm, optic tracts, or a lesion in the occipital lobe may manifest as a visual field deficit and

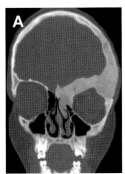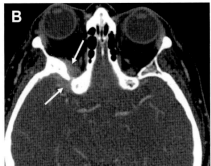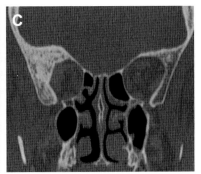

Fig. 20. Fibrous dysplasia and sphenoid wing meningioma pitfall. Patient 1: a 10-year-old child with slowly progressive left proptosis. (A) Coronal unenhanced CT in bone detail shows an expansile bone lesion involving the left frontal bone, crista galli, and middle turbinate with ground-glass appearance and relative sparing of the cortex characteristic of fibrous dysplasia. Patient 2: a 54-year-old patient with right proptosis. (B) Axial contrast-enhanced CT shows hyperostosis and mild expansion of the right sphenoid wing with extraosseous contiguous soft tissue masses located in the posterior orbit and middle cranial fossa (arrows), consistent with a sphenoid wing meningioma. (C) Coronal unenhanced CT in bone detail shows enlargement and sclerosis of the right sphenoid wing that could be mistaken for fibrous dysplasia if the images are not carefully analyzed.

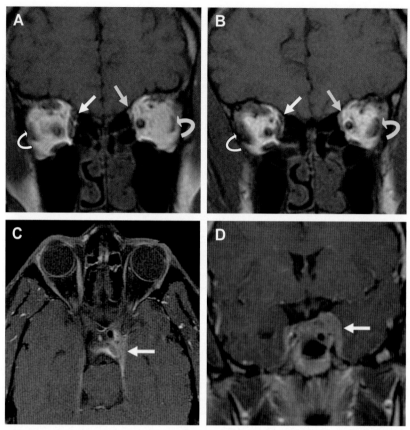

Fig. 21. Extraocular muscle denervation caused by cavernous sinus meningioma. A 34-year-old patient with oph-thalmoplegia. (*A, B*) Coronal T1W MR images show atrophy of the left extraocular muscles innervated by the third cranial nerve (superior, medial, and inferior rectus), as well as atrophy of the left superior oblique muscle (*yellow arrow*) compared with the right side (*white arrow*) and the left lateral rectus muscle (*yellow curved arrow*) compared with the right (*white curved arrow*), representing fourth and sixth cranial nerve palsies, respec-tively. (*C*) Axial and (*D*) coronal enhanced fat-suppressed T1W MR images show a homogeneously enhancing left cavernous sinus mass (*arrow*) consistent with a meningioma. On the axial image (*C*), the left globe is deviated.

require imaging to identify the disorder. Clinical assessment places the lesion as prechiasmatic, chiasmatic, or postchiasmatic by the pattern of visual field defect or additional symptoms (ie, proptosis) and allows directed imaging of the orbit, sella, and/or brain. Suprasellar masses such as a pituitary macroadenoma, meningioma, or aneu-rysm are usually readily differentiated with dedi-cated thin-section MR imaging of the sella.

A third cranial nerve palsy can be clinically characterized as pupillary sparing or pupillary involving. The parasympathetic fibers from the Edinger-Westphal nucleus are located on the periphery of the third nerve through the interpe-duncular cistern. An extrinsic mass compressing the nerve, such as a posterior communicating artery aneurysm, may result in parasympathetic dysfunction and an abnormally dilated pupil. An acute third nerve palsy with pupillary involvement must be evaluated for an aneurysm with CT angi-ography or MR angiography as initial imaging. Sparing of these parasympathetic fibers is more often seen with disorders involving the core of the third nerve such as ischemia or diabetic cranial neuropathy. Acute neuroimaging does not need to be performed for a complete, pupil-sparing third nerve palsy in the presence of vascular risk factors.[50]

The long length of the fourth (trochlear) and sixth (abducens) cranial nerves makes them prone to multiple disorders that result in stretching of the nerves (hydrocephalus, hemorrhage, increased intracranial pressure).[51] Permanent dysfunction may develop in these nerves and, at later time of imaging, no identifiable disorder is present. An important unique dysfunction of lateral gaze known as intranuclear ophthalmoplegia is most commonly related to a demyelinating lesion in the dorsal pons affecting the medial longitudinal fasciculus, which connects nuclei for the third and sixth cranial nerves assisting in coordinated movement of the extraocular muscles.

Extraocular muscle atrophy may uncommonly be caused by denervation. The third cranial nerve innervates the superior, medial, and inferior rectus muscles, the inferior oblique muscle, and the levator palpebrae superioris muscle. The fourth cranial nerve innervates the superior oblique muscle, whereas the sixth cranial nerve innervates the lateral rectus muscle. Congenital hypoplasia or absence of the sixth cranial nerve is uncommon but can be seen with Moebius syndrome or Duane syndrome and, on imaging, shows a small lateral rectus muscle and inability to identify the sixth cranial nerve. A combination of cranial nerve 3, 4, and 6 dysfunction or denervation atrophy should raise suspicion for a mass located in the cavernous sinus or near the orbital apex (**Fig. 21**). Disorders may include inflammation caused by orbital pseudotumor/Tolosa-Hunt syndrome; cavernous sinus thrombosis; or tumors such as meningiomas, schwannomas, metastatic disease, lymphoma, or central skull base primary bone tumors (chordoma, chondrosarcoma). Imaging should lead to development of a narrow differential diagnosis with further recommendations if a specific diagnosis cannot be made.

SUMMARY

Evaluation of orbital disorders requires integration of clinical history with assessment of the orbital structures. Although it is important to describe the location of a lesion with respect to the muscle cone, it is perhaps more helpful when creating a differential to evaluate orbital lesions to establish whether they alter a normal structure, whether there is an aberrant lesion in the orbit, or whether the disorder is from the bony orbit or tissues around the orbit.

REFERENCES

1. Aiken AH, Mukherjee P, Green AJ, et al. MR imaging of optic neuropathy with extended echo-train acquisition fluid-attenuated inversion recovery. AJNR Am J Neuroradiol 2011;32(2):301–5.

2. Kirsch E, von Arx G, Hammer B. Imaging in Graves' orbitopathy. Orbit 2009;28(4):219–25.

3. Ozgen A, Ariyurek M. Normative measurements of orbital structures using CT. AJR Am J Roentgenol 1998;170(4):1093–6.

4. Miller NR. Primary tumours of the optic nerve and its sheath. Eye 2004;18:1026–37.

5. Ozgen A, Aydingoz U. Normative measurement of orbital structures using MRI. J Comput Assist Tomogr 2000;24(3):493–6.

6. Lagreze WA, Lazarro A, Weigel M, et al. Morphometry of the retrobulbar human optic nerve: comparison between conventional sonography and ultrafast magnetic resonance sequences. Invest Ophthalmol Vis Sci 2007;48(5):1913–7.

7. Ettl A, Salomonowitz E, Koornneef L, et al. High-resolution MR imaging anatomy of the orbit. Correlation with comparative cryosectional anatomy. Radiol Clin North Am 1998;36(6):1021–45.

8. Tamboli DA, Harris MA, Hogg JP, et al. Computed tomography dimensions of the lacrimal gland in normal Caucasian orbits. Ophthal Plast Reconstr Surg 2011;27(6):453–6.

9. Lerdlum S, Boonsirikamchai P, Setsakol E. Normative measurements of extraocular muscle using computed tomography. J Med Assoc Thai 2007; 90(2):301–12.

10. Lee JS, Lim DW, Lee SH, et al. Normative measurements of Korean orbital structures revealed by computerized tomography. Acta Ophthalmol Scand 2001;79:197–200.

11. Barkovich AJ. Pediatric neuroimaging. 4th edition. Philadelphia: Lippincott Williams and Wilkins; 2005.

12. Binning MJ, Liu JK, Kestle JR, et al. Optic pathway gliomas: a review. Neurosurg Focus 2007;23(5):E2.

13. Pereira LS, McCulley TJ. Perineural arachnoidal gliomatosis: case report. Arq Bras Oftalmol 2008;71(4): 595–8.

14. Kornreich L, Blaser S, Schwarz M, et al. Optic pathway glioma: correlation of imaging findings with the presence of neurofibromatosis. AJNR Am J Neuroradiol 2001;22(10):1963–9.

15. Pau D, Al Zubidi N, Yalamanchili S, et al. Optic neuritis. Eye 2011;25:833–42.

16. Saeed P, Rootman J, Nugent RA, et al. Optic nerve sheath meningiomas. Ophthalmology 2003;110(10): 2019–30.

17. Purvin V, Kawasaki A, Jacobson DM. Optic perineuritis: clinical and radiographic features. Arch Ophthalmol 2001;119(9):1299–306.

18. Albert & Jakobiec's principles & practices of ophthalmology. 3rd edition. Philadelphia: Saunders Elsevier; 2008.

19. Douglas RS, Gupta S. The pathophysiology of thyroid eye disease: implications for immunotherapy. Curr Opin Ophthalmol 2011;22:385–90.

20. Gould DJ, Roth FS, Soparkar C. The diagnosis and treatment of thyroid-associated ophthalmopathy. Aesthetic Plast Surg 2012;36(3):638–48. DOI:10.1007/s00266-011-9843-4.

21. Bahn RS. Graves' ophthalmopathy. N Engl J Med 2010;362(8):726–38.

22. Weber AL, Romo LV, Sabates NR. Pseudotumor of the orbit. Clinical, pathologic, and radiologic

evaluation. Radiol Clin North Am 1999;37(1): 151–68.

23. Sepahdari AR, Aakalu VK, Setabutr P, et al. Indeterminate orbital masses: restricted diffusion at MR imaging with echo-planar diffusion-weighted imaging predicts malignancy. Radiology 2010;256(2): 554–64.

24. Ahn Yuen SJ, Rubin P. Idiopathic orbital inflammation. Distribution, clinical features, and treatment outcome. Arch Ophthalmol 2003;121:491–9.

25. Lacey B, Chang W, Rootman JR. Nonthyroid causes of extraocular muscle disease. Surv Ophthalmol 1999;44(3):187–213.

26. Carlow TJ, Depper MH, Orrison WW Jr. MR of extraocular muscles in chronic progressive external ophthalmoplegia. AJNR Am J Neuroradiol 1998;19: 95–9.

27. Halbach VV, Hieshima GB, Higashida RT, et al. Carotid cavernous fistulae: indications for urgent treatment. AJR Am J Roentgenol 1987;149:587–93.

28. Mafee MF. Orbit: embryology, anatomy, and pathology. In: Som PM, Curtin HD, editors. Head and neck imaging. 4th edition. St Louis(MO): Mosby; 2003. p. 529–654.

29. Smoker WR, Gentry LR, Yee NK, et al. Vascular lesions of the orbit: more than meets the eye. Radiographics 2008;28:185–204.

30. Rubin PA, Remulla HD. Orbital venous anomalies demonstrated by spiral computed tomography. Ophthalmology 1997;104:1463–70.

31. Mafee MF, Edward DP, Koeller KK, et al. Lacrimal gland tumors and simulating lesions. Clinicopathologic and MR imaging features. Radiol Clin North Am 1999;37(1):219–39.

32. Mavrikakis I, Rootman J. Diverse clinical presentations of orbital sarcoid. Am J Ophthalmol 2007; 144(5):769–75.

33. Simon EM, Zoarski GH, Rothman MI, et al. Systemic sarcoidosis with bilateral orbital involvement: MR findings. AJNR Am J Neuroradiol 1998;19(2):336–7.

34. Prabhakaran VC, Saeed P, Esmaeli B, et al. Orbital and adnexal sarcoidosis. Arch Ophthalmol 2007; 125(12):1657–62.

35. Atlas SW, Grossman RI, Savino PJ, et al. Surface-coil MR of orbital pseudotumor. AJNR Am J Neuroradiol 1987;8:141–6.

36. Weis E, Rootman J, Joly TJ, et al. Epithelial lacrimal gland tumors. Pathologic classification and current understanding. Arch Ophthalmol 2009;127(8): 1016–102.

37. Mafee MF, Pai E, Philip B. Rhabdomyosarcoma of the orbit. Evaluation with MR Imaging and CT. Radiol Clin North Am 1998;36(6):1215–27.

38. Lee JH, Lee MS, Lee BH, et al. Rhabdomyosarcoma of the head and neck in adults: MR and CT Findings. AJNR Am J Neuroradiol 1996;17:1923–8.

39. Lope LA, Hutcheson KA, Khademian ZP, et al. Magnetic resonance imaging in the analysis of pediatric orbital tumors: utility of diffusion-weighted imaging. J AAPOS 2010;14(3):257–62.

40. MacArthur CJ, McGill TJ, Healy GB. Pediatric head and neck rhabdomyosarcoma. Clin Pediatr 1992; 31(2):66–70.

41. Bairey O, Kremer I, Rakowsky E, et al. Orbital and adnexal involvement in systemic non-Hodgkin's lymphoma. Cancer 1994;73(9):2395–9.

42. Demirci H, Shields CL, Karatza EC, et al. Orbital lymphoproliferative tumors: analysis of clinical features and systemic involvement in 160 cases. Ophthalmology 2008;115:1626–31.

43. Miyamoto J, Tatsuzawa K, Owada K, et al. Usefulness and limitations of fluorine-18-fluorodeoxyglucose positron emission tomography for the detection of malignancy of orbital tumors. Neurol Med Chir 2008;48:495–9.

44. Chung EM, Specht CS, Schroeder JW. Pediatric orbit tumors and tumorlike lesions: neuroepithelial lesions of the ocular globe and optic nerve. Radiographics 2007;27:1159–86.

45. Kadom N, Sze RW. Radiological reasoning: leukocoria in a child. AJR Am J Roentgenol 2008;191:s40–4.

46. Mafee MF, Karimi A, Shah JD, et al. Anatomy and pathology of the eye: role of MR Imaging and CT. Radiol Clin North Am 2006;44:135–57.

47. Chung EM, Murphey MD, Specht CS, et al. From the archives of the AFIP: pediatric orbit tumors and tumorlike lesions: osseous lesions of the orbit. Radiographics 2008;28:1193–214.

48. Selva D, White VA, O'Connell JX, et al. Primary bone tumors of the orbit. Surv Ophthalmol 2004;49(3): 328–42.

49. Curtin HD, Rabinov JD. Extension to the orbit from paraorbital disease. The sinuses. Radiol Clin North Am 1998;36(6):1201–13.

50. Yanovitch T, Buckley E. Diagnosis and management of third nerve palsy. Curr Opin Ophthalmol 2007;18: 373–8.

51. Chi SL, Bhatti MT. The diagnostic dilemma of neuroimaging in acute isolated sixth nerve palsy. Curr Opin Ophthalmol 2009;20:423–9.

Patterns of Perineural Tumor Spread in Head and Neck Cancer

Gul Moonis, MD[a,b,*], Mary Beth Cunnane, MD[a],
Kevin Emerick, MD[c], Hugh Curtin, MD[a]

KEYWORDS

- Perineural tumor spread • Trigeminal nerve • Facial nerve • Adenoid cystic carcinoma
- Skin cancer metastases

KEY POINTS

- Perineural tumor may extend in a retrograde or antegrade direction and can have skip lesions. Inspection of the entire course of the nerve should be performed.
- Perineural tumor spread (PNS) is most common along branches of the trigeminal and facial nerves.
- PNS can spread from the facial to the trigeminal nerve and vice versa via the auriculotemporal or greater superficial petrosal nerves.

PATTERNS OF PERINEURAL SPREAD IN HEAD AND NECK CANCER

Perineural tumor spread (PNS) is a well-recognized entity in head and neck cancers and represents the dissemination of tumor from the primary site via the nerve and neural sheath. It is important to distinguish between perineural invasion and PNS of tumor. Perineural invasion represents small nerve involvement and is a histologic finding at the primary site, present when tumor cells lie within any of the layers of the nerve sheath or when tumor cells surround more than 33% of the circumference of the nerve.[1] Perineural invasion has significant negative prognostic value and correlates with recurrence. Perineural spread, however, describes extension of malignancy beyond the confines of the primary tumor via neural conduits and represents gross, radiologically evident large nerve involvement. It is a mode of metastasis rather than a histologic feature of the primary tumor. PNS most commonly occurs in a retrograde fashion, toward the central nervous system, but also can occur in an antegrade direction. Like perineural invasion, PNS is also considered a poor prognostic factor and suggests aggressive tumor biology.

The common head and neck tumors that spread via the perineural route include cutaneous malignancies, mucosal primaries such as squamous cell carcinoma and salivary gland malignancies (especially adenoid cystic carcinoma), desmoplastic melanoma, nasopharyngeal carcinoma, myeloma, lymphoma, and leukemia. Various theories have been proposed for why PNS occurs; the nerve may represent the line of least resistance through anatomy otherwise difficult to traverse by tumor, or it may be caused by expression of neurotropic growth factors by tumors of the head and neck.[2] Among patients with PNS, 40% are asymptomatic, which puts the onus on the radiologist to be vigilant to its presence.[3] If symptomatic, the patients present with pain, numbness, burning, and dysesthesia along the course of the affected nerve, and motor denervation changes. The latter is most commonly manifested as weakness of the muscles of mastication or facial paralysis. Another

[a] Department of Radiology, Massachusetts Eye and Ear Infirmary, 243 Charles St, Boston, MA 02114, USA;
[b] Department of Radiology, Beth Israel Deaconess Medical Center, 330 Brookline Avenue, Boston, MA 02215, USA; [c] Department of Otorhinolaryngology, Massachusetts Eye and Ear Infirmary, 243 Charles St, Boston, MA 02114, USA
* Corresponding author. Department of Radiology, Beth Israel Deaconess Medical Center, Massachusetts Eye and Ear Infirmary, Boston, MA.
E-mail address: gmoonis@bidmc.harvard.edu

Magn Reson Imaging Clin N Am 20 (2012) 435–446
doi:10.1016/j.mric.2012.05.006
1064-9689/12/$ – see front matter © 2012 Elsevier Inc. All rights reserved.

common presentation is multiple cranial neuropathies, which indicate involvement of the cavernous sinus and is an ominous sign.

Detection of PNS has important therapeutic implications. Accurate diagnosis of PNS allows complete tumor resection in some cases, and in others allows recognition of unresectable disease before a major ablative surgery is performed. It enables radiation fields to be expanded for complete tumor coverage. PNS also has prognostic significance; in the case of adenoid cystic carcinoma, perineural invasion detected histologically in a larger "named" nerve and skull base involvement predicted much worse rates of local control at 5 years: 12.5% compared with 90% in patients who were named nerve-negative.[4] However, PNS in adenoid cystic carcinoma does not significantly impact long-term survival, which is more dependant on tumor size, TNM staging, histologic subtype, and expression of p53.[5]

In general, PNS occurs along branches of the facial and trigeminal nerves, although spread along the sixth cranial nerve[6] and the greater auricular nerve[7] has also been described. The greater auricular nerve originates from the cervical plexus and is composed of branches of spinal nerves C2 and C3. It provides sensory supply to the skin over the parotid gland, mastoid process, and outer ear. Additionally, the facial and trigeminal nerves have various interconnections that serve as conduits for widespread dissemination of neoplasm.

Relevant Anatomy

The trigeminal nerve arises from the pons and travels through the prepontine cistern to enter the Meckel cave, a cerebrospinal fluid–filled arachnoidal recess posterolateral to the cavernous sinus (**Fig. 1**). The trigeminal gasserian ganglion resides along the lateral and anterior wall of the Meckel cave. Within the Meckel cave, the nerve divides into ophthalmic, maxillary, and mandibular divisions (**Fig. 2**). From the Meckel cave, the ophthalmic and maxillary divisions travel through the lateral wall of the cavernous sinus (**Fig. 3**). The ophthalmic division (V1), the smallest division of cranial nerve V, divides into the nasociliary, frontal, and lacrimal nerves just before it enters the orbit via the superior orbital fissure. The frontal nerve is the largest branch and divides into the supratrochlear and supraorbital branches, which provide sensory innervation to the skin of the forehead and upper eyelid and the mucosa of the frontal sinus. The nasociliary nerve supplies the nasoethmoid mucosa. The lacrimal nerve provides sensory innervation for the lacrimal gland, conjunctiva, and the lateral upper eyelids. From the cavernous sinus, the

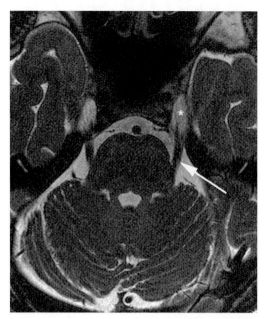

Fig. 1. Cranial nerve V anatomy. Axial 3-dimensional constructive interference in steady state (CISS) image shows the cranial nerve V traveling in the prepontine cistern (*arrow*) before entering the Meckel cave (*asterisk*).

maxillary division (V2) enters the pterygopalatine fossa (PPF) via the foramen rotundum (**Fig. 4**). Within the PPF, V2 gives rise to greater and lesser palatine branches, the zygomatic nerve (sensory to the skin of the temporal region and cheek), and the posterior superior alveolar nerve (supplying the maxillary sinus) before continuing on as the infraorbital nerve in the infraorbital canal (**Fig. 5**). The infraorbital nerve gives off the anterior and middle superior alveolar nerves to the maxillary teeth and gingiva before emerging from the infraorbital foramen to supply the skin of the midface and lateral nose. The greater and lesser palatine nerves descend from the PPF to the hard palate via the descending palatine canals (**Fig. 6**).

The mandibular division (V3) exits the skull base via the foramen ovale without entering the cavernous sinus (see **Fig. 4**B). It enters the masticator space, giving off branches to the muscles of mastication, the lingual nerve (sensory to tongue), auriculotemporal nerve (sensory to temporal scalp, secretomotor to parotid gland), and buccal nerve (sensory to buccal mucosa and molar teeth), and continues as the inferior alveolar nerve, which enters the mandibular canal and supplies the mandibular teeth and gingiva. At the level of the second premolar, the inferior alveolar nerve gives off the mental nerve, which exits via the mental foramen on the lateral aspect of the mandibular body and supplies the skin of the chin and lower

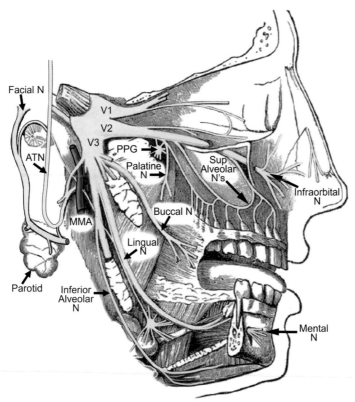

Fig. 2. Cranial nerve V anatomy. Cranial nerve V divides into the ophthalmic (V1), maxillary (V2), and mandibular (V3) branches in the Meckel cave. V1 passes through the cavernous sinus lateral wall and enters the orbit via the superior orbital fissure. V2 passes through the cavernous sinus and exits the skull via foramen rotundum. V3 exits the skull via foramen ovale and enters the masticator space, where it gives off sensory and muscular branches. The auriculotemporal nerve arises from V3 via two roots that encircle the middle meningeal artery and then form a single root, which enters the parotid gland and intermingles with branches of cranial nerve VII. ATN, auriculotemporal nerve; MMA, middle meningeal artery; N, nerve; PPG, pterygopalatine ganglion.

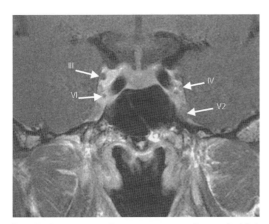

Fig. 3. Cavernous sinus anatomy. Coronal high-resolution postgadolinium image shows cranial nerve III (oculomotor), IV (trochlear), VI (abducens), and V2 (maxillary) traveling through the cavernous sinus. Cranial nerve V1 (ophthalmic) is not well seen on this image.

lip. The auriculotemporal nerve anatomy is described in greater detail in subsequent paragraphs. Tumor anywhere within the dermatomal distribution of the trigeminal nerve can perineurally spread via the pathways mentioned earlier through the skull base foramina into the cranial cavity.

The facial nerve arises from the pons, and its fibers loop around the abducens nucleus to form the facial colliculus in the anterior wall of the fourth ventricle. It crosses the cerebellopontine angle cistern (cisternal segment) and enters the internal auditory canal, where it resides in the superior anterior compartment (canalicular segment). The labyrinthine segment lies between the canalicular segment and the first genu and is so named because of its intimate relationship to the inner ear (labyrinth) (**Fig. 7**A). The tympanic segment travels posterolaterally from the first genu under the lateral semicircular canal (best appreciated on coronal images) (see **Fig. 7**B). From the second

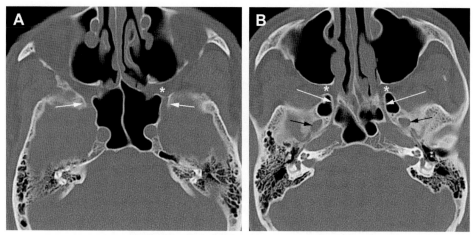

Fig. 4. Cranial nerve V anatomy. Axial CT (*A*) image shows the foramen rotundum (*arrows*) though which V2 travels after exiting from the cavernous sinus. It continues forward and enters the pterygopalatine fossa (*asterisk*). At a slightly inferior level (*B*), the vidian canal (*white arrows*) can be seen extending forward from the foramen lacerum. Foramen ovale resides in the sphenoid wing (*black arrows*). Asterisks indicate the pterygopalatine fossa.

genu, close to the pyramidal process, the nerve travels straight down in the mastoid bone (mastoid segment) and exits the skull via the stylomastoid foramen to enter the parotid gland. The facial nerve has five branches in the parotid gland: temporal, zygomatic, buccal, marginal mandibular, and cervical. Presence of a perineural venous plexus can cause normal enhancement beyond the first genu of the nerve. If the enhancement is thick and asymmetric, even in the parts of the nerve that can normally enhance, one should suspect pathology in the appropriate clinical setting. Any enhancement of the nerve proximal to the first genu is very suspicious.

Connections exist between the facial and trigeminal nerve that facilitate tumor traveling between these nerves. The greater superficial petrosal nerve is a branch of the facial nerve that provides parasympathetic innervation to the lacrimal gland, palate, nasal cavity, and nasopharynx. It contains facial nerve fibers originating in the nervus intermedius, exits the geniculate ganglion at the facial hiatus, passes close to the Meckel cave, and joins with the deep petrosal

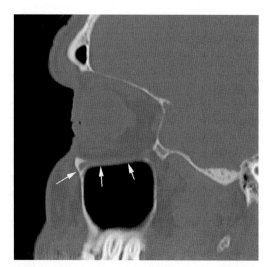

Fig. 5. Cranial nerve V anatomy. The infraorbital foramen and fissure is noted on this sagittal CT image (*arrows*). Skin cancers in the infraorbital region can travel along this pathway to the pterygopalatine fossa.

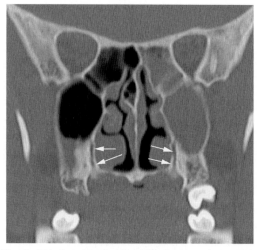

Fig. 6. Palatine canals. The palatine canals carrying the greater and lesser palatine nerves extend superiorly toward the pterygopalatine fossa from the hard palate (*arrows*).

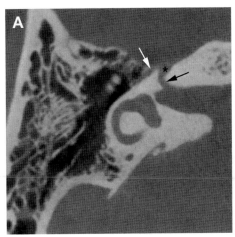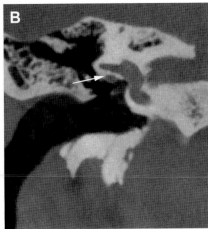

Fig. 7. CN VII anatomy. Axial cone beam CT image (*A*) shows the labyrinthine segment (*black arrow*) extending into the geniculate ganglion (*asterisk*). The proximal tympanic segment is also noted (*white arrow*). On the coronal image (*B*) the tympanic segment of the facial nerve (*arrow*) is seen traveling below the lateral semicircular canal.

nerve to form the vidian nerve, which passes through the vidian canal to the pterygopalatine fossa where its preganglionic fibers synapse in the pterygopalatine ganglion. Some of the post-ganglionic fibers join branches of V2 in the PPF (**Fig. 8**).[8] PNS along the greater superficial petrosal nerve (GSPN) usually occurs after the tumor has reached the PPF, from where retrograde extension via the vidian nerve to GSPN can occur (**Fig. 9**). Also, tumor in the Meckel cave may extend directly to the GSPN because of their proximity.

The auriculotemporal nerve arises as two roots from the posterior division of V3 soon after it exits the skull base via the foramen ovale. The two roots encircle the middle meningeal artery (see **Fig. 2**) and then converge to form a single nerve, which passes into the parotid gland along the posterior border of the mandibular ramus/condylar head. The nerve gives off intraparotid secretomotor branches and eventually provides sensory innervation to the auricle and skin of the temporal region. Rami of the auriculotemporal nerve connect it to the facial nerve within the parotid gland.[9] Tumor may spread from cranial nerve V to VII (or vice versa) along this route (**Fig. 10**).

Finally, the chorda tympani (branch of cranial nerve VII in the temporal bone) joins the lingual nerve (V3 branch) after it exits from the skull and supplies sensation to the anterior two-thirds of the tongue and secretomotor innervation to the submandibular and sublingual glands (see **Fig. 2**).

Fat is generally present where the cranial nerves exit from skull base foramen. These fat pads can be seen at the superior orbital fissure (V1), the PPF (V2), inferior to the foramen ovale (V3; the trigeminal fat pad), and the stylomastoid foramen. Obliteration of these juxtaforaminal fat pads is a key element in detecting PNS.

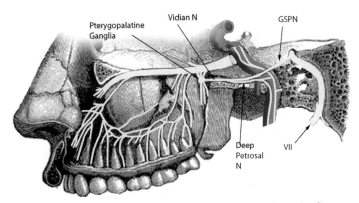

Fig. 8. Greater superficial petrosal nerve (GSPN) anatomy. The GSPN arises from the first genu of the facial nerve in the temporal bone, travels anteriorly and joins with the deep petrosal nerve to form the vidian nerve in the vidian canal. The vidian nerve then joins V2 branches in the pterygopalatine ganglion residing in the pterygopalatine fossa. N, nerve.

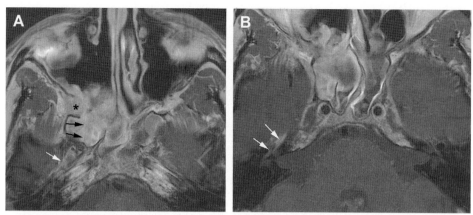

Fig. 9. PNS along the GSPN in a patient with a history of maxillary sinus squamous cell carcinoma. Axial T1-weighted postgadolinium image (*A*) shows tumor in the PPF (*asterisk*), enlargement of the vidian N (*black arrows*), and enhancement along the foramen lacerum (*white arrow*). (*B*) Enhancement extends back to the GSPN and proximal tympanic segment of the facial nerve (*arrows*); this is one of the connections between the cranial nerves V and VII, which facilitate PNS between the nerves.

Imaging approach

CT better detects the bony changes associated with PNS, but MRI is by far the preferred study for evaluation of PNS. CT findings that should raise concern for PNS include obliteration of juxtaforaminal fat pads and fat planes along the paths of cranial nerves, and foraminal enlargement and destruction (see **Fig. 10**; **Fig. 11**). Attention should be specifically directed to the pterygopalatine fossa, the foramen ovale, and the stylomastoid foramen. Although MRI is more sensitive for detecting PNS, patients frequently present for imaging without a history of primary tumor, and recognition of these findings on CT can diagnose the cause of symptoms and indicate a likely site of tumor origin. High-resolution MRI (3 mm sections, small field of view) can then be performed for the most accurate depiction of the extent of PNS. Precontrast T1-weighted images are helpful in detecting obliteration of fat along the nerves or in the juxtaforaminal fat. Fat is your friend![10] At the authors' institution, high-resolution postgadolinium 3-mm axial and coronal images without fat suppression are performed. Other head and neck radiologists advocate postgadolinium images with fat suppression for evaluation of PNS, but one must be aware of artifacts associated with fat suppression at the skull base when reviewing the images. On MRI, obliteration of fat planes and foraminal enlargement may also be appreciated,

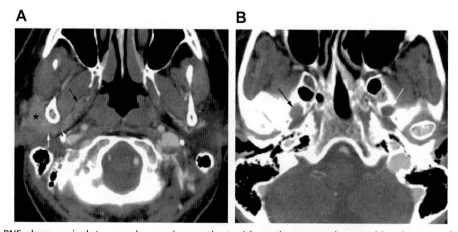

Fig. 10. PNS along auriculotemporal nerve in a patient with carcinoma ex pleomorphic adenoma of the right parotid gland. Axial contrast-enhanced CT (*A*) shows a mass in the superficial lobe of the right parotid gland (*asterisk*). Curvilinear soft tissue thickening is seen along the back of the mandibular ramus (*white arrows*) indicating tumor involving the auriculotemporal nerve, which continues anteromedially to join the trunk of V3 in the masticator space (*black arrow*). (*B*) Enlargement of the right foramen ovale is seen (*black arrow*) with loss of fat compared with the left (*white arrow*).

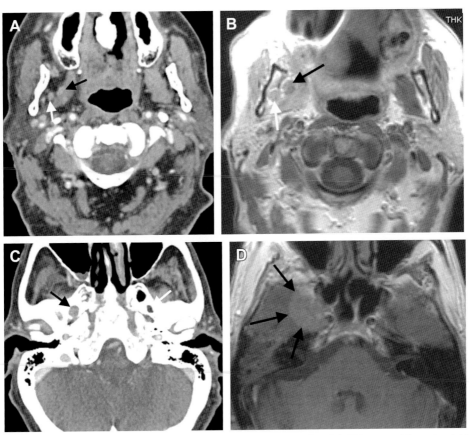

Fig. 11. PNS from adenoid cystic carcinoma of the submandibular gland. Axial CT image with contrast (*A*) shows thickening and enlargement of the right lingual nerve (*black arrow*) and inferior alveolar nerve (*white arrow*). The same findings are seen on the axial T1-weighted image with gadolinium (*B*). Tumor extension to the foramen ovale is seen (*black arrow*), which is enlarged with replacement of the normal fat on axial CT image with contrast. Normal left foramen ovale (*white arrow*) (*C*). Tumor extension is noted into the right Meckel cave and middle cranial fossa (*arrows*) on the axial T1-weighted postgadolinium image (*D*).

but subtler findings of nerve enhancement and nerve enlargement also may be seen.[11] Intracranial findings of PNS along the trigeminal nerve include bulging of the wall of the cavernous sinus, enhancement of nerves in the cavernous sinus or basal cistern, and enhancing soft tissue in the Meckel cave (see **Fig. 11**; **Figs. 12** and **13**).[12] Intracranial findings of PNS along the facial nerve include enhancement in the internal auditory canal and in the cerebellopontine angle cistern. The radiologist should be aware of skip lesions with PNS and should perform an inspection of the nerve in its entirety and look for antegrade lesions. Once tumor has accessed the PPF from any route, antegrade PNS may occur along the infraorbital nerve (see **Fig. 13**). Similarly, once tumor reaches the cavernous sinus or Meckel cave via V3, it can easily spread antegrade along V1 and V2 and retrograde to the pons. One should also look for secondary signs, such as denervation changes in the

muscles supplied by the nerves (**Fig. 14**). On MRI, denervated muscles undergo a characteristic pattern of change. Acute changes (<1 month) cause T2 hyperintensity and enhancement with increased volume. Subacute changes (up to 12–20 months) are heralded by increase in T1 hyperintensity because of fat deposition but no volume loss. Chronic changes (after 12–20 months) are characterized by increased fatty atrophy and volume loss of the affected muscle.[13] Although PNS may be evident on CT, in the authors' opinion MRI using skull base protocol (including axial thin-section non–fat saturated T1-weighted images) should be the preferred modality for complete evaluation and should be performed even if the CT is positive for PNS.

Knowledge of the site of primary tumor allows careful examination of the nearest large nerve for nerve enhancement, nerve thickening, and foraminal enlargement. **Table 1** provides a

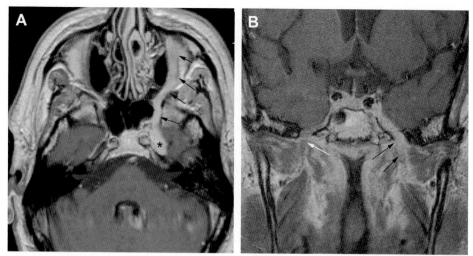

Fig. 12. PNS along V2 in a patient with desmoplastic melanoma of the cheek. Axial postcontrast T1-weighted image (*A*) shows thickening and enlargement of V2 (*arrows*) extending to PPF, foramen rotundum, and Meckel cave (*asterisk*). The coronal postgadolinium image (*B*) shows PNS into the left V3 (*black arrows*) via foramen ovale. Note the normal right V3 (*white arrow*).

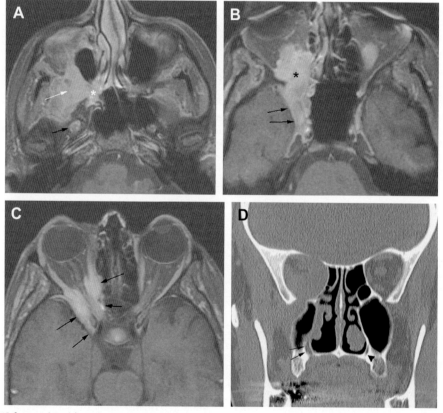

Fig. 13. PNS from adenoid cystic carcinoma of the hard palate via the palatine nerves. Axial T1-weighted postga-dolinium image (*A*) shows tumor in the PPF (*white asterisk*) and pterygomaxillary fissure/masticator space (*white arrow*). Enlargement and enhancement of the right foramen ovale is seen (*black arrow*) from direct involvement of V3 via the masticator space. (*B*) PNS into the infraorbital nerve (*asterisk*) via antegrade spread from the PPF is noted. Tumor spread is also seen into the cavernous sinus (*black arrows*). At a slightly higher level, axial T1-weighted postgadolinium image (*C*) shows tumor extending into the orbit via direct extension from the PPF with encasement of the optic nerve. The enlargement of the right palatine canals (*black arrows*) is better appre-ciated on the coronal CT image (*D*); note the normal sized left palatine canal (*black arrowhead*).

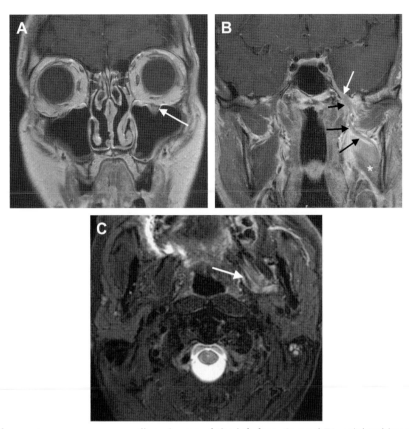

Fig. 14. PNS from cutaneous squamous cell carcinoma of the left face. Coronal T1-weighted image postgadolinium (*A*) shows a thickened enlarged infraorbital nerve (*arrow*). (*B*) Tumor extended retrogradely to the PPF and cavernous sinus with antegrade spread into the left V3 (*black arrows*), which exits the skull base via the foramen ovale (*white arrow*). Also note the enhancement of the left muscles of mastication (*asterisk*), with increased T2 signal (*white arrow*) on the axial T2-weighted images (*C*) compatible with acute denervation changes.

comprehensive list of primary tumors and nerves at risk. If the primary site is a cutaneous malignancy of the skin of the nose or cheek, attention should be directed to the infraorbital nerve (see **Figs. 12** and **14**). For orbital primaries, one should inspect the supratrochlear nerve/supraorbital nerves with attention to the orbital apex/superior orbital fissure/cavernous sinus for potential spread along V1 (ophthalmic nerve). If the primary site is the palate, then the greater and lesser palatine foramina and PPF should be evaluated carefully (see **Fig. 13**). Retromolar trigone cancers can involve the lingual or inferior alveolar nerve, and inspection of the V3 trunk is essential. Submandibular tumors should prompt inspection of the lingual and hypoglossal nerves (see **Fig. 11**), and mandibular tumors should prompt inspection of the inferior alveolar nerve. V2 involvement is seen with maxillary sinus tumors. Ethmoid sinus or medial orbital tumors may spread along V1 (ophthalmic N) branches (**Fig. 15**). The facial and auriculotemporal nerves

should be examined in all parotid malignancies (see **Fig. 10**; **Fig. 16**). Nasopharyngeal carcinoma can involve V3 through either perineural spread or direct extension to the main trunk of V3 in the masticator space. Nasopharyngeal carcinoma can also directly extend to the PPF and then involve V2 perineurally (**Fig. 17**).

In all cases, the combined V3 trunk should be evaluated within the trigeminal fat pad to the level of foramen ovale. Evaluation of a parotid tumor should include inspection of the stylomastoid foramen and the path of the auriculotemporal nerve posterior to the mandibular ramus into the trigeminal fat pad and foramen ovale.

Radiologists, treating physicians, and patients must be aware that after treatment, the imaging findings of PNS may persist indefinitely despite clinical evidence for improvement. Evidence of radiographic or clinical progression will thus become the indicator of recurrent tumor in the setting of previously noted PNS on imaging, not the mere persistence of enhancing nerves.

Table 1
Major head and neck tumors and their at-risk nerves for PNS

Primary Tumor	At-Risk Distal Nerve Branch for PNS	At-Risk Main Trunk for PNS
Cutaneous malignancy, forehead	Supratrochlear, supraorbital branch of frontal nerve	V1
Cutaneous malignancy, ear	Greater auricular nerve, auriculotemporal nerve	VII
Cutaneous malignancy, temple, upper lateral face	Zygomatic nerve Frontal nerve	V2, VII
Cutaneous malignancy, cheek	Infraorbital nerve, branches, zygomatic nerve, distal facial nerve	V2, VII
Cutaneous malignancy, nose	Infraorbital nerve	V2
Cutaneous malignancy, upper lip	Infraorbital nerve Buccal branches of facial nerve	V2, VII
Cutaneous malignancy, lower lip, chin	Mental nerve Marginal mandibular nerve	V3, VII
Floor of mouth	Lingual nerve	V3
Submandibular gland	Lingual nerve, hypoglossal nerve	V3, X11
Mandible	Inferior alveolar nerve	V3
Retromolar trigone	Lingual nerve, inferior alveolar nerve	V3
Buccal cancer	Buccal branches	V3, VII
Base of tongue	Hypoglossal nerve	XII
Palate	Greater and lesser palatine nerves	V2, PPF
Maxillary sinus	Superior alveolar nerve	V2
Ethmoid sinus	Nasociliary nerve, optic nerve	V1, II, III, IV, abducens
Frontal sinus	Supraorbital nerve	V1
Parotid gland	Facial nerve branches, auriculotemporal nerve	V3, VII
Nasal cavity	PPF via sphenopalatine foramen	V2

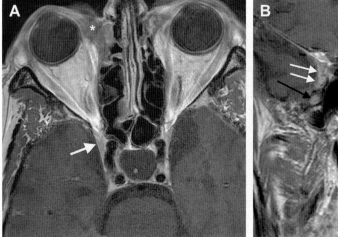 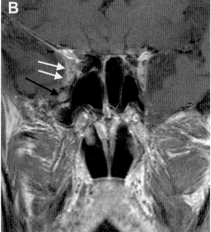

Fig. 15. PNS from lacrimal sac adenoid cystic carcinoma. Axial T1-weighted postgadolinium image (*A*) shows the primary lesion in the right lacrimal sac (*asterisk*) and enlargement of the right cavernous sinus (*arrow*). The coronal postgadolinium (*B*) image shows the PNS to the orbital apex (*white arrows*) and foramen rotundum (*black arrow*).

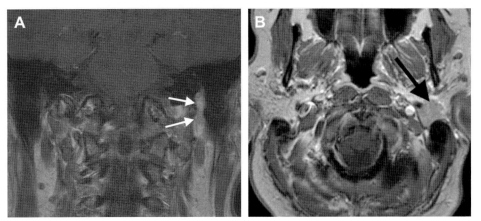

Fig. 16. PNS from adenoid cystic carcinoma of the parotid. Coronal T1-weighed image after contrast (*A*) shows a thickened enhancing left mastoid segment of the facial nerve (*arrows*). (*B*) Axial T1-weighted image with gadolinium shows the primary neoplasm in the parotid (*arrow*) extending into the stylomastoid foramen, which was pathologically proven to be adenoid cystic carcinoma.

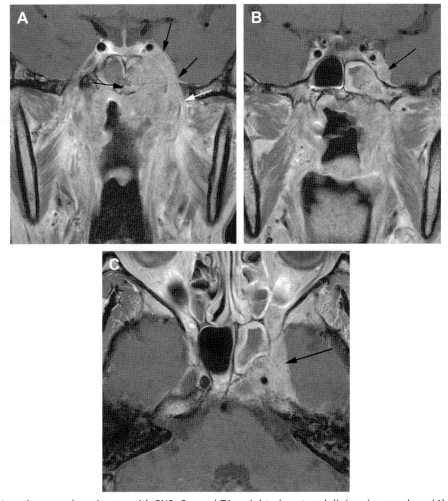

Fig. 17. Nasopharyngeal carcinoma with PNS. Coronal T1-weighted post gadolinium images show (*A*) left nasopharyngeal carcinoma with direct extension to the V3 trunk in the masticator space (*white arrow*) and into the Meckel cave and sphenoid sinus (*black arrows*). (*B*) Coronal T1-weighted post gadolinium images shows tumor extension into the sphenoid sinus, enlargement of the left cavernous sinus, and PNS along V2 (*black arrow*). PNS along V2 (*arrow*) is also well seen on the axial postgadolinium T1-weighted image (*C*) that also shows involvement of the Meckel cave and encasement of the internal carotid artery.

The imaging differential for PNS includes viral neuritis, carcinomatosis, sarcoid, meningioma, schwannoma, and rhinocerebral mucormycosis, and imaging findings may be very similar. In most cases clinical history itself is the most useful factor in differentiating these entities. At initial imaging presentation, PNS is recognized by the presence of tumor outside of the confines of the cranium, whereas in leptomeningeal carcinomatosis, sarcoid tumor, and meningioma the bulk of disease will lie in the intracranial compartment. In the case of a schwannoma disease along the nerve tends to be bulkier and the nerve acts as the epicenter of the disease process. Patients with invasive fungal sinus disease have a much more acute presentation than do patients with perineural tumor spread and disease will be clustered about the paranasal sinuses with inflammatory change in the sinuses themselves.

Multiple studies have attempted to assess the diagnostic ability of MRI for PNS. In general, research is somewhat hampered by the low prevalence of tumors demonstrating PNS, with multiple reports featuring small numbers of patients. In addition, the presence of PNS into the skull base often mitigates against surgery in many centers, precluding histologic confirmation of imaging findings. Most studies attempt to determine the sensitivity and specificity of imaging for PNS in a population of patients known to have cancer. In this group, with higher pretest probability than the general population, MRI performs well, with reported sensitivities of 100%; however, the extent of PNS is typically underestimated.[14,15]

SUMMARY

Knowledge of the anatomy of the nerves commonly involved with PNS in the head and neck and appropriate use of imaging modalities will enable early detection and positively impact management of head and neck cancer. In searching for PNS, "fat is your friend," and special attention should be paid to the T1-weighted images.

REFERENCES

1. Liebig C, Ayala G, Wilks J, et al. Perineural invasion in cancer: a review of the literature. Cancer 2009; 115(15):3379–470.
2. Gandour-Edwards R, Kapadia SB, Barnes L, et al. Neural cell adhesion molecule in adenoid cystic carcinoma invading the skull base. Otolaryngol Head Neck Surg 1997;117(5):453–8.
3. Catalano PJ, Sen C, Biller HF. Cranial neuropathy secondary to perineural spread of cutaneous malignancies. Am J Otol 1995;16(6):772–7.
4. Tarsitano A, Pizzigallo A, Gessaroli M, et al. Intraoperative biopsy of the major cranial nerves in the surgical strategy for adenoid cystic carcinoma close to the skull base. Oral Surg Oral Med Oral Pathol Oral Radiol Endod 2011, May 5. [Epub ahead of print].
5. da Cruz Perez D, de Abreu Alves F, Nobuko Nishimoto I, et al. Prognostic factors in head and neck adenoid cystic carcinoma. Oral Oncol 2006; 42(2):139–85.
6. Lian K, Bartlett E, Yu E. Perineural tumor spread along the sixth cranial nerve: CT and MR imaging. AJNR Am J Neuroradiol 2011;32(9):E178.
7. Ginsberg L, Eicher S. Great auricular nerve: anatomy and imaging in a case of perineural tumor spread. AJNR Am J Neuroradiol 2000;21(3): 568–639.
8. Ginsberg L, De Monte F, Gillenwater A. Greater superficial petrosal nerve: anatomy and MR findings in perineural tumor spread. AJNR Am J Neuroradiol 1996;17(2):389–482.
9. Schmalfuss I, Tart R, Mukherji S, et al. Perineural tumor spread along the auriculotemporal nerve. AJNR Am J Neuroradiol 2002;23(2):303–14.
10. Curtin HD. Detection of perineural spread: fat is a friend. AJNR Am J Neuroradiol 1998;19(8): 1385–6.
11. Majoie C, Hulsmans F, Verbeeten B, et al. Perineural tumor extension along the trigeminal nerve: magnetic resonance imaging findings. Eur J Radiol 1997;24(3):191–396.
12. Laine FJ, Braun IF, Jensen ME, et al. Perineural tumor extension through the foramen ovale: evaluation with MR imaging. Radiology 1990;174(1): 65–71.
13. Fischbein NJ, Kaplan MJ, Jackler RK, et al. MR imaging in two cases of subacute denervation change in the muscles of facial expression. AJNR Am J Neuroradiol 2001;22(5):880–4.
14. Gandhi MR, Panizza B, Kennedy D. Detecting and defining the anatomic extent of large nerve perineural spread of malignancy: comparing "targeted" MRI with the histologic findings following surgery. Head Neck 2011;33(4):469–75.
15. Nemzek WR, Hecht S, Gandour-Edwards R, et al. Perineural spread of head and neck tumors: how accurate is MR imaging? AJNR Am J Neuroradiol 1998;19(4):701–6.

Aggressive Inflammatory and Neoplastic Processes of the Paranasal Sinuses

Michael J. Hartman, MD*, Lindell R. Gentry, MD

KEYWORDS

- Sinus • Nasal • Neoplasms • Infection • Aggressive

KEY POINTS

- A thorough knowledge of the anatomy of the sinonasal region and adjacent structures is essential for proper evaluation.
- Magnetic resonance (MR) imaging is a vital imaging modality for the assessment of aggressive and neoplastic diseases affecting the nasal cavity and paranasal sinuses.
- MR imaging is much superior to computed tomography at separating tumor from inflammatory mucosal disease, depicting the full extent of disease involvement, and evaluating perineural tumor spread.

INTRODUCTION

Most radiology practices receive daily requests to perform diagnostic imaging studies in patients with sinus symptoms. Most problems that require evaluation will be caused by common inflammatory diseases that require little or no acute treatment. Importantly, however, the patients' symptoms may occasionally have other causes, such as a more aggressive inflammatory process or a malignant neoplasm. There is often a significant overlap in the presenting symptoms of benign inflammatory, aggressive inflammatory, and neoplastic paranasal sinus diseases. Some patients with underlying neoplasms may even be mistakenly treated with one or more courses of antibiotics before imaging is obtained and other possibilities are considered. In an immunocompromised host, more aggressive causes must be considered as soon as possible because any delay in diagnosis may lead to significant morbidity or even mortality.

Many patients with neoplasms present with advanced disease at diagnosis because of the failure to consider this possibility until late in the course.

Additionally, given the capacious nature of the sinuses, tumors can grow large before becoming symptomatic. Sinonasal neoplasms tend to present at an advanced stage and have a poor overall prognosis. Clinically, they have nonspecific presenting signs, including nasal stuffiness, bleeding, pain, and numbness. Pain and numbness may herald the onset of perineural tumor spread by the lesion. Cancers of the head and neck account for approximately 4% of all malignancies.[1] Sinonasal tumors make up 3% to 4% of head and neck cancers.[1–3] There are several tissue types that are normally found in the sinonasal cavity, including epithelial (neuroendocrine, schneiderian, squamous, olfactory), mesenchymal (bone, cartilage, fibrous), muscle, nervous, and vascular. Because of this, there is a wide spectrum of neoplasms that may originate in the sinonasal cavity. Most sinus cancers are squamous cell carcinoma (80%)[4] and these most commonly involve the maxillary sinus (36%–80%) followed by the nasal cavity (25%–44%) and ethmoid sinuses (10%).[5,6] The sphenoid and frontal sinuses are rare sites of origin.

Department of Radiology, University of Wisconsin Hospital, Madison, WI 53711, USA
* Corresponding author.
E-mail address: mhartman@uwhealth.org

Magn Reson Imaging Clin N Am 20 (2012) 447–471
http://dx.doi.org/10.1016/j.mric.2012.05.001

The purpose of this article is to explore the differentiating imaging features of aggressive inflammatory versus neoplastic lesions of the paranasal sinuses. A secondary focus is to look at common patterns of spread of aggressive sinus lesions to adjacent structures.

IMAGING

Computed tomography (CT) and magnetic resonance (MR) imaging can be considered complimentary diagnostic studies for the evaluation of aggressive inflammatory and neoplastic diseases of the sinuses (**Figs. 1** and **2**). CT is typically the first diagnostic test used for the evaluation of the paranasal sinuses. With thin slices and multiplanar reformations, CT does a satisfactory job at evaluating most disease processes involving the sinuses. CT is excellent at evaluating the bony anatomy, orbital fat, bony cortex, and for depicting the internal architecture of some fibro-osseous (see **Fig. 1**) and other bony lesions (see **Fig. 2**). MR imaging is a better choice for identifying the full extent of aggressive sinonasal disease that spread into the orbit, skull base, brain, and cavernous sinus. It is more definitive than CT for separating tumor from inflammatory mucosal disease and retained secretions. MR imaging is superior to CT for detecting the full extent of perineural spread of tumors. In many cases, CT and

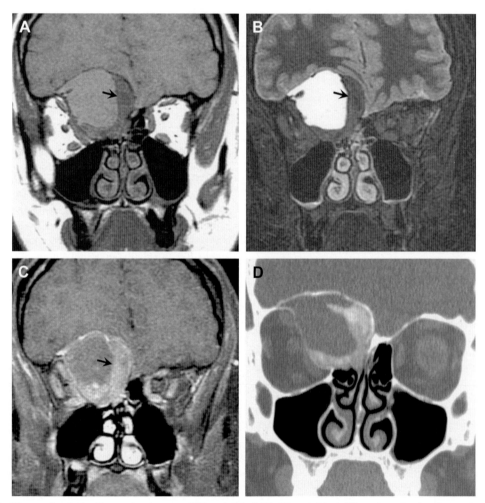

Fig. 1. Fibrous dysplasia: Noncontrast coronal T1-weighted (*A*), T2-weighted (*B*), and contrast-enhanced coronal T1-weighted (*C*) MR images demonstrate an expansile mass of the ethmoid sinuses displacing the brain superiorly and compressing the orbital apex. The superolateral portion of the mass is hyperintense on both T1- and T2-weighted images, which suggests a mucoproteinaceous fluid collection. The medial portion of the mass is hypointense on noncontrast scans and demonstrates nonspecific, fairly homogeneous enhancement (*arrows*). Coronal noncontrast CT image (*D*) is much more specific with typical imaging features of fibrous dysplasia. Fibrous dysplasia should always be considered in the differential diagnosis of any enhancing sinonasal mass.

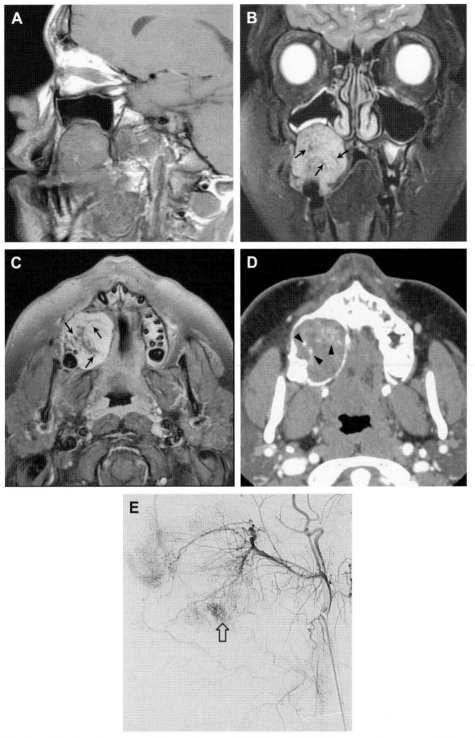

Fig. 2. Maxillary alveolus schwannoma: Noncontrast sagittal T1-weighted (A), noncontrast coronal T2-weighted (B), and contrast-enhanced axial T1-weighted (C) MR images demonstrate an expansile mass of the maxillary sinus and alveolus. These images reveal multiple rounded and linear areas of hypointensity suspicious for flow voids within vessels (arrows). Axial contrast-enhanced CT image (D) confirms numerous small intralesional vessels (arrowheads). Lateral external carotid angiogram (E) demonstrates intralesional tumor blush (open arrow) indicating a significantly vascular neoplasm.

MR imaging play complimentary roles. Important things to evaluate include bone remodeling versus destruction, presence of calcification, inherent T1 and T2 signal intensity, lesion cellularity (**Fig. 3**), degree of contrast enhancement, vascularity, and the involvement of the orbital, premaxillary, and retromaxillary fat. Detecting spread into the orbit, skull base, cavernous sinus, and brain as well as the presence of perineural tumor spread will usually alter the type of treatment. The accurate assessment of tumor spread will also influence the discussion of viable treatment options and overall disease prognosis with patients. Cerebral angiography or MR angiography may be helpful in the management of vascular sinonasal masses (see **Fig. 2**; **Fig. 4**). The radiologist's job is to separate nonaggressive inflammatory sinus disease from more aggressive inflammatory or neoplastic processes. Patients can then undergo a biopsy for the final diagnosis and appropriate treatment.

A recommended CT protocol includes the acquisition of thin (0.5–1.5 mm) axial images that are reconstructed in both soft tissue and bone algorithms (see **Fig. 2**). These images are then used to generate thin (1.25–2.5 mm), 2-dimensional reconstructions in the coronal and sagittal planes (see **Fig. 1**). A typical MR imaging protocol includes axial, coronal, and sagittal noncontrast T1-weighed images, axial diffusion-weighted images, and axial and coronal noncontrast T2-weighted images. Postcontrast axial, coronal, and sagittal T1-weighted images are then obtained using fat suppression.

ANATOMY

The paranasal sinuses are present to a varying degree in newborns. The maxillary and ethmoid sinuses are usually present at birth, whereas the frontal and sphenoid sinuses are absent. The sinuses undergo varying rates of maturation, with each of the sinuses showing time periods of more rapid development. The paranasal sinuses reach near maturity by 12 years of age, with maximal size attained by early adulthood. Sinus opacification is typically not considered of clinical significance until the age of 2 to 3 years. The paired maxillary sinuses develop within the maxillary bones and contain 4 recesses: alveolar, zygomatic, palatine, and infraorbital. The mucosa is lined by ciliated epithelium that propels secretions to the ostia of each sinus. The drainage pathway of the maxillary sinus is via the ostiomeatal unit, which is centered about the uncinate process and is comprised of the maxillary ostium, infundibulum, hiatus semilunaris, and middle meatus. An accessory ostium may be seen in approximately 20% to 30% of patients. Innervation is via maxillary nerve branches, including the anterior, middle, and posterior superior alveolar nerves. Arterial supply is primarily via the posterior superior alveolar artery and the infraorbital and greater palatine arteries.

The ethmoid sinuses consist of several pneumatized 3-18 air cells within each ethmoid bone. These cells are divided into anterior and posterior cell groups by the basal lamella. The agger nasi cell lies anterior to the frontal sinus drainage pathway and may be a source of frontal sinus obstruction. Additional inconstant air cells include frontal infundibular cells (Bent-Kuhn types 1–4).[7] The lateral border of the ethmoid sinus is formed by the lamina papyracea, which is also the medial wall of the orbits. The roof of the ethmoid sinuses is covered by the fovea ethmoidalis, a projection of the frontal bone. Adjacent to the upper medial wall of the ethmoid sinus is the medial and lateral lamella of the cribriform plate of the ethmoid bone. The appearance of the cribriform plate has been classified into Keros types 1 to 3 according to the depth that it extends into the nasal cavity.[8] Innervation is from the anterior and posterior ethmoid nerves that are branches of the nasociliary nerve, which arises from the V1 portion (ophthalmic division) of the trigeminal nerve. The blood supply is via the anterior and posterior ethmoidal arteries, which are branches of the ophthalmic artery.

The frontal sinus is typically the last sinus to aerate. Up to 4% of the population may not develop a frontal sinus. It is variable in size, ranging from nonpneumatized to hyperpneumatized (involving almost all of the frontal bone). A variable number of bony septations may be present in the frontal sinus. Drainage is via the frontal recesses into the middle meatus. Innervation is from branches of the supraorbital nerves, which are branches of the ophthalmic nerve (V1). The blood supply is from the supraorbital and anterior ethmoidal arteries.

The sphenoid sinus lies within the sphenoid bone just posterior to the nasal cavity. It may contain variable bony septa. The sphenoid sinus can be hypoplastic in size or hyperpneumatized with aeration of the lateral pterygoid recesses and even the greater sphenoid wing. Drainage is via the sphenoid ostia into the sphenoethmoidal recess of the posterosuperior nasal cavity. Several important structures lie in close proximity to the sphenoid sinus. These structures include the internal carotid arteries; cavernous sinuses; and cranial nerves III, IV, V1, V2, and VI. The optic nerves lie superomedial to the sphenoid sinuses.

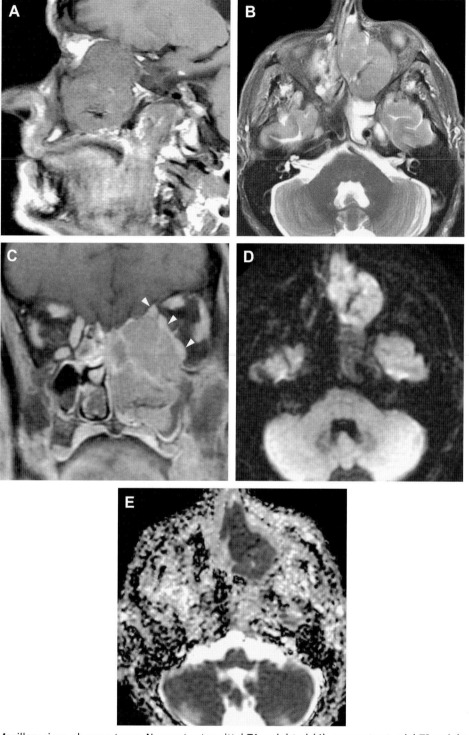

Fig. 3. Maxillary sinus plasmacytoma: Noncontrast sagittal T1-weighted (*A*), noncontrast axial T2-weighted (*B*), and contrast-enhanced coronal T1-weighted (*C*) MR images demonstrate an expansile mass of the maxillary sinus with extension into the ethmoid sinuses and medial orbit. The lesion abuts and displaces the superior oblique and the medial and inferior rectus muscles (*arrowheads*). The hypointense signal intensity on the T2-weighted image and evidence of restricted diffusion on the diffusion-weighted images (*D*) and Apparent diffusion coefficient maps (*E*) indicates that the neoplasm has a high cellularity.

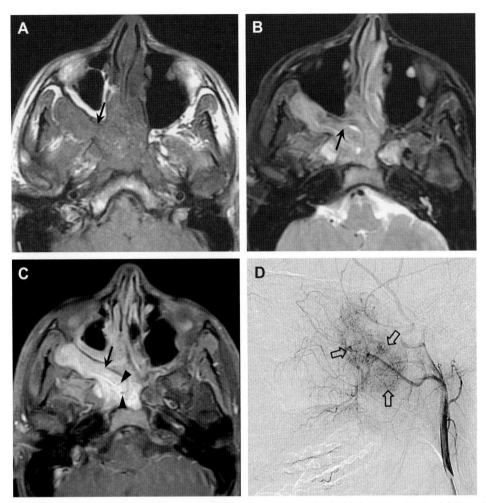

Fig. 4. Juvenile nasopharyngeal angiofibroma: Noncontrast axial T1-weighted (*A*), noncontrast axial T2-weighted (*B*), and contrast-enhanced axial T1-weighted (*C*) MR images demonstrate a multi-compartmental mass centered in the pterygopalatine fossa (*arrows*) and posterior nasopharynx. The expansile lesion is located in the typical location of a juvenile nasopharyngeal angiofibroma. Also present are a few subtle rounded and linear areas of hypointensity suspicious for flow voids (*arrowheads*). Lateral external carotid angiogram (*D*) demonstrates intralesional tumor blush (*open arrows*) supplied by branches of the internal maxillary artery confirming a highly vascular neoplasm.

The floor of the anterior cranial fossa, sella turcica, and pituitary gland are located superiorly. The vidian nerve courses along the floor of the sinus. It is occasionally located entirely within the sinus lumen on a thin bony stalk when the pterygoid recess is hyperpneumatized. The foramen rotundum lies along the inferolateral aspect of the sinus. Innervation of the sphenoid sinus is from the posterior ethmoidal nerves and postganglionic parasympathetic fibers of the facial nerve. The blood supply is primarily via the posterior ethmoidal and pterygovaginal arteries.

The pterygopalatine fossa is located posterosuperior to the medial wall of the maxillary sinus and is a central way station for potential perineural spread. It is in communication with the nasal cavity medially via the sphenopalatine foramen, infrazygomatic masticator space laterally via the pterygomaxillary fissure, orbit anteriorly via the superior and inferior orbital fissures, cavernous sinus and middle cranial fossa posteriorly via the foramen rotundum, facial nerve genu posteriorly via the pterygoid canal, and palate inferiorly via the descending pterygopalatine canal.

Lymph node drainage of the sinuses can be through anterior channels, including the facial, parotid, submandibular, and upper internal jugular chain nodes, or posterior drainage to the retropharyngeal nodes. Nodal involvement is most common with maxillary sinus cancers (approximately 15%), uncommon with ethmoid involvement, and almost never seen with sphenoid or frontal sinus tumors.

TUMOR STAGING

Staging of sinus neoplasms is most commonly based on the 2010 American Joint Committee on Cancer (AJCC) staging manual (**Boxes 1–3**). TNM staging is divided into a maxillary sinus staging and a nasal cavity and ethmoid sinus staging. Frontal and sphenoid sinus cancers are rare enough that no TNM staging exists. Final staging of any malignancy should be a combination of clinical, radiologic, and pathologic staging. Melanoma has a separate staging system, which is discussed later.

Maxillary sinus staging historically involved the use of the Ohngren's line. This line was drawn on a lateral radiograph connecting the medial canthus of the orbit and the angle of the mandible. It divided the maxillary sinus into anteroinferior and posterosuperior segments. Posterosuperior disease had a poorer prognosis because of its closer proximity to the skull base, orbit, and other critical structures. Current TNM staging is depicted in **Boxes 1–3**.

The assessment for lymph node involvement includes evaluating size, shape, central or

---

Box 1
Primary tumor staging of maxillary sinus neoplasms

T1: Tumor limited to maxillary sinus mucosa with no erosion or destruction of bone

T2: Tumor causing bone erosion or destruction, including extension into the hard palate or middle nasal meatus, except extension to posterior wall of maxillary sinus and pterygoid plates

T3: Tumor invades any of the following: bone of the posterior wall of the maxillary sinus, subcutaneous tissues, floor or medial wall of orbit, pterygoid fossa, ethmoid sinuses

T4a (moderately advanced local disease): Tumor invades anterior orbital contents, skin of cheek, pterygoid plates, infratemporal fossa, cribriform plate, sphenoid or frontal sinuses

T4b (very advanced local disease): Tumor invades any of the following: orbital apex, dura, brain, middle cranial fossa, cranial nerves other than maxillary division of trigeminal nerve (V2), nasopharynx, or clivus

---

Box 2
Primary tumor staging of nasal cavity and ethmoid sinus neoplasms

T1: Tumor restricted to any one subsite, with or without bony invasion

T2: Tumor invading 2 subsites in a single region or extending to involve an adjacent region within the naso-ethmoidal complex, with or without bony invasion

T3: Tumor extends to involve the medial wall or floor of the orbit, maxillary sinus, palate, or cribriform plate

T4a (moderately advanced local disease): Tumor invades any of the following: anterior orbital contents, skin of nose or cheek, minimal extension to anterior cranial fossa, pterygoid plates, sphenoid, or frontal sinuses

T4b (very advanced local disease): Tumor invades any of the following: orbital apex, dura, brain, middle cranial fossa, cranial nerves other than maxillary division of trigeminal nerve (V2), nasopharynx, or clivus

---

Box 3
Local and regional metastatic spread of sinus malignancies

Nodal staging[a]

NX: Regional lymph nodes cannot be assessed

N0: No regional lymph node metastasis

N1: Metastasis in a single ipsilateral lymph node, 3 cm or less in greatest dimension

N2a: Metastasis in a single ipsilateral lymph node, more than 3 cm, but not more than 6 cm in greatest dimension

N2b: Metastasis in multiple ipsilateral lymph nodes, none more than 6 cm in greatest dimension

N2c: Metastasis in bilateral or contralateral lymph nodes, none more than 6 cm in greatest dimension

N3: Metastasis in a lymph node, more than 6 cm in greatest dimension

Distant metastasis

M0: No distant metastasis

M1: Distant metastasis

[a] A modifier for the presence or absence of extracapsular disease may be used (ECS±). Extracapsular spread does not affect staging.

peripheral hypodensity, and enhancement, and the evaluation for the presence or absence of extracapsular extension. The AJCC nodal staging system for sinus neoplasm is depicted in **Box 3**. Note that N3 nodal disease requires the enlargement of a single node and not a conglomerate of multiple nodes. Imaging assessment for tumor spread to nodes is difficult in daily practice with sensitivity and specificity in the moderate range. Sensitivity and specificity measurements based on a nodal size of 10 mm, in one study, were 88% and 39% for CT and 81% and 48% for MR imaging.[9] It is, therefore, important to use other imaging signs of nodal metastasis (enhancement, central hypointensity, T1- or T2-weighted signal inhomogeneity) in addition to nodal size when calling a node positive. In practice, the decision as to whether or not to treat the neck for nodal spread will not be completely based on imaging findings or clinical examination alone. If the probability for nodal disease involvement for a given T-stage of a tumor is high (>20%–30%), the neck will often be treated electively regardless of whether there is clinical or radiographic evidence of nodal spread. Positron emission tomography (PET) imaging can be helpful in the characterization of the primary tumor and any metastatic nodes. The accuracy of nodal assessment by PET compared with CT and MR imaging is approximately 67% to 90% sensitive and 81% to 94% specific for PET and CT and MR imaging are approximately 64% to 82% sensitive, 75% to 85% specific and 67% to 80% sensitive, 77% to 79% specific, respectively.[10,11] Similarly, PET is useful for the pretreatment detection of distant metastasis in high-risk patients, evaluation of posttreatment response of the primary tumor, and for subsequent posttreatment surveillance for recurrence.[12–14] Posttreatment PET is preferably performed at least 12 weeks after therapy to help minimize the postsurgical and postradiation inflammatory changes that can lead to false-positive results.

INFECTIOUS/INFLAMMATORY

Sinus inflammatory disease can have an aggressive appearance, especially if complications occur (**Box 4**). These aggressive appearances typically involve direct contiguous spread of the infection into adjacent spaces and structures. This spread can occur with either bacterial or fungal sinusitis. There can be involvement of the adjacent bone (osteomyelitis), orbit (subperiosteal abscess), or the brain and its coverings (subdural/epidural abscess, cerebritis, meningitis, cavernous sinus thrombosis). The spread of disease can be from direct extension or along neurovascular channels. Complications of sinus disease are more common in younger patients, children and adolescents. These complications include an orbital subperiosteal abscess seen mostly in children and intracranial infections (epidural, subdural, and intraparenchymal abscesses) in adolescents and young adults. Aggressive granulomatous and fungal causes are covered specifically.

Granulomatosis with polyangiitis (Wegener's granulomatosis) is a rare multisystem autoimmune disease of unknown cause (see **Box 4**). It involves the lungs (95%), paranasal sinuses (90%), kidneys

---

> **Box 4**
> **Aggressive sinonasal diseases**
>
> *Infectious/inflammatory*
>
> Aggressive bacterial
>
> Sinonasal polyposis (allergic, cystic fibrosis)
>
> Pseudotumor
>
> *Granulomatous*
>
> Granulomatosis with polyangiitis (Wegener)
>
> Sarcoidosis
>
> *Fungal*
>
> Aspergillus
>
> Mucormycosis
>
> Allergic fungal sinusitis
>
> *Benign neoplastic*
>
> Inverted papilloma
>
> Juvenile nasopharyngeal angiofibroma
>
> Fibro-osseous lesions (especially fibrous dysplasia)
>
> Nerve sheath tumors
>
> Meningioma
>
> *Malignant neoplastic*
>
> Squamous cell carcinoma
>
> Sinonasal undifferentiated carcinoma
>
> Esthesioneuroblastoma
>
> Minor salivary gland neoplasms (adenoid cystic, mucoepidermoid, adenocarcinoma)
>
> Verrucous carcinoma
>
> Neuroendocrine (carcinoid, small cell)
>
> Melanoma
>
> Lymphoma
>
> Sarcomas (chondrosarcoma, rhabdomyosarcoma, Ewing)

(85%), nasopharynx (65%), and joints (65%).[15] Pathophysiologic analysis shows noncaseating multinucleated giant cell granulomas and necrotizing vasculitis in small and medium-sized blood vessels. A serologic marker, c-ANCA, is a specific marker used to establish the diagnosis. The incidence is purported to be 3 cases per 100,000 individuals in the United States.[16] It has a slight male predominance with a male-to-female ratio of approximately 1.5:1.0. It can occur at any age but is typically found in those aged between 35 and 55 years. Before treatment with corticosteroids and cyclophosphamide was introduced, 1-year survival was approximately 20% and after the introduction of this treatment, remission occurred in 75% of cases. Sinonasal Wegener presents with nasal

septal perforation, bone erosion/destruction, irregular calcifications, and soft tissue masses (**Fig. 5**). Bone destruction can sometimes be punctate in nature occurring along the course of traversing arteries. On imaging, no defining characteristics are present; however, Wegener should be considered in patients presenting with painful mucosal thickening in conjunction with bone destruction and orbital involvement. The main differential considerations for a destructive lesion of the sinonasal tract are lymphoma and squamous cell carcinoma (SCCA).

Fungal sinusitis in its aggressive form is typically caused by aspergillosis or mucormycosis. Mucormycosis is a term used to describe fungal infections caused by organisms in the order Mucorales. The

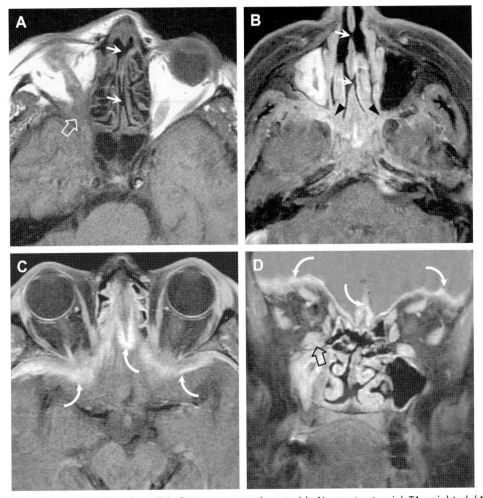

Fig. 5. Granulomatosis with polyangiitis (Wegener granulomatosis): Noncontrast axial T1-weighted (*A*) and gadolinium-enhanced axial (*B, C*) and coronal (*D*) T1-weighted MR images demonstrate multifocal areas of destruction of the nasal septum (*arrows*). There is extension to involve the orbital apex and inferior rectus muscles (*open arrows*), bilateral pterygopalatine fossa (*arrowheads*), and the dura (*curved arrows*) of the anterior and middle cranial fossae.

species *Mucor, Rhizopus,* and *Absidia* are most often implicated. Mucormycosis may involve the sinonasal cavity, central nervous system (CNS), lungs, subcutaneous tissue, and gastrointestinal tract.[17] The rhinocerebral form is the most common type.[18,19] Most individuals are regularly exposed to mucormycosis given the ubiquitous presence of these organisms in organic matter and soil. It is only when a person is immunocompromised that it usually presents a problem. In immunocompromised patients, the organism is aggressive and often invades structures adjacent to the sinuses, including the orbit, skull base, cavernous sinus, and brain, by spreading along fascial planes and neurovascular structures. The spread of the infection tends to occur rapidly, making prompt diagnosis important to reduce morbidity and mortality. MR imaging is particularly well suited to evaluate mucormycosis because of the disease's propensity for multi-compartmental spread or invasion. Early signs of invasion include mucosal thickening with extraocular muscle thickening and proptosis, usually progressive; the visualization of a discrete orbital mass is uncommon.[20] Necrotic tissue is a common accompaniment of mucormycosis infection and is best detected as nonenhancing areas on T1-weighted postcontrast scans.[21] To maximize patient survival, surgery is urgently indicated to

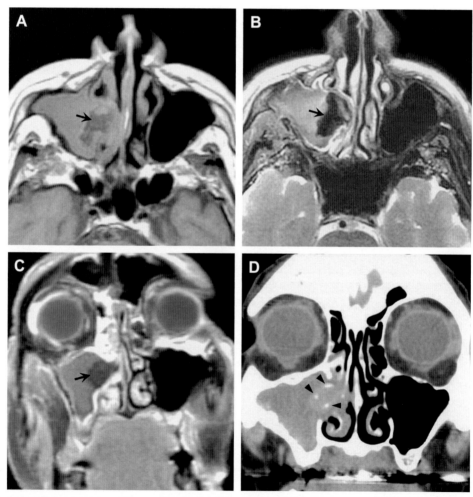

Fig. 6. Aspergillus mycetoma: Noncontrast axial T1-weighted (*A*), noncontrast axial T2-weighted (*B*), and contrast-enhanced coronal T1-weighted (*C*) MR images demonstrate a hypointense mass along the medial wall of the maxillary sinus (*arrows*). The hypointense nature of the mass on all pulse sequences is suggestive of fungal mycetoma or densely calcified mass. There are trapped secretions filling the remainder of the maxillary sinus and peripheral enhancement of the sinus walls but no enhancement of the lesion itself. Coronal contrast-enhanced CT image (*D*) confirms numerous small intralesional punctate calcifications (*arrowheads*) typical of a fungal mycetoma.

remove all infected and necrotic tissue. Despite aggressive treatment, mortality is still about 50% and in some instances, including disseminated disease, mortality can approach 100%.[20]

Aspergillus is a genus consisting of several hundred different mold species. They tend to grow in aerobic environments and within tissues that have a high sugar or carbohydrate content. Aspergillus infections have several presentations in the sinonasal region, including fungal mycetoma (**Fig. 6**), allergic fungal sinusitis (AFS), infiltrative fungal sinusitis, and fulminant invasive fungal sinusitis. The radiographic findings of the less-aggressive forms of fungal sinusitis (fungal mycetoma, AFS) are not the focus of this article because the infection is primarily confined to the sinus lumen in these cases. Imaging characteristics of the more-invasive forms of fungal sinusitis (infiltrative and fulminant invasive) can often resemble malignant neoplasms. They must be differentiated from these neoplasms because the former can rapidly progress to death or severe morbidity over the course of hours. Invasive fungal disease usually has both a soft tissue component that involves the sinus mucosa and adjacent soft tissues and the contents of the sinus lumen. The soft tissue infection usually has a nonspecific, fairly homogeneous, isodense attenuation on CT.

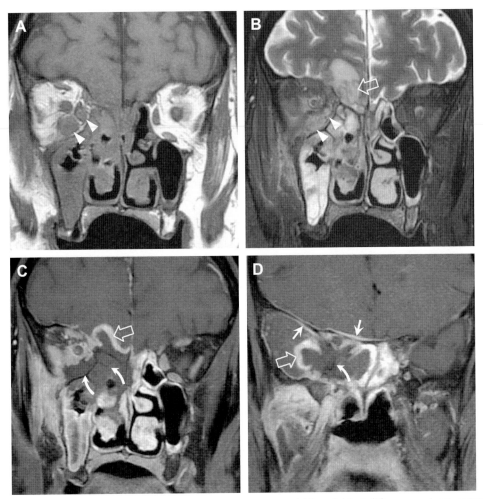

Fig. 7. Invasive Aspergillus fungal sinusitis: Noncontrast coronal T1-weighted (A), noncontrast coronal T2-weighted (B), and contrast-enhanced coronal T1-weighted (C, D) MR images demonstrate ill-defined soft tissue fullness of the right nasal cavity, maxillary sinus, and soft tissues of the face. The aggressive nature is indicated by orbital cellulitis with edema and swelling of the medial and inferior rectus muscles (*arrowheads*). There is invasion of the pachymeninges (*arrows*) and the frontal and temporal lobes (*open arrows*) demonstrating intense peripheral enhancement. There is a lack of enhancement of the orbital apex and cavernous sinus (*curved arrows*) signifying nonviable necrotic tissue.

There may be areas of sinus wall thickening caused by preexisting chronic sinusitis and subtle areas of bone destruction. Locally infiltrative fungal sinusitis usually involves only 1 or 2 sinuses and demonstrates homogenous contrast enhancement, lack of sinus expansion, and bone erosion localized to the area of extrasinus extension. There may be spread of the aggressive infection outside the sinus lumen without obvious bone destruction in many cases because the disease may follow natural foramina and fissures. The MR imaging appearance of mucosal infection and early spread of infection into adjacent soft tissue spaces may be fairly nonspecific, so a high index of suspicion is required. Significant edema related to the infection is often the earliest key to detecting the inflammatory nature of the lesion. There may also be an associated inflammatory component within the sinus lumen. Depending on the viscosity of the sinus contents, these secretions are usually isointense to hyperintense on T1-weighted scans and generally hypointense on T2-weighted MR imaging sequences.

Early in the course of infection, MR imaging enhancement is fairly homogeneous in areas of tissue invasion. Later, as tissue necrosis develops, there may be a lack of enhancement. This observation is important because these areas of necrosis must be surgically removed because antibiotics will not reach the necrotic tissue (**Fig. 7**). Locally infiltrative fungal sinusitis and fulminant invasive fungal sinusitis share many

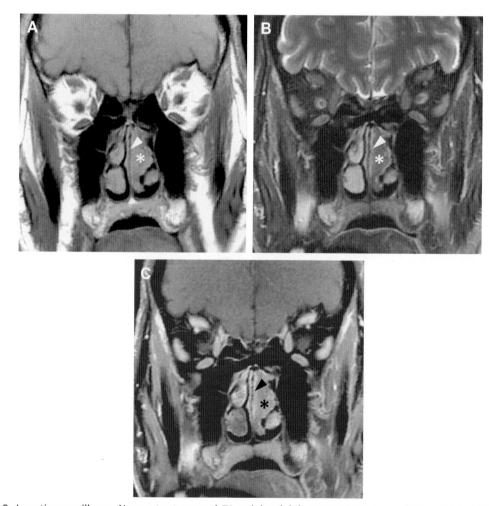

Fig. 8. Inverting papilloma: Noncontrast coronal T1-weighted (*A*), noncontrast coronal T2-weighted (*B*), and contrast-enhanced coronal T1-weighted (*C*) MR images demonstrate a fairly well-demarcated mass lesion of the nasal cavity (*asterisks*). The hypointense appearance of the lesion on the T2-weighted scan differentiates this lesion from an inflammatory polyp. There is invasion of the nasal septum, however, indicating local aggression (*arrowheads*).

imaging features, although the infection typically progresses much more rapidly in the latter.

Rarely, sinonasal polyposis and AFS can have an aggressive appearance. AFS usually involves multiple sinuses, demonstrates fairly homogeneous increased CT attenuation of the sinus contents, and often demonstrates some degree of sinus expansion. Occasionally, there will be thinning of the sinus walls that may be suggestive of an aggressive lesion. MR imaging demonstrates a variable appearance, depending on the viscosity of the sinus contents. The intraluminal secretions typically show heterogeneous isointensity/hyperintensity on T1-weighted scans and hypointensity on T2-weighted sequences. Occasionally, the signal intensity of luminal contents may be so hypointense on T2-weighted images that it may mimic air. Enhancement is minimal to absent except for the mucosal lining of the sinuses. Sinonasal polyposis may rarely be so expansile that it too can mimic malignancy. Extreme expansion of the sinuses from polyposis can lead to marked thinning of the sinus walls and protrusion into the orbit and anterior skull base.

BENIGN NEOPLASMS

Inverted papilloma is an uncommon benign tumor of the nasal cavity and paranasal sinuses accounting for up to 4% of primary nasal tumors.[22]

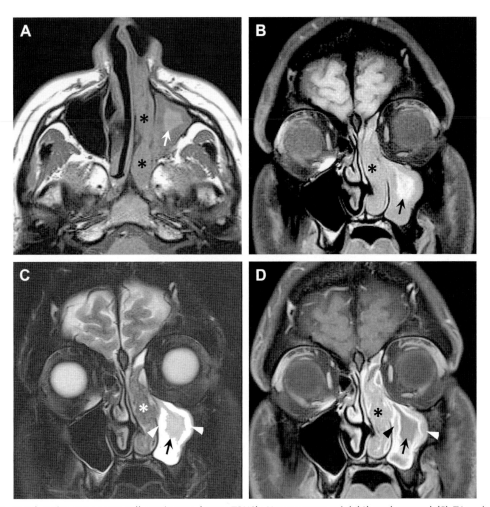

Fig. 9. Nasal cavity squamous cell carcinoma (stage T2N0): Noncontrast axial (*A*) and coronal (*B*) T1-weighted images and a noncontrast coronal T2-weighted (*C*) MR image demonstrate a mass lesion (*asterisks*) confined to the nasal cavity and ethmoid sinuses. The T1- and T2-weighted images allow separation of the neoplasm from trapped secretions in the maxillary sinus (*arrows*). The contrast-enhanced coronal T1-weighted image (*D*), in conjunction with the T2-weighted image, allows differentiation of inflammatory mucosal thickening (*arrowheads*) from tumor.

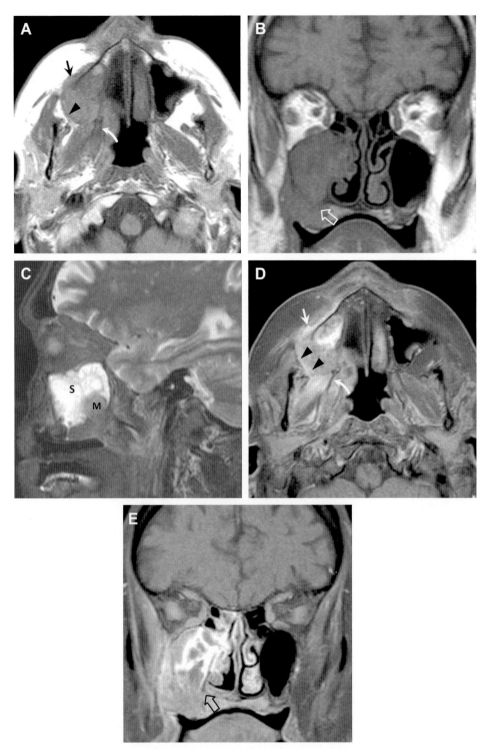

Fig. 10. Maxillary sinus squamous cell carcinoma (T4aN0): Noncontrast axial (*A*) and coronal (*B*) T1-weighted images as well as a noncontrast sagittal T2-weighted (*C*) MR image demonstrate a mass (M) lesion of the maxillary sinus. The T2-weighted image best allows separation of the neoplasm from trapped secretions (S) in the maxillary sinus. The contrast-enhanced axial (*D*) and coronal (*E*) T1-weighted images reveal invasion of the premaxillary (*arrows*) and retro-maxillary fat (*arrowheads*), pterygoid plates, and pterygoid musculature (*curved arrows*), indicating a T4a stage. There is extensive invasion of the hard palate near the greater palatine foramen (*open arrows*).

It occurs primarily in men in the fourth to sixth decades of life. Inverted papilloma has malignant potential, with SCCA developing in approximately 7% to 15% of patients.[23,24] Despite its benign classification, it can behave aggressively, with destruction and invasion of local structures, and should be treated like a malignant lesion. Recurrence rates are widely variable, dependent on the extent of disease and resection, but are estimated to be between 13% and 67%.[22,23,25] It characteristically arises from the lateral nasal cavity wall but extension into the adjacent maxillary or ethmoid sinuses is not uncommon. It may also extend intracranially through the cribriform plate. On imaging, an inverted papilloma is usually seen as a solid mass (**Fig. 8**). It is classically described as having a cerebriform appearance on contrast-enhanced studies, although this is not always present. Its appearance is similar to malignant lesions and, therefore, histologic diagnosis is required. Krouse[26] proposed a staging system for inverting papillomas in 2000. Stage I neoplasms are limited to the nasal cavity alone. Stage II tumors are limited to the ethmoid sinuses and medial and superior portions of the maxillary sinuses. Stage III cancers involve the lateral or inferior aspects of the maxillary sinuses or extend into the frontal or sphenoid sinuses. Stage IV tumors are those that spread outside the confines of the nose and sinuses.

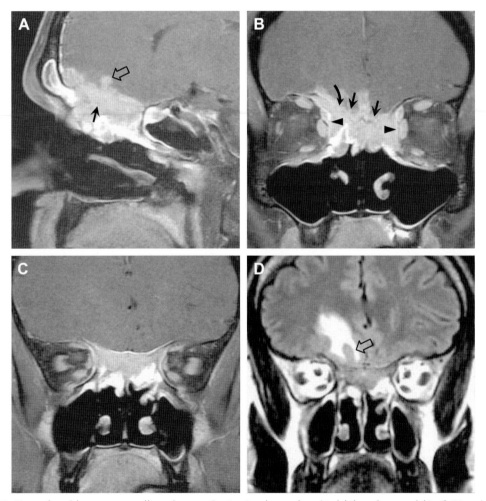

Fig. 11. Nasoethmoid squamous cell carcinoma: Contrast-enhanced sagittal (*A*) and coronal (*B, C*) T1-weighted images and a contrast-enhanced coronal T2–fluid attenuated inversion recovery (FLAIR) image (*D*) demonstrate an extensive neoplasm of the nasal cavities and ethmoid sinuses bilaterally. There is invasion of the orbits (*arrowheads*), extension through the cribriform plates (*arrows*), and destruction of the right fovea ethmoidalis (*curved arrow*). Frontal lobe invasion (*open arrows*) is best seen on the sagittal image and adjacent to the adjacent vasogenic edema on the T2-FLAIR image.

Meningioma is a benign tumor of arachnoid cap cells. Occurrences outside of the CNS are rare, accounting for less than 2% of all meningiomas.[27] The extracranial meningioma of the sinonasal cavity composes approximately 25% of extracranial meningiomas.[28] They can occasionally mimic an aggressive sinonasal neoplasm. Multiple theories have been proposed for the ectopic location of these lesions. Extracranial involvement may be the result of arachnoid rests outside of the CNS, direct extension, or rarely, metastasis from a malignant meningioma. They maintain their typical appearance of isointensity on T1-weighted scans and slight hypointensity on T2-weighted images and show marked contrast enhancement.

Fibrous dysplasia is a benign lesion in which normal bone is replaced by a mixture of collagen, fibroblasts, and irregular bony trabeculae. It is most commonly monostotic but can be polyostotic, especially when associated with the McCune-Albright syndrome. There may be disease progression over time, but lesion stability tends to occur by early adulthood. Lesions are typically of no clinical significance but can be disfiguring or lead to cranial nerve compromise. In these instances, surgery or sometimes radiation therapy is used. Otherwise, these lesions are treated conservatively because they have no malignant potential. Fibrous dysplasia can have an appearance on MR imaging that can mimic an

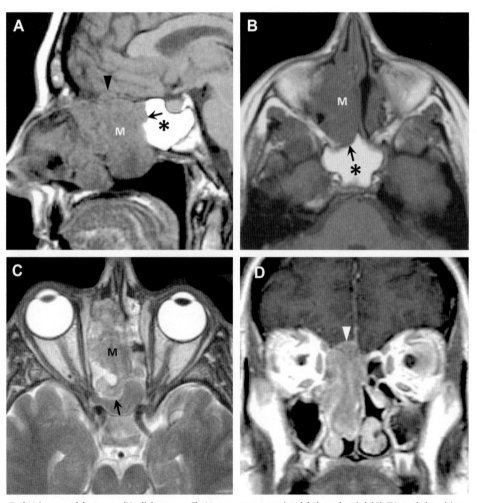

Fig. 12. Esthesioneuroblastoma (Kadish stage C): Noncontrast sagittal (A) and axial (B) T1-weighted images and a noncontrast axial T2-weighted (C) image demonstrate a mass lesion of the nasal cavity and right ethmoid sinuses (M). There is invasion of the anterior aspect of the sphenoid sinus (arrows) trapping T1-hyperintense proteinaceous secretions (asterisks) within the sphenoid sinus. The highly cellular nature of the neoplasm is indicated by its hypointense T2-weighted signal intensity. The contrast-enhanced coronal (D) T1-weighted image reveals diffuse enhancement of the lesion and invasion of the cribriform plate (arrowhead) confirming the Kadish C staging.

aggressive neoplasm (see **Fig. 1**). On MR imaging, these lesions can have a variable T1 and T2 appearance and typically show a moderate degree of contrast enhancement. They can, in some instances, look aggressive because there may be expansion of the sinus, obscuration of the outer cortex of the sinus that may mimic bone destruction, protrude into the orbit or cranial cavity, and may demonstrate extensive contrast enhancement. It is important to keep this lesion in mind in cases of skull base and sinonasal lesions. A confirmatory CT scan is easy to obtain and usually clinches the diagnosis, demonstrating its typical ground-glass appearance (see **Fig. 1**).

MALIGNANT SINONASAL TUMORS

SCCA is the most common sinonasal malignancy, accounting for about 60% to 90% of lesions.[6,29,30] Of these, up to 80% occur in the maxillary sinus. Primary frontal and sphenoid sinus tumors are rare. Typical patients are men of at least 50 years of age. The major risk factors include environmental factors, including nickel exposure, chromium pigment, and woodworking, and a subgroup identified as human papilloma virus (HPV) positive. Tobacco use is also a causative factor. MR imaging is excellent at differentiating SCCA from sinus inflammatory disease (**Figs. 9 and 10**). The typical MR imaging appearance of

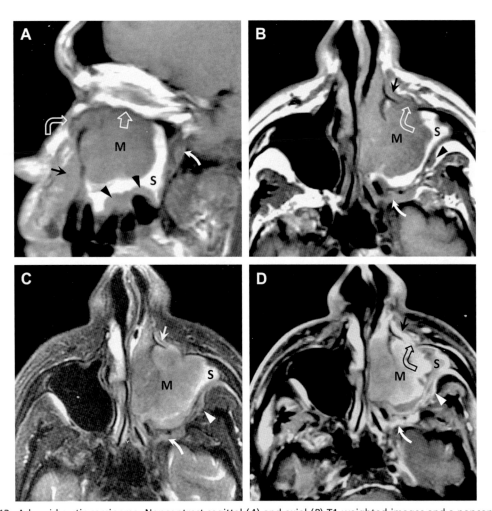

Fig. 13. Adenoid cystic carcinoma: Noncontrast sagittal (*A*) and axial (*B*) T1-weighted images and a noncontrast axial T2-weighted (*C*) image demonstrate a solid mass that nearly fills the maxillary sinus (M). Inferolateral to the neoplasm are trapped secretions that are hyperintense on the T1-weighted images (S). Tumor invasion of the anterior wall of the maxillary sinus (*arrows*) and floor of the orbit (*open arrow*) indicates a T3 stage. The contrast-enhanced axial (*D*) T1-weighted image reveals enhancement of the tumor and several areas of perineural tumor spread. There is spread along the infraorbital nerve (*curved open arrows*), posterior superior alveolar nerves (*arrowheads*), and the main trunk of the maxillary nerve within the pterygopalatine fossa (*curved arrows*).

SCCA is T1 isointensity, T2 hypointensity caused by high cellularity, and solid enhancement. Sinus inflammatory disease will typically be isointense to slightly hyperintense on T1-weighted images, hyperintense on T2-weighted scans, and show peripheral enhancement. The main goals of imaging are to first determine that a lesion is not inflammatory sinus disease (mucosal thickening, polyps, mucus retention cyst) and secondly, to determine the extent of disease, including perineural tumor spread. MR imaging is excellent for delineating the submucosal extent of the disease, intracranial involvement (**Fig. 11**), orbital extension, and perineural spread. Staging is based on the AJCC TNM staging criteria with separate staging systems for maxillary sinus cancer and nasal cavity/ethmoid sinus cancer (see **Boxes 1–3**). Primary frontal and sphenoid sinus neoplasms are rare enough that an AJCC staging classification has not been developed. Nodal staging is based on size, number, and laterality (see **Box 3**). Despite aggressive multimodality treatment, including surgery, radiation, and possibly chemotherapy, the 5-year survival is approximately 25% to 64%.[5,6,30,31] HPV positive status tends to result in a slightly better overall 5-year survival: 80% versus 31%.[32]

Sinonasal undifferentiated carcinoma (SNUC) is a highly malignant, aggressive neoplasm. It is of neuroendocrine origin along the spectrum of esthesioneuroblastoma. It is typically locally advanced on presentation with frequent involvement

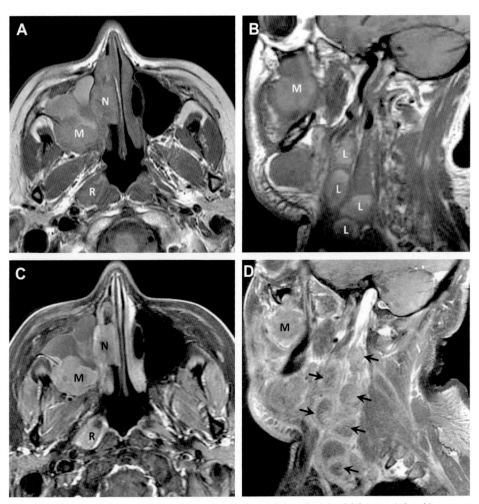

Fig. 14. Melanotic maxillary sinus melanoma: Noncontrast axial (*A*) and sagittal (*B*) T1-weighted images and axial (*C*) and sagittal (*D*) contrast-enhanced T1-weighted fat-suppressed images demonstrate masses within the nasal cavity (N) and maxillary sinus (M). The primary tumor and multiple metastatic retropharyngeal (R) and cervical (L) lymph nodes have a T1-hyperintense appearance on noncontrast images consistent with the melanotic nature of the tumor. Sagittal T1-weighted scan reveals multiple abnormal matted level 2 to 4 lymph nodes (*arrows*).

of the adjacent orbit and cranial cavity. Up to 30% of people will have nodal disease on presentation.[33] Metastases to lung or bone are rare. Mortality is high, with 5-year survival data reported from 15% to 63%.[34,35] Survival for patients is 47% to 64% at 2 years with aggressive multimodality treatment. It presents in middle age as a sinonasal mass most commonly in the upper nasal cavity or ethmoid region. No characteristic imaging findings are present, although a soft tissue mass with bone destruction is most common. There is frequent involvement of adjacent structures, including the orbit, skin, and skull base, at the time of presentation. CT imaging can help to assess for bony destruction, including the lamina papyracea and cribriform plate regions. MR imaging is valuable for the assessment of deep extension of the mass into the orbit and skull base and for perineural tumor spread. A heterogeneous enhancement pattern is typical. PET is useful for assessing regional and distant disease.

Olfactory neuroblastoma (esthesioneuroblastoma) is a malignant tumor of neuroendocrine origin arising from the olfactory neuroepithelium (**Fig. 12**). It is thought to be along the spectrum of other neuroendocrine malignancies, including the aforementioned SNUC. It has a bimodal incidence of occurrence in the second and sixth decades of life. Clinical presentation includes nasal stuffiness, decreased smell, pain, and occasionally epistaxis. On imaging, one finds a heterogeneous mass centered high in the nasal vault near the cribriform plate. It is typically hypointense on T1-weighted images and intermediate to high signal intensity on T2-weighted scans and demonstrates marked enhancement. It may cross the cribriform plate to extend intracranially. Peripheral cysts of the intracranial portion of the mass may occur and are highly suggestive of olfactory neuroblastoma. There are multiple grading systems for this tumor, including the Kadish[36] and Hyams systems. Kadish stage A tumors are limited to the nasal cavity, stage B tumors are limited to the nasal cavity and paranasal sinuses, and stage C lesions extend beyond the nasal cavity and paranasal sinuses. Morita published a revised Kadish system in 1993 to also include a stage D indicating distant metastases. TNM staging is defined as the following: T1: tumor involving nasal cavity or paranasal sinuses (excluding sphenoid) with sparing of the most superior ethmoid air cells; T2: tumor involving the nasal cavity or paranasal sinuses (including the sphenoid), with extension to or erosion of the cribriform plate; T3: tumor extending into the orbit or protruding into the anterior cranial fossa, without dural invasion; T4: tumor involving the brain; nodal staging of N0: no nodal metastasis; N1: any form of cervical nodal metastasis; metastasis staging of M0: no metastasis; M1: distant metastasis present. The treatment is typically surgical excision. This treatment may be followed by radiation for more advanced disease, with possibly adjuvant chemotherapy. Advanced-stage tumors tend to respond poorly. Overall survival at 5 years has been reported at a mean of 45%,[37] with the highest overall survival found of 93%.[35]

Adenoid cystic carcinoma accounts for 10% of salivary gland neoplasms (**Fig. 13**). It is the most common minor salivary gland neoplasm, representing approximately 33% of lesions. It accounts for up to 15% of sinonasal tumors, with most cases occurring in the maxillary sinus (50%), nasal cavity (33%), and less than 5% involving the sphenoid or frontal sinuses. This tumor is typically a slow-growing but relentless tumor characterized by its propensity for perineural spread, including skip lesions. It also has a tendency to recur even years after the initial diagnosis and treatment. Five-year overall survival is reported to be approximately 65% and 15-year survival of approximately 30%. Up to 40% of patients will have metastatic disease to the lungs, which also tends to be a slow-growing process with which people can survive for years. Surgery is the primary treatment because the tumor does not tend to respond well to radiation or chemotherapy. On imaging, it is crucial to look for perineural tumor spread given the sinuses are in close proximity to many neural structures that communicate with the orbits,

---

Box 5
Primary tumor, nodal disease, and metastasis staging of head and neck melanoma

T3: Mucosal disease

T4a: Moderately advanced disease

   Tumor involving deep soft tissue, cartilage, bone, or overlying skin

T4b: Very advanced disease

   Tumor involving brain, dura, skull base, lower cranial nerves (IX, X, XI, XII), masticator space, carotid artery, prevertebral space, or mediastinal structures

NX: Regional lymph nodes cannot be assessed

N0: No regional lymph node metastases

N1: Regional lymph node metastases present

M0: No distant metastasis

M1: Distant metastasis present

cavernous sinuses, and the brain. These structures include the infraorbital and posterior superior alveolar nerves, which run within the walls of the maxillary sinus, and the vidian and maxillary nerves along the walls of the sphenoid sinus. The anterior and posterior ethmoidal branches of the ophthalmic nerve may also be involved by ethmoid sinus lesions. All of these nerves can access the pterygopalatine fossa or superior orbital fissure, which can, in turn, allow the spread to the cavernous sinus. Although any sinonasal malignancy can have perineural spread, adenoid cystic carcinoma has the highest propensity. Assessment for perineural tumor spread should be undertaken regardless of the histology, however. Other

minor salivary gland malignancies that may affect the sinuses include mucoepidermoid carcinoma, undifferentiated carcinoma, and adenocarcinoma. Adenocarcinoma is common in woodworkers and has a predilection for the ethmoid air cells.

Melanoma accounts for 3% to 5% of sinonasal malignancies. It most commonly arises in the nasal cavity and less frequently from the maxillary or ethmoid regions (**Fig. 14**). Epistaxis is a common presenting symptom. It typically occurs in men older than 40 years of age. Most sinonasal melanomas are melanotic, which can aid in imaging diagnosis. Melanotic melanomas appear as hyperintense on precontrast T1 imaging and hypointense on T2 imaging and show avid contrast

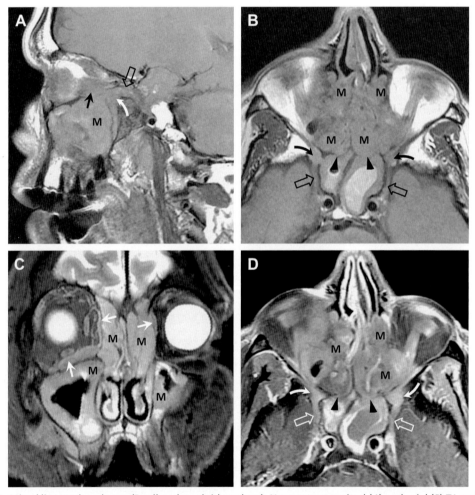

Fig. 15. Mixed lineage lymphoma (B cell and myeloid markers): Noncontrast sagittal (*A*) and axial (*B*) T1-weighted and coronal T2-weighted images (*C*) demonstrate extensive bilateral soft tissue masses (M) filling the nasal cavity, ethmoid sinuses, and maxillary sinuses. There is bilateral orbital invasion (*arrows*) and extension through the anterior walls of the sphenoid sinus (*arrowheads*). There is perineural tumor spread into the pterygopalatine fossa (*curved arrows*) and along the maxillary nerves (*open arrows*), best seen on the axial T1-weighted contrast-enhanced image (*D*). Note that the inflammatory mucosal disease within the sphenoid sinus enhances more intensely than the tumor.

enhancement. Six percent to 25% of patients present with lymph node involvement at diagnosis.[38] The treatment of choice is wide local excision with or without postoperative radiation. Despite aggressive therapy, the overall 5-year survival for head and neck mucosal melanoma is approximately 30%.[39,40] Given its aggressive behavior, a separate staging has been developed. To reflect this, the AJCC TNM staging of melanomas begins at T3 (**Box 5**).

Lymphoma is the second most common malignancy of the head and neck.[41] Non-Hodgkin lymphoma is by far the most common type. Historically, sinonasal lymphoma has had several names, including lethal midline granuloma,

idiopathic midline destructive disease, and lymphomatoid granulomatosis, among others. The main cell types are B cell and natural killer/T cell. It typically presents with nondescript sinus symptoms in middle-aged to elderly men. The nasal cavity and maxillary sinus are most commonly involved, with rare involvement of the frontal or ethmoid sinuses (**Fig. 15**). The workup for systemic disease should be performed if the initial diagnosis of lymphoma is made in the paranasal sinuses. Additionally, posttransplant lymphoproliferative disease should be suspected in transplant patients. On imaging, it demonstrates homogeneous, variable signal intensity with prominent enhancement. Bone remodeling or frank erosion

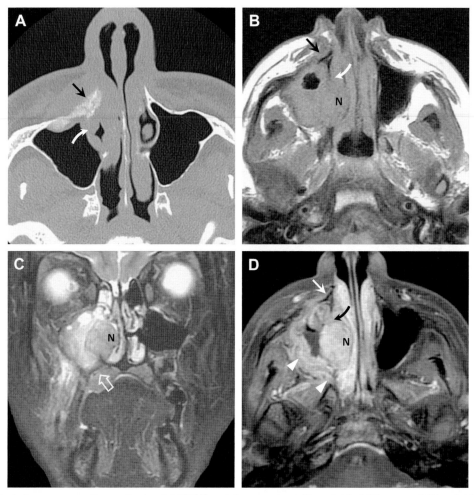

Fig. 16. Ewing sarcoma: Noncontrast axial CT (*A*), axial noncontrast T1-weighted (*B*), coronal T2-weighted (*C*), and axial contrast-enhanced T1-weighted (*D*) images demonstrate a mass lesion involving the frontal process of the maxilla (*arrows*), nasal cavity (N), and the medial wall of the maxillary sinus (*curved arrows*). The MR images best detect perineural spread of the lesion along the greater palatine nerve (*open arrows*) and extension to involve the retromaxillary fat and pterygopalatine fossa (*arrowheads*). The CT scan, however, reveals spiculated periosteal new bone formation and expansion of the frontal process, which is more helpful in suggesting a primary bone neoplasm.

may be present. Chemotherapy and radiotherapy are the typical treatment.

Ewing sarcoma most commonly involves the pelvis and long bones. It is approximately 4% to 10% of malignant bone neoplasms and is most frequently seen in the second decade of life. Four percent to 7% of cases involve the head and neck region.[42,43] Primary sinonasal is rare, with most cases involving the skull base or mandible. It is classified as a primitive neuroectodermal tumor. Given its propensity for bone involvement, CT is a useful evaluation (**Fig. 16**). MR imaging can help assess the degree of soft tissue involvement and evaluate for perineural spread. Histopathologic analysis is needed for definitive diagnosis. The treatment is typically multimodality, including surgery, chemotherapy, or radiotherapy depending on extent of the disease.

Rhabdomyosarcoma is the most common soft tissue sarcoma of children. It accounts for approximately 50% of these tumors and 3.5% to 5.0% of all childhood cancers. The head and neck region is the most common area to be involved by rhabdomyosarcoma, accounting for approximately 40% of cases.[44,45] The sinonasal area is a common area of involvement. It is typically locally aggressive and frequently presents with a perineural spread (**Fig. 17**) and distant metastasis (lung most commonly). On imaging, it has aggressive features, including invasion of tissue planes and bone destruction.

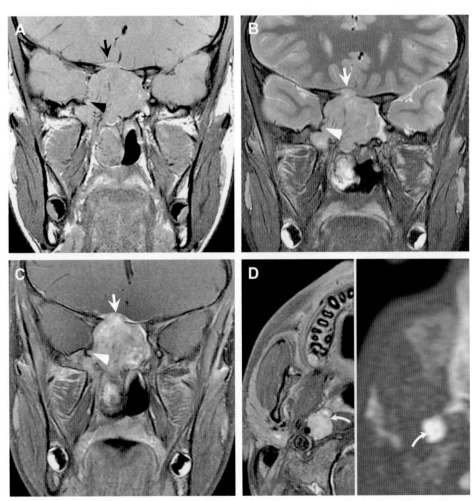

Fig. 17. Embryonal rhabdomyosarcoma nasal cavity: Noncontrast coronal T1-weighted (*A*) and coronal T2-weighted (*B*) images demonstrate a mass involving the sphenoid sinuses. The hypointense signal on the T2-weighted imaged is likely caused by the high cellularity of the lesion. There is erosion of the planum sphenoidale with epidural spread of tumor (*arrows*). A coronal contrast-enhanced T1-weighted image (*C*) also reveals involvement of the maxillary nerve within foramen rotundum (*arrowheads*). Contrast-enhanced axial T1-weighted and diffusion-weighted images (*D*) reveal tumor spread to a lateral retropharyngeal node (*curved arrows*).

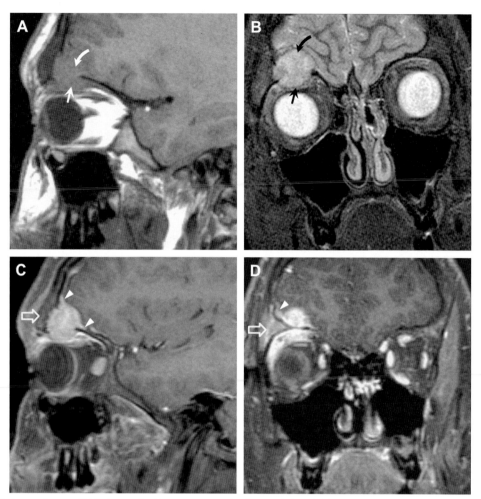

Fig. 18. Langerhans cell histiocytosis: Noncontrast sagittal T1-weighted (*A*) and coronal T2-weighted (*B*) images demonstrate a soft tissue mass likely originating within the frontal bone with extension into the orbit (*arrows*) and epidural space (*curved arrows*). Contrast-enhanced sagittal (*C*) and coronal (*D*) T1-weighted images show homogeneous enhancement of the lesion and the adjacent bone (*open arrows*). There is periosteal and dural enhancement (*arrowheads*), suggesting an aggressive process.

Langerhans cell histiocytosis has no known cause. It is characterized by the proliferation of histiocytic cells and can present as either a single-organ or multisystem disease. Epstein-Barr virus has been suggested as a possible contributing factor.[46] It can occur at any age but is mostly seen in children. Head and neck involvement is not uncommon, occurring in 74% in one study (**Fig. 18**).[47] Isolated sinonasal involvement (see **Fig. 18**) is rare, with only case reports identified in the literature.[48]

REFERENCES

1. Muir MB, Weiland L. Upper aerodigestive tract cancers. Cancer 1995;75:147–53.

2. Myers LL, Nussenbaum B, Bradford CR, et al. Paranasal sinus malignancies: an 18-year single institution experience. Laryngoscope 2002;112: 1964–9.

3. Goldenberg D, Golz A, Fradis M, et al. Malignant tumors of the nose and paranasal sinuses: a retrospective review of 291 cases. Ear Nose Throat J 2001;80:272–7.

4. Loevner LA, Sonners AI. Imaging of neoplasms of the paranasal sinuses. Magn Reson Imaging Clin N Am 2002;10:467–93.

5. Raghavan P, Phillips CD. Magnetic resonance imaging of sinonasal malignancies. Top Magn Reson Imaging 2007;18:259–67.

6. Resto VA, Deschler DG. Sinonasal malignancies. Otolaryngol Clin North Am 2004;37:473–87.

7. Bent JP, Cuilty-Siller C, Kuhn FA. The frontal cell as a cause of frontal sinus obstruction. Am J Rhinol 1994;8:185–91.

8. Keros P. On the practical value of differences in the level of the lamina cribrosa of the ethmoid. Z Laryngol Rhinol Otol 1962;41:809–13.

9. Curtin HD, Ishwaran H, Mancuso AA, et al. Comparison of CT and MR imaging in staging of neck metastases. Radiology 1998;207:123–30.

10. Wu L, Xu J, Liu M, et al. Value of magnetic resonance imaging for nodal staging in patient's with head and neck squamous cell carcinoma: a meta-analysis. Acad Radiol 2012;19:331–40.

11. Adams S, Baum RP, Stuckensen T, et al. Prospective comparison of 18F-FDG PET with conventional imaging modalities (CT, MR, US) in lymph node staging of head and neck cancer. Eur J Nucl Med 1998;25:1255–60.

12. Nayak JV, Walvekar RR, Andrade RS, et al. Deferring planned neck dissection following chemoradiation for stage IV head and neck cancer: the utility of PET-CT. Laryngoscope 2007;117:2129–34.

13. Wang Y, Liu R, Chu P, et al. Positron emission tomography in surveillance of head and neck squamous cell carcinoma after definitive chemoradiotherapy. Head Neck 2009;31:442–51.

14. Lyford-Pike S, Ha PK, Jacene HA, et al. Limitations of PET/CT in determining need for neck dissection after primary chemoradiation for advanced head and neck squamous cell carcinoma. ORL J Otorhinolaryngol Relat Spec 2009;71:251–6.

15. Lohrmann C, Uhl M, Warnatz K, et al. Sinonasal computed tomography in patients with Wegener's granulomatosis. J Comput Assist Tomogr 2006;30: 122–5.

16. Hoffman GS, Kerr GS, Leavitt RY, et al. Wegener granulomatosis: an analysis of 158 patients. Ann Intern Med 1992;116:488–98.

17. Hilal AA, Taj-Aldeen SJ, Mirghani AH. Rhinoorbital mucormycosis secondary to Rhizopus oryzae: a case report and literature review. Ear Nose Throat J 2004;83:556–62.

18. Pillsbury HC, Fischer ND. Rhinocerebral Mucormycosis. Arch Otolaryngol 1977;103:600–4.

19. Weprin BE, Hall WA, Goodman J, et al. Long term survival in rhinocerebral mucormycosis. J Neurosurg 1998;88:570–5.

20. Spellberg B, Edwards J Jr, Ibrahim A. Novel perspectives on mucormycosis: pathophysiology, presentation, and management. Clin Microbiol Rev 2005;18:556–69.

21. Safder S, Carpenter JS, Roberts TD, et al. The "Black Turbinate" Sign: an early MR imaging finding of nasal mucormycosis. AJNR Am J Neuroradiol 2010;31:771–4.

22. Anari S, Carrie S. Sinonasal inverted papilloma: narrative review. J Laryngol Otol 2010;124:705–15.

23. Phillips PP, Gustafson RO, Facer GW. The clinical behavior of inverting papilloma of the nose and paranasal sinuses: report of 112 cases and review of the literature. Laryngoscope 1990;100: 463–9.

24. Lee JT, Bhuta S, Lufkin R, et al. Isolated inverting papilloma of the sphenoid sinus. Laryngoscope 2003;113:41–4.

25. Jardine AH, Davies GR, Birchall MA. Recurrence and malignant degeneration of 89 cases of inverted papilloma diagnosed in a non-tertiary referral population between 1975 and 1995: clinical predictors and p53 studies. Clin Otolaryngol 2000; 25:363–9.

26. Krouse JH. Development of a staging system for inverted papilloma. Laryngoscope 2000;110:965–8.

27. Thompson LD, Gyure KA. Extracranial sinonasal tract meningiomas: a clinicopathologic study of 30 cases with a review of the literature. Am J Surg Pathol 2000;24:640–50.

28. Rushing EJ, Bouffard JP, McCall S, et al. Primary extracranial meningiomas: an analysis of 146 cases. Head Neck Pathol 2009;3:116–30.

29. Hermans R, De Vuysere S, Marchal G. Squamous cell carcinoma of the sinonasal cavities. Semin Ultrasound CT MR 1999;20:150–61.

30. Lopez F, Llorente JL, Garcia-Inclan C, et al. Genomic profiling of sinonasal squamous cell carcinoma. Head Neck 2011;33:145–53.

31. Kerner C, Poeschl PW, Wutzl A, et al. Surgical treatment of squamous cell carcinoma of the maxilla and nasal sinuses. J Oral Maxillofac Surg 2008;66: 2449–53.

32. Alos L, Moyano S, Nadal A, et al. Human papillomaviruses are identified in a subgroup of sinonasal squamous cell carcinomas with favorable outcome. Cancer 2009;115:2701–9.

33. Tanzler ED, Morris CG, Orlando CA, et al. Management of sinonasal undifferentiated carcinoma. Head Neck 2008;30:595–9.

34. Gallo O, Graziana P, Fini-Storchi O. Undifferentiated carcinoma of the nose and paranasal sinuses: an immunohistochemical and clinical study. Ear Nose Throat J 1993;72:588–95.

35. Rosenthal DI, Barker JL Jr, El-Naggar AK, et al. Sinonasal malignancies with neuroendocrine differentiation. Cancer 2004;101:2567–73.

36. Kadish S, Goodman M, Wang CC. Olfactory neuroblastoma. A clinical analysis of 17 cases. Cancer 1976;37:1571–6.

37. Dulguerov P, Abdelkarim SA, Calcaterra TC. Esthesioneuroblastoma: a meta-analysis and review. Lancet Oncol 2001;2:683–90.

38. Moreno MA, Hanna EY. Management of mucosal melanomas of the head and neck: did we make any progress? Curr Opin Otolaryngol Head Neck Surg 2010;18:101–6.

39. Clifton N, Harrison L, Bradley PJ, et al. Malignant melanoma of nasal cavity and paranasal sinuses: report of 24 patients and literature review. J Laryngol Otol 2011;125:479–85.

40. Moreno MA, Roberts DB, Kupferman ME, et al. Mucosal melanoma of the nose and paranasal sinuses, a contemporary experience from the M. D. Anderson Cancer Center. Cancer 2010;116:2215–23.

41. Harnesberger HR, Bragg D, Osborn AG, et al. Non-Hodgkin's lymphoma of the head and neck: CT evaluation of nodal and extranodal sites. AJR Am J Roentgenol 1987;149:785–91.

42. Hafezi S, Seethala RR, Stelow EB, et al. Ewing's family of tumors of the sinonasal tract and maxillary bone. Head Neck Pathol 2011;5:8–16.

43. Vaccani JP, Forte V, de Jong AL, et al. Ewing's sarcoma of the head and neck in children. Int J Pediatr Otorhinolaryngol 1999;48:209–16.

44. Callender TA, Weber RS, Janjan N, et al. Rhabdomyosarcoma of the nose and paranasal sinuses in adults and children. Otolaryngol Head Neck Surg 1995;112:252–7.

45. Herrmann BW, Sotelo-Avila C, Eisenbeis JF. Pediatric sinonasal rhabdomyosarcoma: three cases and a review of the literature. Am J Otolaryngol 2003;24:174–80.

46. Shimakage M, Sasagawa T, Kimura M, et al. Expression of Epstein-Barr virus in Langerhans' cell histiocytosis. Hum Pathol 2004;35:862–8.

47. Nicollas R, Rome A, Belaich H, et al. Head and neck manifestation and prognosis of Langerhans' cell histiocytosis in children. Int J Pediatr Otorhinolaryngol 2010;74:669–73.

48. Yu G, Huang F, Kong L, et al. Langerhans cell histiocytosis of the sphenoid sinus: a case report. Turk J Pediatr 2010;52:548–51.

MR Assessment of Oral Cavity Carcinomas

Mari Hagiwara, MD[a],[*], Annette Nusbaum, MD[a],
Brian L. Schmidt, DDS, MD, PhD[b]

KEYWORDS

- Oral cavity ● Squamous cell carcinomas ● Minor salivary gland neoplasms ● MR Imaging ● Staging

KEY POINTS

- Surgical resection with 1-cm tumor-free margins is the primary treatment for oral cavity carcinomas.
- Accurate preoperative planning is critical to achieve adequate surgical margins and thereby minimize the risk for tumor recurrence.
- MR imaging is particularly advantageous in the evaluation of the oral cavity, because it provides a better-detailed depiction of normal oral structures and has reduced dental artifact compared with CT.
- Placement of a rolled 2 × 2–in gauze adjacent to the tumor just before the MR examination separates the mucosal surfaces and significantly improves tumor delineation.
- Evaluation of tumor depth and size, bone invasion, lymph node metastases, and perineural tumor spread is essential for all oral cavity carcinomas.

INTRODUCTION

Head and neck carcinomas account for 5% of all cancers, with approximately half of those arising from the oral cavity.[1] Globally, the annual estimated incidence for oral cavity cancers is approximately 275,000, with oral cavity carcinomas constituting up to 25% of all new cancers in high-risk countries, such as India and Pakistan.[2] Squamous cell carcinomas (SCCs) account for more than 90% of oral cavity cancers, with the remainder of oral cavity malignancies including salivary gland tumors (mucoepidermoid carcinoma, adenoid cystic carcinoma, polymorphous low-grade adenocarcinoma, and adenocarcinoma not otherwise specified), lymphomas, metastases, melanomas, and sarcomas.[3] These cancers are typically not distinguishable on imaging.

Oral cavity carcinomas most frequently occur in older men, although recently the incidence among young men and women has increased.[1,4,5] Risk factors include tobacco and alcohol use, betel quid (most commonly in Asia), and a vitamin-poor diet.[1,2,6] Sun exposure with ultraviolet radiation is a major risk factor for carcinomas of the lips. Human papilloma virus (HPV) infections have been implicated in a small percentage of oral cavity carcinomas, although not nearly to the same degree as with oropharyngeal carcinomas.[1,4,7] HPV does not entirely account for the increasing incidence of oral cavity carcinomas in the younger population.[1,4]

Oral cavity carcinomas present as white or red lesions involving the oral mucosa, occasionally with ulceration or exophytic components.[1] Most patients with oral cavity carcinomas present with pain, which often limits oral function.[8] Other clinical findings and symptoms include loose teeth, oral bleeding, dysarthria, dysphagia, and palpable lymphadenopathy.[1] Most, if not all, oral cavity

[a] Department of Radiology, NYU School of Medicine, 660 1st Avenue, 2nd floor Radiology, New York, NY 10016, USA; [b] Department of Oral & Maxillofacial Surgery, Bluestone Center for Clinical Research, New York University College of Dentistry, 421 First Avenue, Room 233W, New York, NY 10010, USA
* Corresponding author.
E-mail address: Mari.Hagiwara@nyumc.org

Magn Reson Imaging Clin N Am 20 (2012) 473–494
http://dx.doi.org/10.1016/j.mric.2012.05.003
1064-9689/12/$ – see front matter Published by Elsevier Inc.

SCCs arise from premalignant oral cavity lesions including erythroplakia, leukoplakia, erythroleuko-plakia and proliferative verrucous leukoplakia.[8,9]

Surgical resection with 1-cm tumor-free margins is the primary treatment for oral cavity carci-nomas.[8] Close or positive surgical margins are strongly associated with poor prognosis and locoregional recurrence.[8] Indications for adjuvant radiation therapy or chemoradiotherapy include advanced-stage tumors, positive or close surgical margins, perineural invasion, extensive bone inva-sion, and nodal metastases with extracapsular spread.[8,10] Adjuvant radiation therapy, however, does not seem to improve local control rates in patients with positive surgical margins.[8] Radiation therapy alone may be performed for patients who are not surgical candidates, although the recur-rence rate is high for both the primary lesion and neck disease.[8,10] Radiation therapy is also as-sociated with significant morbidity, including os-teoradionecrosis and speech and swallowing dysfunction.[8]

The diagnosis of oral cavity cancer is typically known at imaging; the mucosal extent is best eval-uated through visual inspection and manual palpa-tion. Preoperative imaging is essential for tumor staging and appropriate treatment planning. Care-fully performed and interpreted imaging can assist in determining the depth of invasion, involvement of critical structures, including bone and the internal carotid artery, and the presence of lymph node metastases. Clear surgical margins are a primary determinant of patient outcome; accu-rate preoperative planning is critical to achieve adequate surgical margins and thereby minimize the risk for tumor recurrence. An accurate assess-ment of the size of the cancer and the required resection volume also allows the surgical team to plan appropriately for reconstruction. MR imaging is particularly advantageous in evaluation of the oral cavity. MR imaging provides a better-detailed depiction of normal oral structures and has reduced dental artifact compared with CT. In addition, advanced MR imaging techniques, in-cluding spectroscopy, diffusion-weighted imaging, and perfusion imaging, are currently being investi-gated to better delineate true tumor extent, more accurately determine lymph node metastases, and predict treatment response.

IMAGING ANATOMY

The oral cavity includes the lips, maxillary and mandibular gingiva, buccal mucosa, hard palate, anterior two-thirds of the tongue, floor of the mouth, and retromolar trigone. The vestibule is the space posterior and medial to the lips and cheek, respectively, and anterior and lateral to the gingiva and teeth. Posteriorly, the oral cavity is separated from the oropharynx by the circum-vallate papillae, the anterior tonsillar pillars, and the junction of the hard and soft palates. The circumvallate papillae are easily identified on clin-ical examination but not delineated on imaging. The circumvallate papillae divide the tongue into the oral tongue, which lies in the oral cavity, and the base of tongue, which lies in the oropharynx.

The gingiva covers the buccal (outer) and lingual or palatal (inner) surfaces of the maxillary and mandibular alveolar ridges. The gingiva covering the buccal surfaces is continuous with the buccal mucosa lining the inner lips and cheeks at the gin-givobuccal sulcus. The gingiva covering the lingual surface of the maxilla is continuous with the mucosa covering the hard palate. The hard palate forms the roof of the oral cavity and posteriorly attaches to the soft palate, which lies in the oropharynx. Coronal and sagittal T1-weighted images best depict the hypointense cortices and central hyperintense marrow of the osseous hard palate. A variable amount of T1 hyperintense submucosal fat can be seen along the inferior margin of the hard palate. A high concentration of minor salivary glands is present in the submu-cosal space of the hard palate and can occasion-ally be seen as small enhancing foci (**Fig. 1**F).

The floor of the mouth is a U-shaped space located inferior to the oral tongue and covered superiorly by squamous mucosa. The paired mylo-hyoid muscles provide the primary support for the floor of mouth, originating from the mylohyoid ridge along the inner surface of the mandible and attaching to a fibrous median raphe medially and to the hyoid bone posteriorly. On imaging, the my-lohyoid muscles are best delineated in the coronal plane, forming a sling between the right and left inner margins of the mandible (see **Fig. 1**A, B). In the axial plane, the muscles appear as linear struc-tures, near-parallel and deep to the mandibular bodies; the mylohyoid muscles can also be readily identified in this plane, forming a "lollipop" config-uration with the submandibular glands, with the "stick of the lollipop" formed by the mylohyoid muscle, and the "candy of the lollipop" formed by the submandibular gland (see **Fig. 1**C). The paired geniohyoid muscles and anterior bellies of the digastric muscles provide additional support for the floor of mouth, located immediately supe-rior and inferior to the mylohyoid muscle, respec-tively. These muscles are best depicted in the coronal plane (see **Fig. 1**A).

The mylohyoid sling separates the sublingual space superiorly and medially from the subman-dibular space inferiorly and laterally. The posterior margin of the mylohyoid muscles is a free border that allows communication between the sublingual and submandibular spaces. The superficial portion of the submandibular gland lies within the submandibular space, with a small deep portion extending around the posterior margin of the mylohyoid muscle into the sublingual space. The duct of the submandibular gland courses anteriorly within the sublingual space and drains into the subfrenular region near midline (see **Fig. 1**D). The sublingual space contains the deep portion of the submandibular gland, Wharton's (submandibular) duct, sublingual gland, anterior portion of the hyoglossus muscle, hypoglossal and lingual nerves, and lingual artery and vein. The submandibular space is a predominantly fat-filled space that contains the superficial portion of the submandibular gland, anterior belly of the digastric muscle, facial artery and vein, and submandibular and submental nodes.

The oral tongue is composed of a midline fibrofatty lingual septum and four interdigitating intrinsic tongue muscles, including the superior longitudinal, inferior longitudinal, transverse, and vertical/oblique muscles. These intrinsic muscles cannot be distinguished from one another on imaging. There are also four paired extrinsic tongue muscles with origins external to the tongue, including the genioglossus, hyoglossus, styloglossus, and palatoglossus muscles. Involvement of these extrinsic muscles by carcinoma upstages the tumor to T4a. The genioglossus muscles arise from the genial tubercle along the inner surface of the mandible and superiorly interdigitate with the intrinsic tongue musculature. These muscles are easily identified on imaging as fan-shaped muscles forming the bulk of the tongue on sagittal T1-weighted images and as rectangular muscles on either side of the midline fatty lingual septum on coronal and axial images (see **Fig. 1**A, C, E). The hyoglossus, styloglossus, and palatoglossus muscles are located laterally, with attachments to the hyoid bone, styloid process, and soft palate, respectively. The hyoglossus muscles are depicted in the coronal and axial planes as thin rectangular muscles parallel and medial to the mylohyoid muscles and lateral to the genioglossus muscles (see **Fig. 1**B, C). Because the neurovascular bundles are closely related to the hyoglossus muscles,[11] involvement of the hyoglossus muscle by tumor is a strong marker for neurovascular invasion.

The retromolar trigone is a triangular area just posterior to the mandibular and maxillary third molars, immediately anterior to the mandibular ramus. The retromolar trigone lies immediately medial to the pterygomandibular raphe, which is a fascial band connecting the buccinator muscle anteriorly with the superior pharyngeal constrictor muscle posteriorly (**Fig. 2**). Superiorly, the pterygomandibular raphe attaches to the hamulus of the medial pterygoid plate, and inferiorly, the raphe attaches to the mandibular body near the posterior margin of the mylohyoid ridge. The pterygomandibular raphe has been implicated in the route of tumor spread from the retromolar trigone.[12]

MR IMAGING

MR imaging provides superior soft tissue contrast and better depicts the detailed anatomy of the oral cavity compared with CT, and therefore can more accurately delineate the borders and extent of infiltration of oral cavity carcinomas. MR imaging also has the advantage of reduced metallic artifact from dental amalgam, which often hampers evaluation of the primary carcinoma with CT images. In addition, MR is the preferred imaging modality in the evaluation of perineural tumor spread and bone marrow invasion, which are important factors in treatment planning.

MR imaging should be performed with a dedicated neck coil and should include small field of view (FOV) images (14–18 cm) with thin sections (3–4 mm) dedicated to the oral cavity, and large FOV (20 cm) images of the entire neck to evaluate for nodal metastases (**Box 1**). Small FOV images of the oral cavity should include thin-section axial and coronal T1-weighted images and axial and coronal thin-section postcontrast T1-weighted images, the latter with or without fat suppression. Fat suppression increases conspicuity of the enhancing tumor and enables distinction of tumor from the normal T1 hyperintense fat present throughout the oral cavity. However, fat saturation causes increased artifact from dental amalgam and soft tissue/air interfaces (**Fig. 3**C, D). Fat saturation also increases the time of acquisition, which may increase motion artifact.[12] Frequency-selective fat-saturated T2-weighted images or short time inversion recovery (STIR) images should also be performed through the oral cavity and neck. At the authors' institution, a coronal STIR sequence with a small FOV is obtained of the oral cavity, and an axial T2-weighted, frequency-selective fat-saturated sequence with a large FOV is obtained of the entire neck to evaluate for nodal metastases.

Although MRI significantly reduces dental artifact compared with CT, extensive dental hardware may produce susceptibility artifact that can still obscure the primary tumor. Avoidance of gradient-echo (GRE), use of lower field strength magnets, reduction in echo train length (ETL) and echo time (TE), and increase in bandwidth are techniques that can minimize dental artifact (**Box 2**).[13] Frequency-selective fat saturation increases artifact from dental amalgam. As a result, a STIR sequence, which is not as affected by magnetic field inhomogeneities produced by metallic hardware, may be preferred over a frequency-selective fat-saturated T2-weighted sequence (see **Fig. 3**C, E).[13] In addition, postcontrast images without fat saturation in at least one plane may be helpful in patients with extensive dental work; although there is decreased conspicuity of the lesion without fat saturation, the gray signal of the enhancing tumor is typically distinguishable from the surrounding T1 hyperintense fat (see **Fig. 3**D, F, G).[12]

Because the structures within the oral cavity abut one another when imaged with the mouth closed, delineation of tumor depth may be problematic, particularly for evaluation of small mucosal tumors and tumors in certain locations, such as the gingiva and buccal mucosa. For CT examinations, the

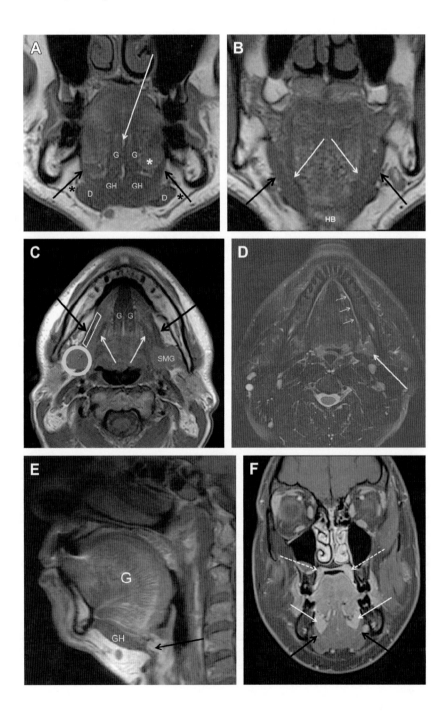

"puffed cheek" method of distending the cheeks has been successfully used, although the longer scanning times of MR imaging make it more difficult for the patient to maintain the same degree of distension throughout the examination.[14–16] Placement of a rolled 2 × 2–in gauze adjacent to the tumor just before the MR examination has been shown to effectively separate the mucosal surfaces and significantly improve tumor delineation, with gauze having a similar appearance to air.[15] This technique is particularly useful for the evaluation of buccal carcinomas (see Fig. 3; Fig. 4).

On noncontrast T1-weighted images, tumors demonstrate isointense to hypointense signal to muscle. The variable fat content of the oral cavity musculature and the interspersed fat between the muscles enables distinction from tumor, despite the similar signal intensities of tumor to muscle.[12] Disruption of the fat planes is a good indicator for invasion, and tongue lesions in particular are clearly delineated if the intrinsic fat content is high.[11,12] Oral cavity carcinomas demonstrate hyperintense signal on T2-weighted images and enhance on postgadolinium T1-weighted images.[17] Although the conspicuity of lesions is greater with T2-weighted and contrast-enhanced T1-weighted images, the extent of tumor may be overestimated, especially with T2-weighted images, because of the similar signal characteristics of surrounding edema and inflammation.[3,12,18]

Tumor thickness is an important component of tumor staging and has been shown to strongly correlate with the presence of nodal metastases, risk of local recurrence, and overall survival.[19–23]

Several studies have shown MR imaging to have high sensitivity for the evaluation of tumor depth and muscle invasion, with higher sensitivity and specificity compared with CT and positron emission tomography (PET)/CT.[18–20,24–26]

Accurate preoperative determination of bone involvement is essential in treatment planning and staging; bone involvement upstages the tumor to at least a T4a. Oral cavity carcinomas invade bone at sites of abutment and can invade the bone through the cortex, or more commonly through the periodontal ligament or at a site of previous tooth extraction.[19,27] Determining the presence and extent of bone invasion is critical to determine the planned osteotomy sites.[28] Segmental mandibulectomy involves removal of a section of the mandible and is required for bone marrow invasion. Marginal mandibulectomy, however, involves removal of only the cortex and a portion of the marrow; mandibular continuity is maintained. This procedure can be used for minor cortical erosion and tumors in close proximity to the mandible.[12,28] However, obtaining a 1-cm margin often leaves a thin residual mandible that is prone to fracture,[8] which is particularly problematic in edentulous patients with mandibular atrophy; this subset of patients often requires a segmental mandibulectomy, even with minimal osseous invasion.

MR imaging is superior in the detection of bone marrow invasion.[19,26,29] CT better demonstrates small cortical bony erosions, but the study is often limited by metallic artifact from dental amalgam.[30] Nonenhanced T1-weighted images best demonstrate the extent of bone marrow invasion, seen

Fig. 1. Normal anatomy. (A) Coronal T1-weighted image shows the fatty lingual septum (white arrow) in midline, with the paired vertically oriented genioglossus muscles (G) and geniohyoid muscles (GH) on either side. The mylohyoid muscles (black arrows) can be seen forming a sling between the right and left inner mandibular surfaces and separate the sublingual space (white asterisk) superiorly and medially from the submandibular space (black asterisks) inferiorly and laterally. The anterior bellies of the digastric muscles (D) lie directly below the mylohyoid sling within the submandibular space. (B) Coronal T1-weighted image more posteriorly shows the mylohyoid muscles (black arrows) inserting upon the hyoid bone (HB) inferiorly. The hyoglossus muscles (white arrows) can be identified just deep and nearly parallel to the mylohyoid muscles. (C) Axial T1-weighted image shows the mandible anteriorly and laterally with central hyperintense fatty marrow. The fatty lingual septum is seen at midline with the paired genioglossus muscles (G) on either side. The mylohyoid muscles (black arrows) are seen laterally, just deep and nearly parallel to the mandibular bodies; note the lollipop configuration of the mylohyoid muscle with the submandibular gland (SMG) posteriorly (outlined with a rectangle and circle on the right side). The hyoglossus muscles (white arrows) are seen in the sublingual spaces parallel to the mylohyoid muscles. (D) Axial short time inversion recovery (STIR) image shows the submandibular gland (large arrow) posteriorly with the thin hyperintense submandibular duct (small arrows) coursing anteriorly and medially within the sublingual space. (E) Sagittal T1-weighted image shows the fan-shaped genioglossus muscle (G) forming the bulk of the tongue. The geniohyoid muscle (GH) is seen just inferiorly extending from the genial tubercle to the hyoid bone (black arrow) posteriorly. The geniohyoid muscle lies just above but is indistinguishable from the mylohyoid muscle on this image. (F) Coronal postcontrast T1-weighted fat-saturated image shows the enhancing sublingual glands (solid white arrows) in the sublingual space superomedial to the mylohyoid sling (black arrows). More superiorly, submucosal enhancement is seen in the hard palate (dashed white arrows) reflecting the high concentration of minor salivary glands in this region.

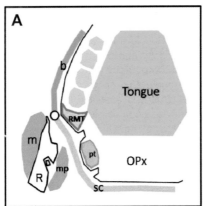
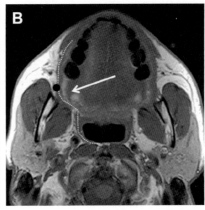

Fig. 2. Normal anatomy of the retromolar trigone. (*A*) The retromolar trigone (RMT) is the small space posterior to the mandibular and maxillary third molars. The pterygomandibular raphe (*white circle*) lies immediately deep to the retromolar trigone and connects the buccinator muscle (b) anteriorly to the superior constrictor muscle (SC) posteriorly. The pterygomandibular raphe has been implicated in the route of spread of tumor from the retromolar trigone. Also note the proximity of the retromolar trigone to the mandibular ramus (R) and inferior alveolar nerve (*small yellow dot drawn within the mandibular foramen*). OPx, oropharynx; pt, palatine tonsil; m, masseter muscle; mp, medial pterygoid muscle. (*B*) The retromolar trigone (*arrow*) can be identified as the space posterior to the maxillary and mandibular molars. The location of the pterygomandibular raphe is approximated by the black dot just deep to the retromolar trigone, connecting the buccinator muscle anteriorly to the superior constrictor muscle posteriorly (*small white dots*). Again, note the proximity of the ascending ramus to the retromolar trigone.

Box 1
Oral cavity MR imaging protocol

Placement of gauze adjacent to lesion, particularly helpful with buccal mucosal carcinomas

Small FOV of oral cavity: 14- to 18-cm FOV, 3- to 4-mm–thick slices

Large FOV of neck: 20-cm FOV, 4- to 5-mm–thick slices

- Large FOV, sagittal precontrast T1-weighted sequence
- Large FOV, axial T2-weighted fat-saturated or STIR sequence
- Small FOV, axial precontrast T1-weighted sequence
- (Small FOV, coronal precontrast T1-weighted sequence—optional)
- Small FOV, coronal T2-weighted fat-saturated or STIR sequence

Injection of intravenous contrast material

- Small FOV, axial postcontrast T1-weighted fat-saturated sequence
- Small FOV, coronal postcontrast T1-weighted fat-saturated sequence
- Large FOV, axial postcontrast T1-weighted fat-saturated sequence

as low signal intensity replacing the high signal of the medullary fat (**Fig. 5**C, D).[29,31] Bone marrow invasion is also depicted as hyperintense signal on fat-suppressed T2-weighted images and enhancement on fat-suppressed postcontrast images. Replacement of the hypointense signal of the bony cortex on T1- and T2-weighted images with the signal intensity of the tumor is a strong indicator for cortical invasion (**Fig. 6**C).[29] Sensitivity and specificity of MR imaging vary widely among studies, with sensitivity ranging from 58% to 100% and specificity ranging from 54% to 97%. Most studies have shown MR imaging to have overall higher sensitivity than CT in evaluating bone involvement, with similar sensitivity to PET/CT.[19,25,26,29–34] MR imaging, however, has lower specificity, with false-positive cases attributed to inflammatory change from dental infections or procedures and to chemical shift artifact from bone marrow fat on T1-weighted MR images.[31,35]

MR also best detects perineural tumor spread, most commonly associated with SCCs and adenoid cystic carcinomas.[36,37] With oral cavity carcinomas, the most common involved nerves are branches of the maxillary (V2) and mandibular (V3) divisions of the trigeminal nerve.[12] Hard palate tumors can spread along the greater palatine nerve (branch of V2) to the pterygopalatine fossa (**Fig. 7**).[37] Tumors invading the mandible and specifically the mandibular canal can spread along the inferior alveolar

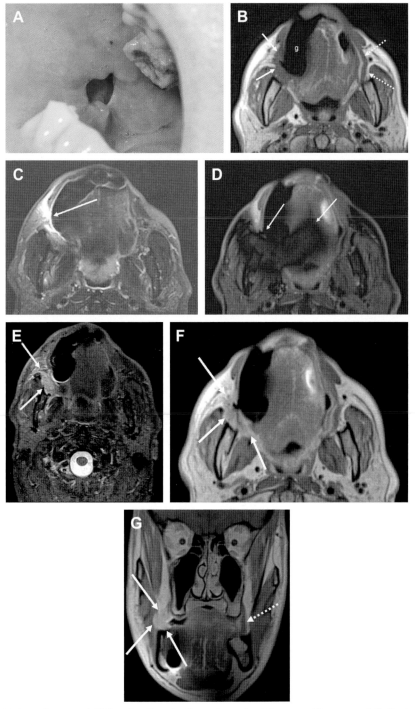

Fig. 3. T2 right buccal mucosal SCC extending to the retromolar trigone, with gauze. (*A*) Photograph shows a surface ulcer that measured 2.2 cm, making this a T2 lesion. (*B*) Axial T1-weighted image shows a T1-isointense mass (*solid arrows*) involving the right buccinator muscle and extending laterally into the buccal space and posteriorly into the retromolar trigone. Replacement of the normal fat in this region can be seen, particularly when compared with the normal left side (*dashed arrows*). During the MR examination, gauze (g) was placed adjacent to the mass, separating the mass and buccal mucosa from the oral tongue and thereby enabling better evaluation of tumor depth. Note the air signal intensity of the gauze. Axial T2-weighted frequency-selective fat-saturated (*C*) and axial postcontrast T1-weighted fat-saturated (*D*) images show extensive artifact from the dental amalgam and gauze (*arrows*) obscuring the mass. Note the decreased artifact and improved lesion visualization on the axial short time inversion recovery (STIR) (*E*) and postcontrast T1-weighted (non–fat-saturated) (*F*) images. The mass is seen as a T2-hyperintense, enhancing mass involving the right buccinator muscle and invading the retromolar trigone (*arrows*). (*G*) Coronal postcontrast T1-weighted (non–fat-saturated) image shows the lesion involving the right buccinator muscle. Despite lack of fat saturation, the gray signal of the tumor (*solid arrows*) can be distinguished from the surrounding fat. Note the normal buccinator muscle on the left side (*dashed arrow*) for comparison.

Box 2
Ways to reduce dental artifact

- Avoidance of GRE
- 1.5T preferable to 3T
- Reduction of ETL and TE
- Increase in bandwidth
- Avoidance of frequency-selective fat-saturation techniques

nerve (branch of V3). Findings of perineural tumor spread include abnormal enhancement and enlargement of the nerves on postcontrast T1-weighted images (see **Fig. 7**F) and obliteration of the hyperintense fat signal in the skull base foramina and pterygopalatine fossa on precontrast T1-weighted images. Perineural tumor spread can be antegrade or retrograde, and therefore the entire course of the nerve should be evaluated, with attention to the pterygopalatine fossa, cavernous sinus, and Meckel's cave. Findings of secondary muscle denervation of the masticator space musculature may also be evident.

Presence of lymph node metastases is one of the most important prognostic factors, with an associated reduction of 50% in patient survival.[10] Carcinomas arising from the oral tongue, floor of mouth, and buccal mucosa have a higher risk of cervical nodal metastases than those from the hard palate and gingiva.[28] Lymphatic drainage is most commonly through the level I and II nodes for oral cavity carcinomas, especially the jugulodigastric nodes. Skip metastases may be seen in level III nodes, although skip metastases to level IV and V are extremely rare.[8] In patients with clinical and radiographic evidence of nodal involvement, a modified radical neck dissection is performed, often with resection of the internal jugular vein and/or sternocleidomastoid muscle. To preserve shoulder function, the spinal accessory nerve is typically preserved unless invaded by tumor.[8]

Findings of nodal involvement on MRI and CT include nodal enlargement and central necrosis (see **Fig. 6**). Although CT more easily detects central necrosis,[28] MRI and CT have similar sensitivity and specificity for evaluating lymph node involvement, with MR sensitivity ranging from 64% to 92% and specificity ranging from 40% to 81%.[26,38] Most studies show that PET/CT is superior to MR in detecting lymph node metastases, although a more recent study by Seitz and colleagues[38] showed similar sensitivity and specificity (88.5% and 75%, respectively, for MRI and

83.8% and 73.9%, respectively, for PET/CT) in 66 patients with oral and oropharyngeal cancers.

Occult nodal micrometastases (ie, no clinical or imaging evidence of lymph node involvement) are present in 21% to 46% of patients with T1 oral cavity tumors, with higher rates in those with T2 through T4 tumors.[8,39] An elective selective neck dissection with resection of nodal levels I, II, and III is indicated if the risk of occult metastases is greater than 20%.[8,40,41] Therefore, selective neck dissections are routinely performed for all oral cavity carcinomas with an N0 neck (**Box 3**).[8,41] The "wait and see" approach with close monitoring of patients without a neck dissection has a high failure rate; 39% to 57% of patients develop nodal metastases with a higher incidence of extracapsular spread, often requiring more radical salvage neck surgery (ie, neck dissection after nodal metastasis has developed).[8,41] Survival for patients who undergo salvage surgery is half that for those who are treated with an elective neck dissection during the initial cancer resection.[42] Radiation therapy of the N0 neck is also associated with poor cancer control rates and significant morbidity.[8]

The exception to this rule is for carcinomas arising from the lips, which have a low risk of nodal metastases. Despite its increased sensitivity for nodal metastases, PET/CT remains limited in the detection of occult metastases and typically does not change patient management.[8,41] Tumors that cross the midline have a high incidence of contralateral occult nodal metastases, and therefore require bilateral nodal dissections. Whether the primary lesion crosses or encroaches the midline is therefore critical to determine preoperatively.

STAGING

Staging of oral cavity carcinomas is based on the American Joint Committee on Cancer TNM system, listed in **Tables 1** and **2**. Staging is determined based on a combination of clinical and imaging findings. T1, T2, and T3 are based on tumor size, and T4 is based on invasion of specific adjacent structures, with T4a subcategorized into lip and oral cavity for moderately advanced local disease (see **Table 1**). Tumor stage strongly correlates with patient prognosis and is a significant predictor for tumor recurrence. However, oral cavity SCC is notorious for its capricious clinical behavior, and even patients with stage 1 can experience local or locoregional treatment failure.

SITE-SPECIFIC FEATURES

Evaluation of tumor depth and size, bone invasion, lymph node metastases, and perineural tumor

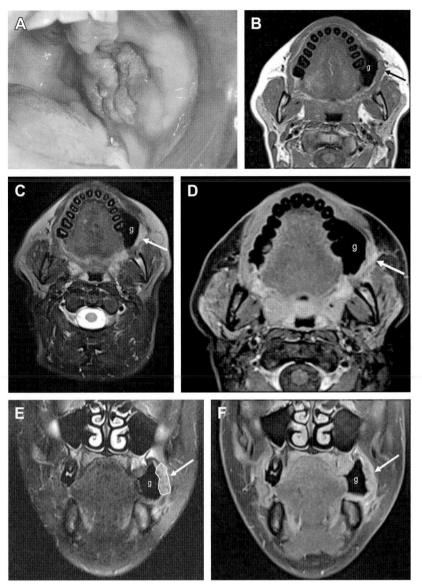

Fig. 4. T2 left buccal mucosal SCC, with gauze. (*A*) Photograph shows an irregular erythematous lesion along the left buccal mucosa, which on palpation measured approximately 3 × 3 cm, making this a T2 lesion. (*B–F*) Axial T1-weighted (*B*), T2-weighted fat-saturated (*C*), and postcontrast T1-weighted fat-saturated (*D*) images and coronal T2-weighted fat-saturated (*E*) and postcontrast T1-weighted fat-saturated (*F*) images show a T1-isointense, T2-hyperintense, enhancing left buccal mass involving the buccinator muscle (*arrows*). The tumor is outlined on Fig. 4E. Placement of gauze (g) between the buccal mucosa and oral tongue enables good visualization of the buccal mass and accurate evaluation of tumor depth.

spread is essential for all oral cavity carcinomas. Patterns of tumor spread and treatment approach depend on the site of origin in the oral cavity, and specific features must be considered based on the site of origin (**Box 4**). The most commonly affected sites in the oral cavity are the oral tongue and floor of mouth.

Oral Tongue

The oral tongue is the most frequently involved site in the oral cavity, accounting for approximately 33% of oral cavity carcinomas.[10] Most oral tongue carcinomas arise from the ventral and lateral portion of the tongue in the middle and posterior thirds (**Figs. 8** and **9**).[11] Tumors may extend

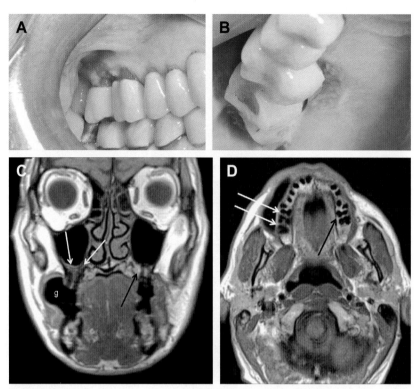

Fig. 5. T4a maxillary gingival SCC with bone invasion. Photographs of the outer buccal gingival view (*A*) and inner palatal gingival view (*B*) show the lesion in the maxillary buccal gingiva, interdental gingiva, and hard palate. Coronal (*C*) and axial (*D*) T1-weighted images show replacement of the normal T1-hyperintense fatty marrow in the right maxillary alveolar ridge (*white arrows*). Note the normal high signal in the left maxillary alveolar ridge for comparison (*black arrows*). The soft tissue component of the tumor was not well delineated on this examination. Gauze (g) had been placed around the tumor laterally.

posteriorly into the base of tongue and glossotonsillar sulcus, inferiorly to the floor of mouth, and medially to the lingual septum and contralateral tongue. From the floor of mouth, tumor may invade the mandible or inferiorly extend through the mylohyoid sling into the submandibular space.

Invasion across the midline lingual septum, involvement of the contralateral neurovascular bundle, and posterior extension to the base of tongue are particularly important factors in surgical planning. Surgical treatments range from transoral wide excision for small (T1 or T2) lesions, to partial, subtotal, or total glossectomy, with or without resection of the base of tongue. Invasion across the midline and involvement of the contralateral neurovascular bundle are contraindications to partial glossectomy and require a subtotal/total glossectomy (see **Fig. 9**). Invasion of the hyoglossus muscle is a good indicator for neurovascular invasion given the proximity of these structures.[11] Controversy exists regarding subtotal and total glossectomy for the treatment of advanced-stage tumors, given the associated morbidity related to speech and swallowing impairment[12,43]; however,

oral function can usually be adequately maintained with microvascular flap reconstruction if a significant portion of the base of tongue is preserved.

The risk of lymph node metastases, including occult metastases, is high given the rich lymphatic drainage of the oral tongue. Bilateral elective neck dissections are indicated in tumors that cross the midline and in tumors where the 1-cm surgical margin crosses the midline.[8,41] Tumor thickness of tongue cancer in particular has been shown to correlate strongly with lymph node metastases.[18,21,22]

Floor of Mouth

Floor of mouth carcinomas account for approximately 18% of oral cavity carcinomas,[10] with most originating anteriorly at the midline.[11] These tumors are particularly difficult to evaluate on clinical examination, and surgeons rely heavily on imaging for surgical planning. Tumors of the floor of mouth may extend superiorly into the ventral oral tongue, inferiorly through the mylohyoid muscle into the submandibular space, anteriorly and laterally into the bordering mandible, and

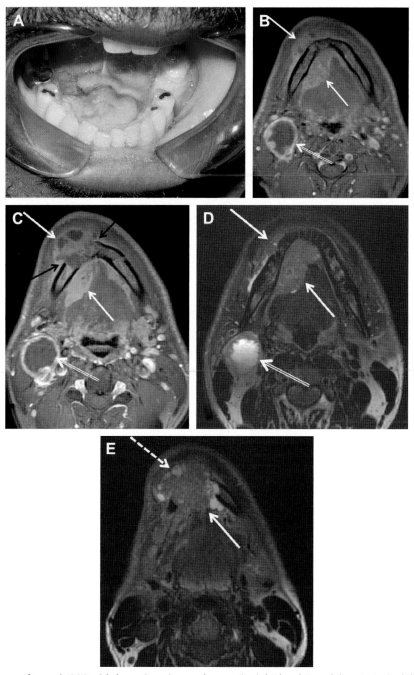

Fig. 6. T4a floor of mouth SCC with bone invasion and necrotic right level II nodal metastasis. (*A*) Photograph shows a large exophytic and ulcerated mass in the right floor of mouth extending across the midline. (*B, C*) Axial postcontrast fat-saturated T1-weighted images from superior to inferior show a large heterogeneously enhancing mass with areas of necrosis in the right floor of mouth (*solid white arrows*) extending across the midline anteriorly. Gross tumor invasion of the mandible with erosion through the outer cortex is seen (*solid black arrows in C*). No evidence was seen on imaging of perineural invasion in the inferior alveolar canal. A large necrotic right level II node is seen posteriorly (*double-lined white arrows*). (*D, E*) T2-weighted fat-saturated images from superior to inferior similarly show a mass in the floor of mouth (*solid arrows*) extending across the midline, with anterior extension through the mandible into the submental region (*dashed white arrow in E*). Note the low T2 signal intensity of most of the mass, indicating hypercellularity. The necrotic right level II node (*double lined white arrow in D*) is also seen.

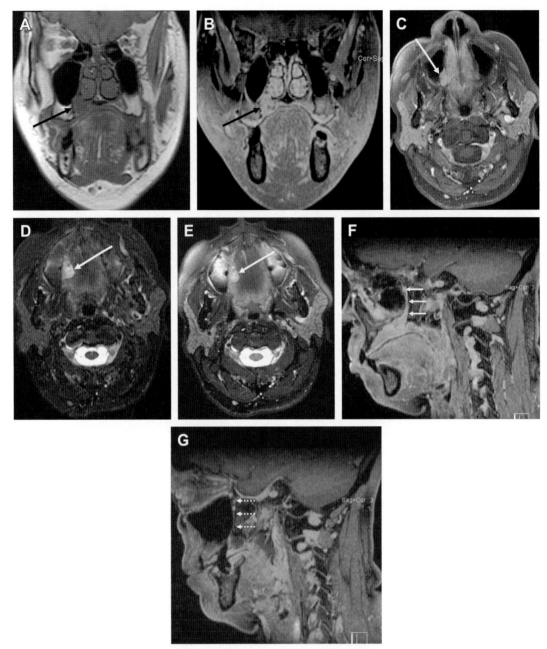

Fig. 7. T4a hard palate adenoid cystic carcinoma with bone invasion and perineural spread. (*A–C*) Coronal T1-weighted (*A*) and coronal (*B*) and axial (*C*) postcontrast fat-saturated T1-weighted images show a T1-isointense enhancing mass (*arrows*) in the posterior right aspect of the hard palate. The tumor involves the region of the greater palatine foramen. (*D, E*) Axial STIR (*D*) and T2-weighted frequency-selective fat-saturated (*E*) images show hyperintense signal within the mass (*arrows*). Note the higher lesion conspicuity on the STIR image and the areas of artifact and poor fat saturation on the frequency-selective fat-saturated image. (*F, G*) Reconstructed parasagittal postcontrast images through the level of the pterygopalatine canal show abnormal thick enhancement of the right greater palatine nerve (*solid arrows in F*) compared with the normal left side (*dashed arrows in G*), indicating perineural tumor spread.

posteriorly into the base of tongue (see **Fig. 6**; **Fig. 10**). Carcinomas arising from the anterior floor of mouth can obstruct the Wharton ducts, and ductal dilatation and findings of submandibular sialadenitis with glandular enlargement and increased enhancement may be evident on imaging. The sublingual glands are more likely to be directly invaded by tumor, although they may also be secondarily obstructed.[12] Involvement of the midline is common and important to determine preoperatively, because it necessitates bilateral nodal dissections.

Retromolar Trigone

Retromolar trigone tumors account for 7% to 12% of oral cavity carcinomas.[10,44] This site is also the second most common site of minor salivary gland tumors (**Figs. 11** and **12**). These cancers tend to rapidly invade the deep soft tissues and have a propensity for mandibular invasion because of the proximity of the retromolar trigone to the ascending ramus. The retromolar trigone is located at the junction of the oral cavity, oropharynx, and masticator space, and carcinomas originating from the retromolar trigone may spread anteriorly along the buccal mucosa and gingiva, posteriorly to the adjacent anterior tonsillar pillar and soft palate, and posterolaterally to the masticator space.[12,45] The pterygomandibular raphe lies immediately deep to the mucosa of the retromolar trigone, and it has been postulated that tumor from the retromolar trigone can spread along the raphe.[12] The pterygomandibular raphe connects the buccinator muscle to the superior constrictor muscle, and extends from the hamulus of the medial pterygoid plate to the posterior mandibular body; the raphe therefore provides access for these tumors to invade the buccinator muscle and buccal space, pterygoid plates and musculature, posterior mandible and maxilla, and the skull base.[28,45] Perineural tumor spread may occur along the inferior alveolar nerve (branch of V3) because of the proximity of the nerve to the retromolar trigone (see **Fig. 12**).[28]

Buccal Mucosa

Although relatively uncommon in North America and Europe, buccal carcinomas account for a large percentage of oral cavity carcinomas in Asia, and is much more common in men than in women.[46,47] This finding is likely related to the common practice of chewing betel quid by men in this region. Buccal carcinomas most commonly arise in the mid and posterior part of the cheek near the occlusal margin, where betel quid is typically retained.[3] Buccal cancer frequently demonstrates aggressive behavior and is associated with a high rate of treatment failure with poor locoregional control.[46,47] Submucosal invasion of the underlying buccinator muscle is common, with potential further spread into the buccal and masticator spaces. Invasion of the Stensen (parotid) duct may occur, which pierces the buccinator muscle at the level of the second maxillary molar. Tumor may also spread craniocaudally to the gingivobuccal sulci and the maxilla and mandible. Placement of gauze is particularly useful for MR evaluation of these tumors, because the gauze separates the buccal mucosa from the adjacent gingiva and enables better tumor delineation (see **Figs. 3** and **4**).[15]

Lymph node drainage is most commonly to the submental, submandibular, and periparotid lymph nodes.[8] Buccal mucosal carcinomas are associated with a high rate of recurrence even in the setting of negative margins. Therefore, postoperative radiotherapy is commonly indicated for these cancers.[8]

Gingiva

Carcinomas of the gingiva account for 10% to 18% of oral cavity cancers, with more frequent involvement of the lower gingiva.[10,48] The gingival mucosa covers the maxillary and mandibular alveolar ridges, and therefore bone invasion is common with gingival tumors; bone invasion is seen in up to 88% of patients (see **Fig. 5**).[48] Lateral invasion into the buccal space is the most common site of tumor spread for both upper and lower gingival tumors and occurs in nearly half of patients.[48] Lower gingival tumors may invade the masticator space posteriorly and invade the floor of mouth medially. Upper gingival tumors are more likely to invade the maxilla and hard palate, necessitating a partial maxillectomy.[45,48]

Hard Palate

SCCs arising from the hard palate are rare. However, the palate contains the highest concentration of minor salivary glands in the aerodigestive tract and is therefore the most common site of origin for minor salivary gland neoplasms.[37] Adenoid cystic carcinoma is the most frequently observed minor salivary gland malignancy, followed by mucoepidermoid carcinoma and adenocarcinoma.[49] Minor salivary

Table 1
Definitions of TNM

Primary Tumor (T)

TX	Primary tumor cannot be assessed
T0	No evidence of primary tumor
Tis	Carcinoma in situ
T1	Tumor 2 cm or less in greatest dimension
T2	Tumor more than 2 cm but not more than 4 cm in greatest dimension
T3	Tumor more than 4 cm in greatest dimension
T4a	Moderately advanced local disease[a] (lip) Tumor invades through cortical bone, inferior alveolar nerve, floor of mouth, or skin of face, that is, chin or nose (oral cavity) Tumor invades adjacent structures only (eg, through cortical bone [mandible or maxilla] into deep [extrinsic] muscle of tongue [genioglossus, hyoglossus, palatoglossus, and styloglossus], maxillary sinus, skin of face)
T4b	Very advanced local disease Tumor invades masticator space, pterygoid plates, or skull base and/or encases internal carotid artery

Regional Lymph Nodes (N)

NX	Regional lymph nodes cannot be assessed
N0	No regional lymph node metastasis
N1	Metastasis in a single ipsilateral lymph node, 3 cm or less in greatest dimension
N2	Metastasis in a single ipsilateral lymph node, more than 3 cm but not more than 6 cm in greatest dimension; or in multiple ipsilateral lymph nodes, none more than 6 cm in greatest dimension; or in bilateral or contralateral lymph nodes, none more than 6 cm in greatest dimension
N2a	Metastasis in single ipsilateral lymph node more than 3 cm but not more than 6 cm in greatest dimension
N2b	Metastasis in multiple ipsilateral lymph nodes, none more than 6 cm in greatest dimension
N2c	Metastasis in bilateral or contralateral lymph nodes, none more than 6 cm in greatest dimension
N3	Metastasis in a lymph node more than 6 cm in greatest dimension

Distant Metastasis (M)

M0	No distant metastasis
M1	Distant metastasis

[a] Note: Superficial erosion alone of bone/tooth socket by gingival primary is not sufficient to classify a tumor as T4.
Used with the permission of the American Joint Committee on Cancer (AJCC), Chicago, Illinois. The original source for this material is the AJCC Cancer Staging Manual, Seventh Edition (2010) published by Springer Science and Business Media LLC, www.springer.com.

gland tumors are more likely to be submucosal in location and may be difficult to detect and evaluate on clinical examination. Because of the proximity of the palatal mucosa to the bony hard palate, bone invasion is commonly present. Bone invasion has been shown to be more radioresistant for tumors arising in the hard palate than those from other oral cavity sites and is associated with a high risk of osteoradionecrosis.[50] Wide local resection is therefore the preferred treatment.[50]

Coronal and sagittal T1-weighted images are particularly useful in evaluation of the hard palate (see **Fig. 7**). Perineural tumor spread along the greater palatine nerve (branch of V2) to the pterygopalatine fossa is also an important concern for hard palate tumors, particularly adenoid cystic carcinomas (see **Fig. 7F**)[37]; careful attention must be paid to the pterygopalatine canal and fossa, along with other sites of retrograde and antegrade spread, including the foramen rotundum, cavernous sinuses, and Meckel's cave. Large tumors can invade the nasal cavity, maxillary sinus, and maxillary alveolar ridge.[3,23]

Lip

Lip carcinomas behave differently from other oral cavity carcinomas and have different staging

Table 2 Anatomic stage/prognostic groups			
Stage 0	Tis	N0	M0
Stage I	T1	N0	M0
Stage II	T2	N0	M0
Stage III	T3	N0	M0
	T1	N1	M0
	T2	N1	M0
	T3	N1	M0
Stage IVA	T4a	N0	M0
	T4a	N1	M0
	T1	N2	M0
	T2	N2	M0
	T3	N2	M0
	T4a	N2	M0
Stage IVB	Any T	N3	M0
	T4b	Any N	M0
Stage IVC	Any T	Any N	M1

From AJCC Cancer Staging Manual, 7th edition. 2010. Published by Springer Science and Business Media LLC. Available at: www.springer.com; used with the permission of the American Joint Committee on Cancer (AJCC), Chicago, Illinois.

Box 4
What the referring physician needs to know

For all sites

- Tumor depth and size
- Involvement of adjacent structures, such as extrinsic tongue muscles
- Bone involvement
- Perineural tumor spread (most commonly V2/V3 involvement)
- Lymph node metastases

Site-specific considerations

Oral tongue

- Invasion across the midline
- Involvement of the contralateral neurovascular bundle (suggested by hyoglossus muscle involvement)
- Inferior extension to floor of mouth
- Posterior extension to base of tongue

Floor of mouth

- Extension to oral tongue or base of tongue
- Invasion across the midline
- Involvement of mandible

Retromolar trigone

- Involvement of mandible, particularly ascending ramus
- Spread through pterygomandibular raphe
- Perineural tumor spread along inferior alveolar nerve (V3)

Buccal mucosa

- Extension to maxilla/mandible
- Extension to facial skin

Gingiva

- Involvement of maxillary/mandibular alveolar ridge (common)

Hard palate

- Bony hard palate invasion
- Perineural spread along greater palatine nerve (V2)

Lip

- Subcutaneous depth
- Bone invasion to maxillary and mandibular alveolar ridges

criteria for T4a lesions. Ultraviolet radiation is the major risk factor, and lip carcinomas are most commonly seen in patients with prolonged and repeated sun exposure.[51] Lip carcinomas typically originate at the vermillion border of the lower lip.[3,12,23] Because of the external location, these tumors are easy to detect and tend to present early at a lower stage.[23] Imaging is typically not necessary for smaller lesions, and is usually reserved for more advanced lesions to evaluate for subcutaneous and intraoral invasion and bone involvement (**Fig. 13**). Sagittal plane images are particularly useful in evaluation of lip carcinomas.[3] Bone invasion may occur along the buccal margin of the maxillary and mandibular alveolar ridges.[45] Lower lip carcinomas may rarely invade the mental nerve, with retrograde perineural extension along the inferior alveolar nerve.[12]

Unlike tumors arising from other sites in the oral cavity, carcinomas arising from the lips are radiosensitive and have similar success rates in patients treated with surgery and those treated with radiation therapy. The risk for lymph node metastases is low for lip carcinomas, particularly with low-grade lesions. Elective lymph node dissections are thus not performed routinely. Lymph node metastases are most frequently seen at levels IA and IB, followed by level II.

ADVANCED MR IMAGING

Advanced imaging techniques, including diffusion-weighted imaging (DWI), perfusion-weighted

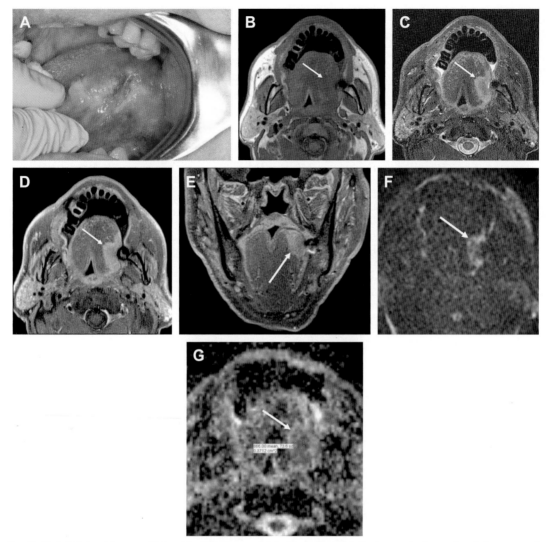

Fig. 8. T2 left lateral tongue SCC, with diffusion-weighted imaging. (*A*) Photograph shows the right tongue is indurated from the anterior one-third to the right tongue base. The surface dimension was approximately 3 × 2 cm, making this a T2 lesion. (*B–E*) Axial T1-weighted (*B*), STIR (*C*), and postcontrast fat-saturated (*D*) images and coronal postcontrast fat-saturated (*E*) images show a T2-hyperintense enhancing mass (*arrows*) in the left posterolateral tongue that does not cross the midline. Diffusion-weighted image (*F*) and corresponding apparent diffusion coefficient map (*G*) show diffusion restriction within this mass, indicating high cellularity (*arrows*).

imaging, and spectroscopy, are currently being investigated as imaging tools that can better delineate true tumor extent, more accurately determine lymph node metastases, distinguish recurrent tumor from posttreatment tissue, and predict treatment response.

DWI

DWI evaluates the relative diffusivity of water protons through tissues. Restricted diffusion is manifested as hyperintense signal on the diffusion-weighted image and signal drop out on the corresponding apparent diffusion coefficient (ADC)

map. Because of its highly cellular nature, head and neck SCCs have been shown to demonstrate restricted diffusion, with ADC values below 0.9 to 1.3 ($\times 10^{-3}$ mm^2/s) in the primary site and in metastatic lymph nodes (see **Fig. 8**F, G).[52,53] DWI also has higher sensitivity and specificity for detecting lymph node metastases compared with CT and conventional MR.[53] In addition, studies have shown DWI to be particularly useful in the posttreatment setting, in which recurrent tumor often cannot be distinguished from posttreatment and inflammatory change on conventional MR imaging. Recurrent tumor demonstrates decreased ADC, reflecting the high cellularity compared with posttreatment

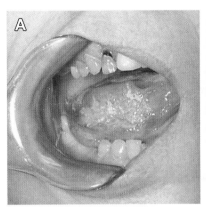
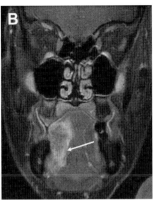
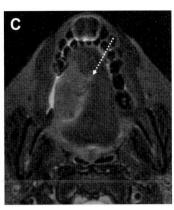

Fig. 9. T4a right lateral tongue SCC crossing midline, with involvement of the genioglossus muscles. (A) Photograph shows an extensive area of mucosal irregularity and leukoplakia involving the right lateral tongue. The patient was unable to move the tongue due to SCC infiltration and pain. (B, C) Coronal T1-weighted postcontrast fat-saturated (B) and axial STIR (C) images show a T2-hyperintense enhancing mass in the right tongue. The coronal image show inferior extension into the floor of mouth/sublingual space (solid white arrow in B) and medial involvement of the genioglossus muscle. The axial image shows extension across the midline (dashed arrow in C). Involvement of the genioglossus muscle makes this a T4a lesion. Extension across the midline is a contraindication for partial glossectomy and requires a subtotal/total glossectomy and bilateral neck dissections.

change, which demonstrates normal to elevated ADC.[52–54]

DWI is also being investigated as an imaging tool to predict and monitor tumor response to chemoradiation. Low ADC values on the baseline pretreatment scan have correlated with treatment response.[55,56] A high degree of ADC increase from the baseline scan compared with scans obtained in the early treatment phase and at the conclusion of chemoradiation also predict better treatment response.[52,55–57]

DWI in the oral cavity may be degraded by susceptibility artifact from dental amalgam; parallel imaging can reduce susceptibility artifact.[52]

Dynamic Perfusion MR Imaging

Perfusion imaging evaluates the degree of vascularity and dynamics of blood flow of a lesion, generating parameters of blood flow, blood volume, permeability, and mean transit time.[52] Several imaging techniques for dynamic perfusion MR

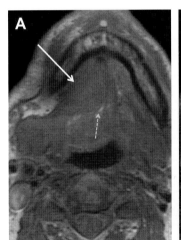
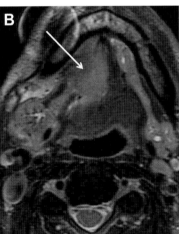
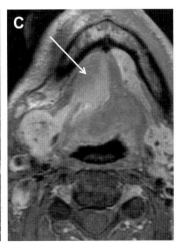

Fig. 10. T4a right floor of mouth SCC crossing midline. Axial T1-weighted (A), T2-weighted (B), and postcontrast T1-weighted (C) images show a T1-isointense, T2-hyperintense enhancing mass in the right floor of mouth (solid arrows) with invasion of the right genioglossus muscle and minimally the left genioglossus muscle. Note the leftward displacement and partial effacement of the T1-hyperintense fatty lingual septum (dashed arrow in A). Involvement of the genioglossus muscles makes this a T4a lesion.

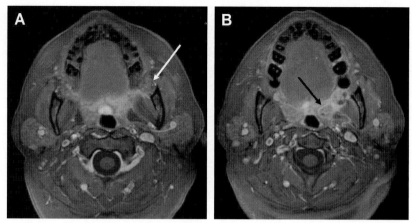

Fig. 11. T2 retromolar trigone mucoepidermoid carcinoma. (*A, B*) Axial postcontrast fat-saturated T1-weighted images from superior to inferior show a heterogeneously enhancing mass in the left retromolar trigone (*white arrow in A*) extending posteriorly to the superior aspect of the left palatine tonsil (*black arrow in B*). The tumor in the retromolar trigone posteriorly abuts the ascending mandibular ramus, although the cortex and bone marrow signal appear preserved.

imaging exist, including T2*-weighted and T1-weighted contrast-enhanced imaging and spin-labeling, which does not require the administration of contrast material. The most commonly used technique is the dynamic susceptibility T2*-weighted contrast-enhanced imaging, which requires administration of a bolus of gadolinium contrast material at a high rate and a series of rapidly acquired images as contrast passes through the capillary bed.[52,58]

Studies have shown malignant head and neck tumors to have statistically significant differences in perfusion parameters compared with normal tissues and benign tumors, with increased perfusion values reflecting the increased degree of angiogenesis of malignant lesions.[52,58] Perfusion MR can also potentially distinguish tumor recurrence from postsurgical change in the treated neck, with recurrent tumor having elevated blood flow and volume relative to posttreatment change.[52,53] Perfusion MR may have a role in predicting treatment response, with tumors of greater vascularity showing greater response to chemoradiation therapy.[52,53]

In the oral cavity, susceptibility artifact from dental amalgam and the soft tissue-air interfaces often limits use of perfusion imaging using the T2*-weighted technique.

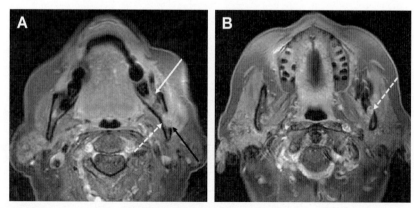

Fig. 12. T4a retromolar trigone SCC with perineural spread along the inferior alveolar nerve and bone invasion. (*A, B*) Axial postcontrast fat-saturated T1-weighted images from inferior to superior show enhancing tumor within the left retromolar trigone (*solid white arrow in A*). More posteriorly, enhancing tumor is seen involving and expanding the left mandibular canal and foramen (*dashed white arrows*), indicating perineural spread along the inferior alveolar nerve. Note the disruption of the buccal cortex overlying the mandibular canal (*black arrow in A*) and extension of tumor into the overlying left masseter muscle.

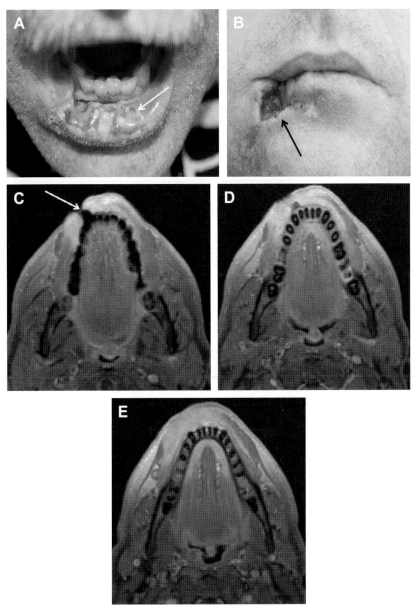

Fig. 13. Lip carcinoma. (*A, B*) Photographs show extensive ulceration and infiltration with erythroleukoplakia of the right lower lip and labial mucosa. Extension across the midline is seen intraorally (*white arrow in A*) and ulceration with breakdown of the skin is seen extraorally (*black arrow in B*). (*C–E*) Axial postcontrast T1-weighted images from superior to inferior show an enhancing mass extending from the skin surface to the buccal surface of the mandible, without evidence of bone invasion. Note the area of ulceration superiorly (*arrow in C*).

Spectroscopy

MR spectroscopy detects the presence of specific metabolites in areas of interest. Studies have shown head and neck malignancies to have elevated choline (Cho)/creatine (Cr) ratios compared with normal tissues and benign tumors.[52,59] Cho is detected by the presence of a spectral peak at 3.2 ppm and is a marker of cell membrane turnover. Cho levels have been shown to correlate

with histologic grading, and the presence of Cho in a treated lesion has been shown to significantly correlate with residual/recurrent tumor after surgery or chemoradiation.[52,59,60] Mixed results have been reported in evaluating the use of spectroscopy to predict treatment response.[52,60]

MR spectroscopy is difficult to perform in the head and neck, and is often severely degraded by patient motion and susceptibility artifact.[59,60]

Contamination of the spectra by a dominant fat peak is also problematic in the tongue, which has a high fat content.[59]

SUMMARY

MR imaging plays an important role in the evaluation of oral cavity carcinomas. MR imaging enables greater detailed depiction of the normal anatomic structures in the oral cavity and has reduced metallic artifact from dental amalgam compared with CT. MR imaging accurately determines the depth of invasion, bone marrow involvement, and presence of perineural spread, which are critical to treatment planning. Advanced MR imaging techniques may potentially better delineate true tumor extent, determine lymph node metastases, and predict treatment response.

REFERENCES

1. Kademani D. Oral cancer. Mayo Clin Proc 2007; 82(7):878–87.
2. Warnakulasuriya S. Living with oral cancer: epidemiology with particular reference to prevalence and life-style changes that influence survival. Oral Oncol 2010;46(6):407–10.
3. Weber AL, Romo L, Hashmi S. Malignant tumors of the oral cavity and oropharynx: clinical, pathologic, and radiologic evaluation. Neuroimaging Clin N Am 2003;13(3):443–64.
4. Patel SC, Carpenter WR, Tyree S, et al. Increasing incidence of oral tongue squamous cell carcinoma in young white women, age 18 to 44 years. J Clin Oncol 2011;29(11):1488–94.
5. Shiboski CH, Schmidt BL, Jordan RC. Tongue and tonsil carcinoma: increasing trends in the U.S. population ages 20-44 years. Cancer 2005;103(9): 1843–9.
6. Johnson NW, Jayasekara P, Amarasinghe AA. Squamous cell carcinoma and precursor lesions of the oral cavity: epidemiology and aetiology. Periodontol 2000 2011;57(1):19–37.
7. Mehta V, Yu GP, Schantz SP. Population-based analysis of oral and oropharyngeal carcinoma: changing trends of histopathologic differentiation, survival and patient demographics. Laryngoscope 2010;120(11): 2203–12.
8. Schmidt BL. Principles of oral cavity management. In: Andersson L, Kahnberg K, Pogrel MA, editors. Oral and maxillofacial surgery. West Sussex (United Kingdom): John Wiley & Sons; 2010. p. 705–34.
9. Hansen LS, Olson JA, Silverman S Jr. Proliferative verrucous leukoplakia. A long-term study of thirty patients. Oral Surg Oral Med Oral Pathol 1985; 60(3):285–98.
10. Kademani D, Bell RB, Bagheri S, et al. Prognostic factors in intraoral squamous cell carcinoma: the influence of histologic grade. J Oral Maxillofac Surg 2005;63(11):1599–605.
11. Sigal R, Zagdanski AM, Schwaab G, et al. CT and MR imaging of squamous cell carcinoma of the tongue and floor of the mouth. Radiographics 1996;16(4):787–810.
12. Forghani R, Smoker WRK, Curtin HD. Pathology of the oral region. In: Som PM, Curtin HD, editors. Head and neck imaging, Volume 2, 5th edition. St Louis (MO): Elsevier; 2011. p. 1643–748.
13. Lee MJ, Kim S, Lee SA, et al. Overcoming artifacts from metallic orthopedic implants at high-field-strength MR imaging and multi-detector CT. Radiographics 2007;27(3):791–803.
14. Fatterpekar GM, Delman BN, Shroff MM, et al. Distension technique to improve computed tomographic evaluation of oral cavity lesions. Arch Otolaryngol Head Neck Surg 2003;129(2):229–32.
15. Dillon JK, Glastonbury CM, Jabeen F, et al. Gauze padding: a simple technique to delineate small oral cavity tumors. AJNR Am J Neuroradiol 2011; 32(5):934–7.
16. Weissman JL, Carrau RL. "Puffed-cheek" CT improves evaluation of the oral cavity. AJNR Am J Neuroradiol 2001;22(4):741–4.
17. Yasumoto M, Shibuya H, Takeda M, et al. Squamous cell carcinoma of the oral cavity: MR findings and value of T1-versus T2-weighted fast spin-echo images. AJR Am J Roentgenol 1995;164(4):981–7.
18. Park JO, Jung SL, Joo YH, et al. Diagnostic accuracy of magnetic resonance imaging (MRI) in the assessment of tumor invasion depth in oral/oropharyngeal cancer. Oral Oncol 2011;47(5):381–6.
19. Vidiri A, Ruscito P, Pichi B, et al. Oral cavity and base of the tongue tumors. Correlation between clinical, MRI and pathological staging of primary tumor. J Exp Clin Cancer Res 2007;26(4):575–82.
20. Lam P, Au-Yeung KM, Cheng PW, et al. Correlating MRI and histologic tumor thickness in the assessment of oral tongue cancer. AJR Am J Roentgenol 2004;182(3):803–8.
21. Okura M, Iida S, Aikawa T, et al. Tumor thickness and paralingual distance of coronal MR imaging predicts cervical node metastases in oral tongue carcinoma. AJNR Am J Neuroradiol 2008;29(1): 45–50.
22. Jung J, Cho NH, Kim J, et al. Significant invasion depth of early oral tongue cancer originated from the lateral border to predict regional metastases and prognosis. Int J Oral Maxillofac Surg 2009; 38(6):653–60.
23. Kirsch C. Oral cavity cancer. Top Magn Reson Imaging 2007;18(4):269–80.
24. Crecco M, Vidiri A, Palma O, et al. T stages of tumors of the tongue and floor of the mouth: correlation

between MR with gadopentetate dimeglumine and pathologic data. AJNR Am J Neuroradiol 1994; 15(9):1695–702.

25. Bolzoni A, Cappiello J, Piazza C, et al. Diagnostic accuracy of magnetic resonance imaging in the assessment of mandibular involvement in oral-oropharyngeal squamous cell carcinoma: a prospective study. Arch Otolaryngol Head Neck Surg 2004; 130(7):837–43.

26. Wiener E, Pautke C, Link TM, et al. Comparison of 16-slice MSCT and MRI in the assessment of squamous cell carcinoma of the oral cavity. Eur J Radiol 2006;58(1):113–8.

27. Brown JS, Lowe D, Kalavrezos N, et al. Patterns of invasion and routes of tumor entry into the mandible by oral squamous cell carcinoma. Head Neck 2002; 24(4):370–83.

28. Stambuk HE, Karimi S, Lee N, et al. Oral cavity and oropharynx tumors. Radiol Clin North Am 2007; 45(1):1–20.

29. Vidiri A, Guerrisi A, Pellini R, et al. Multi-detector row computed tomography (MDCT) and magnetic resonance imaging (MRI) in the evaluation of the mandibular invasion by squamous cell carcinomas (SCC) of the oral cavity. Correlation with pathological data. J Exp Clin Cancer Res 2010;29:73.

30. Gu DH, Yoon DY, Park CH, et al. CT, MR, (18)F-FDG PET/CT, and their combined use for the assessment of mandibular invasion by squamous cell carcinomas of the oral cavity. Acta Radiol 2010;51(10):1111–9.

31. Chung TS, Yousem DM, Seigerman HM, et al. MR of mandibular invasion in patients with oral and oropharyngeal malignant neoplasms. AJNR Am J Neuroradiol 1994;15(10):1949–55.

32. Brown JS, Lewis-Jones H. Evidence for imaging the mandible in the management of oral squamous cell carcinoma: a review. Br J Oral Maxillofac Surg 2001; 39(6):411–8.

33. van den Brekel MW, Runne RW, Smeele LE, et al. Assessment of tumour invasion into the mandible: the value of different imaging techniques. Eur Radiol 1998;8(9):1552–7.

34. Abd El-Hafez YG, Chen CC, Ng SH, et al. Comparison of PET/CT and MRI for the detection of bone marrow invasion in patients with squamous cell carcinoma of the oral cavity. Oral Oncol 2011;47(4):288–95.

35. Imaizumi A, Yoshino N, Yamada I, et al. A potential pitfall of MR imaging for assessing mandibular invasion of squamous cell carcinoma in the oral cavity. AJNR Am J Neuroradiol 2006;27(1):114–22.

36. Gandhi D, Gujar S, Mukherji SK. Magnetic resonance imaging of perineural spread of head and neck malignancies. Top Magn Reson Imaging 2004;15(2):79–85.

37. Ginsberg LE, DeMonte F. Imaging of perineural tumor spread from palatal carcinoma. AJNR Am J Neuroradiol 1998;19(8):1417–22.

38. Seitz O, Chambron-Pinho N, Middendorp M, et al. 18F-Fluorodeoxyglucose-PET/CT to evaluate tumor, nodal disease, and gross tumor volume of oropharyngeal and oral cavity cancer: comparison with MR imaging and validation with surgical specimen. Neuroradiology 2009;51(10):677–86.

39. van den Brekel MW, van der Waal I, Meijer CJ, et al. The incidence of micrometastases in neck dissection specimens obtained from elective neck dissections. Laryngoscope 1996;106(8):987–91.

40. Ng SH, Yen TC, Chang JT, et al. Prospective study of [18F]fluorodeoxyglucose positron emission tomography and computed tomography and magnetic resonance imaging in oral cavity squamous cell carcinoma with palpably negative neck. J Clin Oncol 2006;24(27):4371–6.

41. Cheng A, Schmidt BL. Management of the N0 neck in oral squamous cell carcinoma. Oral Maxillofac Surg Clin North Am 2008;20(3):477–97.

42. Tsang RK, Chung JC, To VS, et al. Efficacy of salvage neck dissection for isolated nodal recurrences in early carcinoma of oral tongue with watchful waiting management of initial N0 neck. Head Neck 2011;33(10):1482–5.

43. Kreeft A, Tan IB, van den Brekel MW, et al. The surgical dilemma of 'functional inoperability' in oral and oropharyngeal cancer: current consensus on operability with regard to functional results. Clin Otolaryngol 2009;34(2):140–6.

44. Crecco M, Vidiri A, Angelone ML, et al. Retromolar trigone tumors: evaluation by magnetic resonance imaging and correlation with pathological data. Eur J Radiol 1999;32(3):182–8.

45. Mukherji SK, Pillsbury HR, Castillo M. Imaging squamous cell carcinomas of the upper aerodigestive tract: what clinicians need to know. Radiology 1997;205(3):629–46.

46. Diaz EM Jr, Holsinger FC, Zuniga ER, et al. Squamous cell carcinoma of the buccal mucosa: one institution's experience with 119 previously untreated patients. Head Neck 2003;25(4):267–73.

47. Lin CS, Jen YM, Cheng MF, et al. Squamous cell carcinoma of the buccal mucosa: an aggressive cancer requiring multimodality treatment. Head Neck 2006;28(2):150–7.

48. Kimura Y, Sumi M, Sumi T, et al. Deep extension from carcinoma arising from the gingiva: CT and MR imaging features. AJNR Am J Neuroradiol 2002; 23(3):468–72.

49. Chijiwa H, Sakamoto K, Umeno H, et al. Minor salivary gland carcinomas of oral cavity and oropharynx. J Laryngol Otol 2009;123(Suppl 31):52–7.

50. Petruzzelli GJ, Myers EN. Malignant neoplasms of the hard palate and upper alveolar ridge. Oncology (Williston Park) 1994;8(4):43–8 [discussion: 50, 53].

51. Scully C, Bagan J. Oral squamous cell carcinoma: overview of current understanding of

aetiopathogenesis and clinical implications. Oral Dis 2009;15(6):388–99.

52. Srinivasan A, Mohan S, Mukherji SK. Biologic imaging of head and neck cancer: the present and the future. AJNR Am J Neuroradiol 2012;33(4):586–94.

53. Shah GV, Wesolowski JR, Ansari SA, et al. New directions in head and neck imaging. J Surg Oncol 2008;97(8):644–8.

54. Abdel Razek AA, Kandeel AY, Soliman N, et al. Role of diffusion-weighted echo-planar MR imaging in differentiation of residual or recurrent head and neck tumors and posttreatment changes. AJNR Am J Neuroradiol 2007;28(6):1146–52.

55. Hatakenaka M, Nakamura K, Yabuuchi H, et al. Pretreatment apparent diffusion coefficient of the primary lesion correlates with local failure in head-and-neck cancer treated with chemoradiotherapy or radiotherapy. Int J Radiat Oncol Biol Phys 2011; 81(2):339–45.

56. Kim S, Loevner L, Quon H, et al. Diffusion-weighted magnetic resonance imaging for predicting and detecting early response to chemoradiation therapy of squamous cell carcinomas of the head and neck. Clin Cancer Res 2009;15(3):986–94.

57. Vandecaveye V, Dirix P, De Keyzer F, et al. Diffusion-weighted magnetic resonance imaging early after chemoradiotherapy to monitor treatment response in head-and-neck squamous cell carcinoma. Int J Radiat Oncol Biol Phys 2011;82(3):1098–107.

58. Razek AA, Elsorogy LG, Soliman NY, et al. Dynamic susceptibility contrast perfusion MR imaging in distinguishing malignant from benign head and neck tumors: a pilot study. Eur J Radiol 2011;77(1):73–9.

59. Shah GV, Fischbein NJ, Patel R, et al. Newer MR imaging techniques for head and neck. Magn Reson Imaging Clin N Am 2003;11(3):449–69, vi.

60. King AD, Yeung DK, Yu KH, et al. Pretreatment and early intratreatment prediction of clinicopathologic response of head and neck cancer to chemoradiotherapy using 1H-MRS. J Magn Reson Imaging 2010;32(1):199–203.

Myocutaneous Flaps and Other Vascularized Grafts in Head and Neck Reconstruction for Cancer Treatment

Kim O. Learned, MD[a],*, Kelly M. Malloy, MD[b],
Laurie A. Loevner, MD[a]

KEYWORDS

- Myocutaneous flaps • Free tissue transfer • Free flap • Pedicled flap • Vascularized flap
- Head and neck cancer • Head and neck reconstruction • Head and neck MR imaging

KEY POINTS

- The workhorse flaps used in oncologic head and neck reconstructions are vascularized tissues composed of skin, subcutaneous fat, and fascia, with or without muscle. These flaps are either pedicled or are revascularized free-tissue grafts by way of microvascular anastomoses.
- MR imaging appearance of a flap reflects its composition and the sequela of denervation or adjuvant chemoradiation.
- Flap failure is assessed clinically without the need for imaging evaluation.
- Neoplasms tend to recur at the interface of the free flap and the recipient surgical bed.
- The expected swelling and enhancement of a normal flap should not be mistaken for neoplasm.

INTRODUCTION

In the United States, the squamous cell carcinoma is the most common head and neck malignancy in adults with a reported incidence of 10.6 per 100,000 cases of oral cavity and pharyngeal cancer (2004–2008 combined years).[1] Five-year relative survival rates of oral and pharyngeal cancer have improved to 65.1% (2001–2007 combined years) from 46% (1950–1954 combined years).[1] Data extracted from the Surveillance, Epidemiology, and End Results database show no significant changes in overall relative survival of sinonasal malignancies; however, the best relative survival was noted in patients treated with surgery or a combination of surgery and radiotherapy.[2] Given the spectrum of pathologies occurring in the head and neck, survival remains difficult to generalize. However, given medical advancements, the growing experience of multidisciplinary approaches to treating head and neck cancer, and the continued innovations in CT and MR imaging techniques, routine posttreatment imaging will become increasingly more common. Assessment for residual or recurrent tumor is the primary goal of follow-up imaging to guide management, monitor treatment response, and determine whether additional surgery or chemoradiation therapy is necessary. The altered anatomy from tumor resection and reconstruction of the surgical bed can present

[a] Neuroradiology Division, Department of Radiology, University of Pennsylvania Health System, University of Pennsylvania Perelman School of Medicine, Hospital of the University of Pennsylvania, 219 Dulles Building, 3400 Spruce Street, Philadelphia, PA 19104, USA; [b] Department of Otorhinolaryngology–Head and Neck Surgery, Hospital of the University of Pennsylvania, University of Pennsylvania Perelman School of Medicine, Ravdin Building 5th Floor, 3400 Spruce Street, Philadelphia, PA 19104, USA
* Corresponding author.
E-mail address: Kim.Learned@uphs.upenn.edu

a challenge to the unfamiliar radiologist. It is paramount that normal reconstructive flaps and grafts not be mistaken for neoplasm. The wide range of flaps and grafts available reflects the individually tailored nature of each reconstruction. The best reconstruction is dictated by the surgeon's experience and the patient's anatomy to maximize the success of defect closure, functional restoration, and cosmesis while minimizing comorbidity. The workhorses for sizable and complex defect reconstruction in oncologic practice are the vascularized tissues including regional pedicled flaps and free-tissue transfer flaps. CT and especially MR imaging offer the advantage of excellent soft tissue definition, which is important in differentiating reconstructive flaps and grafts from neoplasm.

IMPORTANT SURGICAL ANATOMIC CONSIDERATIONS AND FLAP TERMINOLOGY

Broadly speaking, the commonly used vascularized flaps include local-regional flaps and free flaps. The names of the flaps reflect their donor sites, tissue composition, and vascular supply. The local-regional flaps are harvested from the donor sites close to the defect with intact vascular pedicles. They are rotated and transposed to reach the defect for surgical closure. Therefore, the rotated flaps are technically limited by the pedicle vascular length and have to be free of tumor involvement and prior irradiation to ensure their tissue health. Free flaps are transferred from a donor site distant from the primary surgical bed, and the vessels of the flaps are transected and subsequently reanastomosed to available blood

vessels in the recipient bed using microvascular surgical techniques. For head and neck reconstructions, vascular anastomoses are preferentially end-to-end but in some instances end-to-side, and typically use branches of the external carotid artery, such as the facial and superior thyroidal arteries and tributaries of internal jugular or external jugular veins. Less common but viable options for arterial anastomoses include the transverse cervical, superficial temporal, and lingual arteries. Flaps may contain skin paddle, subcutaneous fat, fascia, muscle, or bone. The term "composite flaps" refers to flaps having more than one tissue type, typically containing muscle and bone. For example, a fasciocutaneous flap contains skin, subcutaneous fat, and fascia; a myocutaneous flap contains skin, subcutaneous fat, and muscle; and an osteomyocutaneous flap is myocutaneous flap with an osseous component. There is a plethora of flap options and the commonly used flaps are summarized in **Table 1**.

The type of flap used is dictated by the size and location of the defect, the pedicle length needed, and patient characteristics.[3] Prior chemoradiation may reduce tumor size and extent, but result in less reliable local tissue for reconstruction and poorer wound healing. Free flaps offer a robust blood supply, a wide range of available healthy tissue bulk for ease of contouring, better tissue match for form and function of a given defect, and better wound coverage. Therefore, over the past three to four decades, free-tissue transfers have been used with increasing frequency in salvage surgeries, and are ideal flaps for reconstruction of sizable defects of the upper aerodigestive tract

---

Table 1
Commonly used flaps and their vascular pedicles

Locoregional Flaps[a]	Free Flaps[b]
Nasoseptal flap (nasoseptal branch of sphenopalatine a.)	Radial forearm (radial a. and cephalic v. or venae comitantes)
Pericranial or galeal-pericranial flap (supratrochlear and supraorbital a.)	Anterolateral thigh (perforators of descending branch of lateral circumflex femoral a. and venae comitantes)
Temporalis muscle (deep temporal a.) Temporparietal fascia (superficial temporal a.)	Rectus abdominis (deep inferior epigastric a. and v.)
Pectoralis (pectoral branch of thoracoacromial a.)	Latissimus dorsi (thoracodorsal a. and v.)
Latissimus dorsi (thoracodorsal a.)	Fibular (peroneal a. and venae comitantes)
	Iliac crest (deep circumflex a. and v.)
	Scapular (circumflex scapular a. and v.)

Abbreviations: a, artery; v, vein.
[a] Intact vascular pedicles.
[b] Transected vascular pedicles reanastomosed to external carotid artery branches (facial, thyroidal, superficial temporal, and lingual arteries) and tributaries of internal or external jugular veins.

after cancer resections. Currently, the major flaps used in head and neck reconstruction are radial forearm flaps (RFF), rectus abdominis flaps, anterolateral thigh (ALT) flaps, and latissimus dorsi free flaps.[4] The less bulky RFF is most suitable for most small-to-medium head and neck defects such as small partial glossectomy and maxillectomy defects. The versatile RFF gained popularity because it is thin and easy to roll into a tube graft to repair a pharyngeal defect; conforms to the complex anatomic requirement of oropharyngeal defects, such as base of tongue and lateral oropharynx resections; and provides adequate skin paddle for coverage of mucosal or skin defects. In the setting of large surgical defects, the rectus abdominis and ALT flaps are preferred to RFF. The ALT offers a longer vascular pedicle and larger tissue bulk necessary to reconstruct larger surgical beds, such as total glossectomy and orbital exenteration with maxillectomy.

Pedicled flaps, such as the pectoralis flap, are less popular because of their limited pedicle length and mobility rendering them difficult to reach far defects. In addition, the less pliable nature of these flaps makes it difficult to contour them for optimal use as tube grafts. However, there are specific instances in which these grafts remain quite useful, such as when the local recipient vessels are not available for reanastomosis of a free flap, for reconstruction after free-flap failure, in conjunction with free flap for large dead space and skin defect, in salvage surgery for recurrence, for coverage of the carotid artery with a cervical skin defect, and for pharyngo-cutaneous fistulas.[5]

Typically, vascularized bone flaps are favored to nonvascularized bone grafts for the reconstruction of an irradiated field because the nonvascularized bone grafts rely on a healthy recipient bed for nutrient supply and ultimately flap survival. The cutaneous surface of the flap can be placed externally to replace the lost skin, rolled internally to replace the resected mucosa, and in some instances two skin paddles of the flap are designed to cover cutaneous and mucosal surfaces of a defect. **Table 2** summarizes the general flap choices for common surgical defects.

IMAGING PROTOCOLS

Depending on the reconstruction site, the pathology, and the clinical concern after reconstruction, MR imaging is tailored to provide high-resolution details of the skull base from the top of the orbit to hard palate or to assess the entire neck from skull base through the thoracic inlet (**Box 1**). For example, in a patient with sinonasal carcinoma necessitating orbital exenteration and maxillectomy with reconstruction using ALT and concern for perineural spread of neoplasm, high-resolution MR imaging of the skull base and sinonasal cavity allows optimal distinction of neoplasm from the flap reconstruction. In a patient who has undergone a partial glossectomy and neck dissection reconstructed with an RFF for squamous cell carcinoma with nodal metastases, neck MR imaging provides a comprehensive assessment with excellent soft tissue discrimination of the primary tumor bed and the neck.

ROLE OF MR IMAGING IN THE EVALUATION OF HEAD AND NECK FLAP RECONSTRUCTIONS
Postoperative Complications and Flap Viability

During the critical immediate postoperative period, early recognition of a failing flap and rapid

Table 2 Surgical defects and flap reconstruction options	
Endoscopic reconstruction of small-medium anterior central skull base	Pedicled nasoseptal flap
Open reconstruction of medium-large anterior central skull base	Pericranial or galeal-pericranial flaps
Open reconstruction of lateral skull base, infratemporal fossa, and temporal bone	Pedicled temporalis muscle or temporoparietal fascia
Orbital exenteration, maxillectomy, palatectomy	RFF, ALT, rectus abdominis
Parotidectomy, neck dissection with skin resection	RFF, ALT, alternative rotated pectoralis
Glossectomy, oral cavity resection	RFF, ALT
Mandibulectomy	Fibular, fibular osteocutaneous, iliac, scapular
Total laryngectomy, pharyngectomy	RFF, ATL, alternative rotated pectoralis and jejunal flap or gastro-omental flap

MR imaging of the neck: Precontrast sagittal and axial T1-weighted spin echo, axial STIR, and T2-weighted FSE/TSE, and gadolinium-enhanced axial and coronal T1-weighted with fat saturation (spin echo or FMPSPGR). Slice thickness 5 mm (interleaved). Scan from cavernous sinus to aortopulmonary window.

MR imaging of skull base/paranasal sinuses: axial T2-weighted FSE/TSE with fat saturation of entire head (5 mm thick). Unenhanced axial and coronal T1-weighted spin echo, coronal STIR or T2-weighted FSE/TSE with fat saturation, and gadolinium-enhanced axial, coronal, and sagittal T1-weighted spin echo with fat saturation of the paranasal sinuses (from top of orbits to 2 cm below hard palate, from tip of nose to brainstem, 3 mm thick).

intervention are imperative for successful flap salvage. The gold standard for flap monitoring remains clinical observation of the flap.[4] An implantable Doppler probe secured around the vessel adventitia of a vascular pedicle provides specific information about venous and arterial patency, and is valuable in monitoring flap. MR imaging is not routinely used for the assessment of common complications after flap reconstruction, such as hematomas and other collections, vascular thrombosis, or flap viability. The viability of the vascularized flap has poor correlation with enhancement and the signal characteristics of the flap on imaging.

Occasionally, diagnostic imaging may be indicated to identify a rapidly expanding hematoma that may need evacuation for decompression. In such cases, contrast-enhanced CT or ultrasound are used primarily. In general, the diagnostic performance of contrast-enhanced CT for distinguishing an infected collection from a resolving hematoma or seroma without clinical input has high sensitivity but poor specificity. The edema of the flap and the surgical bed is evident up to 4 to 6 weeks after surgery and can persist for years in patients receiving postoperative irradiation to the surgical bed.[6]

Murray and colleagues[7] reviewed the literature between 1994 and 2005 regarding the morbidity, mortality, and functional outcomes of fasciocutaneous free flap reconstructions of pharyngolaryngoesophageal defects. The cumulative fistula and stricture rates were 13% and 16.1%, respectively. The development and accurate delineation of a fistula is difficult to assess on cross-sectional imaging; however, it can be suggested in experienced hands in the presence of a skin defect and subcutaneous air after the perioperative period. Clinicians uncommonly obtain cross-sectional imaging because most often the presence of a fistula is usually established on clinical examination. Swallow studies may aid in accurately defining pharyngocutaneous fistulas, and in identifying strictures of the reconstructed aerodigestive tract.[8]

Postoperative Evaluation of Flap Reconstruction and Neoplasm

The primary role of MR imaging in the postoperative head and neck is to evaluate the extent of tumor resection, monitor the response to chemoradiation, and assess for tumor recurrence or a new primary tumor. In patients with flap reconstructions, careful assessment of the images for potential complications, such as reconstruction break-down, osteoradionecrosis, fistula, and carotid artery injury including stenosis, should be assessed for routinely.

Knowledge of the normal appearance of reconstructive flaps and altered anatomy of the surgical bed is paramount to accurate imaging assessment. However, there is a wide range of normal imaging appearances of head and neck reconstructions, reflecting the heterogeneities of tumor sites and stages, the treatment philosophy of multidisciplinary teams, and the experience of the reconstructive surgeon. When encountering these complex cases on imaging studies, the radiologist must know what the primary surgery was and how the bed was reconstructed. Image analysis should include identification of the normal flap and delineation of its extent of defect coverage. The normal flap should not be mistaken for a mass and should be correctly outlined. The border between the healthy flap and the recipient resection bed should then be carefully inspected for the presence of tissue concerning for neoplasm. It is valuable to have a baseline imaging study obtained approximately 8 weeks after surgery. Scar tissue retracts, and enlarging or growing tissue at the flap margins should raise suspicion for tumor.

General guidelines for the recognition of the normal MR imaging appearance of fasciocutaneous-myocutaneous flaps are suggested in **Boxes 2** and **3**. The presence of a flap is identified by the replacement of the normal anatomy by a soft tissue mass with unique tissue composition of primarily fat or fat and muscle. The rotated local-regional flaps typically contain bulky muscle, whereas the free flaps are mostly fasciocutaneous flaps without a major muscle component. In general, all flaps contain nonenhancing T1 hyperintense fatty tissue,

Box 2
MR imaging criteria of normal vascularized flaps in head and neck reconstruction

Nasoseptal flap: C-shaped enhancing mucosal flap at the skull base defect

Fasciocutaneous flap: T1 hyperintense fatty graft with variable T2 signal

Myocutaneous or myofasciocutaneous flap: striated muscle component shows T1 intermediate signal similar to adjacent muscle, variable T2 signal, and usually avid enhancement

Osteocutaneous flap: bone stock contoured to the defect using multiple osteostomies and plates and screws

Pedicled temporalis muscle flap: loss of muscle bulk at temporal fossa donor site, intact tendon attachment to coronoid process, ± zygomatic arch osteostomy

Pedicled pectoralis flap: loss of muscle bulk in ipsilateral chest wall and pectoralis muscle draping over clavicle to cover neck defect

Box 3
Pearls and pitfalls of MR imaging evaluation of reconstructive head and neck flaps

Pearls:

- Pedicled or free myocutaneous flaps commonly demonstrate muscle striations and a fatty component.
- Nasoseptal flaps usually enhance on MR imaging performed within 48 hours after surgery with C-shaped configuration over the skull base defect.
- Most flaps gradually loose tissue bulk, whereas neoplasm continues to enlarge.
- Recurrent neoplasm typically occurs at the interface or margin of flaps and recipient native tissues.
- Fistulas may herald tumor recurrence.

Pitfalls:

- Variable T2 signal and enhancement of myocutaneous flaps from denervation and radiation may mimic neoplasm.
- Degree of free flap enhancement has poor correlation with integrity of its vascular reanastomosis.
- Vascularized granulation tissue may mimic neoplasm.

and the MR imaging appearance of the muscle composition is similar for rotated flaps and free flaps with characteristic striation of muscle fibers best depicted on unenhanced T1-weighted images (**Figs. 1** and **2**).[9] The muscular component shows isointensity to other muscles in the neck on T1-weighted images, but variable T2 signal intensity and varying degrees of enhancement relative to adjacent normal muscle (see **Figs. 1** and **2**).[9] Most flaps show persistent T2 hyperintensity and enhancement for months to years after placement, and over serial examinations many flaps may atrophy or lose volume over time. The heterogeneity of T2 signal and enhancement of the muscle component are speculated to reflect the sequela of vascular disruption, neovascularization, or muscular denervation.[9] In addition, the effect of adjuvant radiation to the surgical bed plays a role in the changing appearance of the flaps.

Commonly used rotated flaps can be identified by their unique imaging appearance. In reconstruction of the infratemporal fossa and lateral skull base, the close-by temporalis fascia and temporalis muscle are suitable choices for rotated flaps. The tendinous attachment of the temporalis muscle to the coronoid process of the mandible, the loss of muscle bulk in temporal fossa, and the osteotomy of the zygomatic arch help one identify the transposed temporalis muscle flap (**Fig. 3**).[10,11] The pedicled pectoralis muscle flap is rotated up from its anatomic location along the anterior chest wall and mobilized cranially over the mid-to-medial clavicle to reach the lower neck for reconstruction of the hypopharynx and neck dissection bed (**Fig. 4**).[12] Therefore, absence of the pectoralis muscle in its normal location along the upper anterior chest wall and the flap pedicle tunneled around the clavicle are characteristic findings on imaging studies. In some instances, the bulk of the rotated muscle is nearest the origin of the flap.[6] Pectoralis major flaps are often reserved for second-line or salvage reconstructions, because the combined donor site morbidity with that of extensive often radical neck dissection can be significant.

The flexibility of free-flap harvesting and a wide range of patient body habituses result in variation in size, composition, and contour of these flaps. The commonly used RFF contains a large fat component and is used for smaller defects, such as the oral cavity and maxillectomy beds, whereas the ALT and rectus abdominis flaps provide large tissue bulk and often have sizable muscular component for reconstructing larger defects (see **Fig. 1**; **Figs. 5** and **6**). The lack of rotated vascular pedicle and the previously described unique features of specific transposed flaps help one

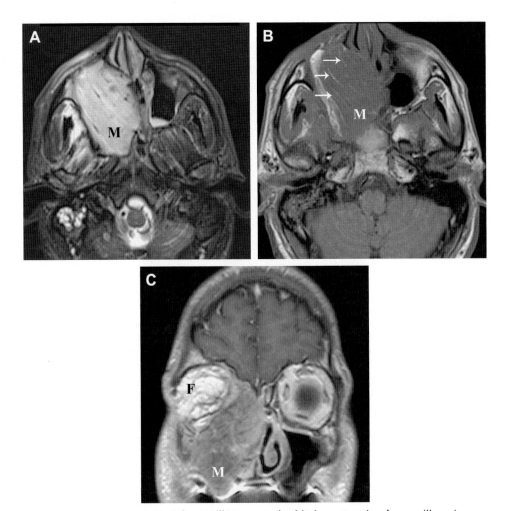

Fig. 1. A 47-year-old man status-post right maxillectomy and orbital exenteration for maxillary sinus squamous cell carcinoma. Reconstruction is performed with ALT flap. Face MR imaging is performed at 3-month follow-up. (*A*) Axial T2-weighted image with fat suppression shows T2 hyperintense striated muscle (M) component of the flap filling the maxillectomy bed. (*B*) Axial T1-weighted image shows T1-isointensity to adjacent muscle and characteristic muscle striation of the flap (*arrows*). (*C*) Coronal enhanced T1-weighted images shows the enhancing muscle component (M) and fatty component (F) of the flap filling the maxilla-orbital defect.

recognize the presence of a free flap. The precise identification on imaging of the arterial and venous anastomoses of free flap pedicles to branches of the external carotid artery and internal or external jugular veins, respectively, is difficult on imaging. Furthermore, the vascular couplers or microscopic sutures that are routinely used in microsurgical technique for the vascular reanastomosis are small and lack visible imaging marker. However, if critical, one can appreciate the vascular anastomosis by applying the knowledge of the surgical principle in head and neck free-tissue transfer. The commonly used external carotid artery branches suitable for reanastomosis are facial-lingual, thyroidal, and superficial temporal arteries. Being limited by the length of the vascular

pedicles, free flaps need to be anastomosed to the closest available vessels at the recipient site. For example, for anterior skull base reconstruction, the RFF pedicle can be anastomosed to the superficial temporal artery (STA) through a temporal burr hole of craniotomy, and for orbital exenteration reconstruction, the RFF pedicle can be tunneled through the cheek to reach the facial vessels at the mandibular border.[13]

Postoperative MR imaging surveillance varies from institution to institution and determining factors include pathology, stage, primary site, and adjuvant treatment. Most patients have postoperative baseline imaging at 2 to 3 months when surgical sequela to the tissues has largely resolved. Denervation intentionally at surgery to

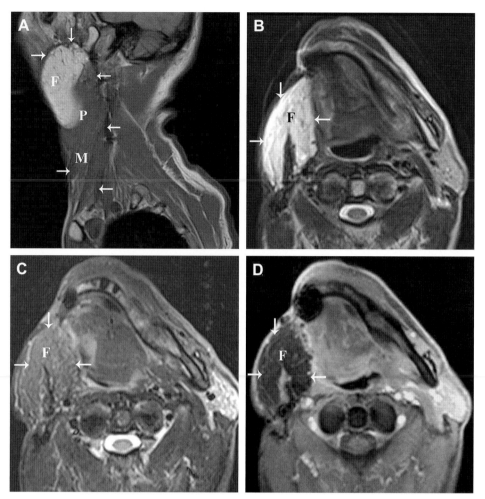

Fig. 2. A 70-year-old man with recurrent retromolar trigone squamous cell carcinoma after resection and reconstruction with an osteocutaneous fibular flap. The patient has undergone salvage surgery and reconstruction using a pectoralis flap. Neck MR imaging is performed at 6-month follow-up. (*A*) Sagittal T1-weighted image shows the pectoralis flap (P, outlined by *arrows*) tunneled over the clavicle to reach the oromandibular defect with the bulky muscle component proximally (M) and fatty component distally (F). (*B–D*) Axial T2, STIR, and fat-saturated enhanced T1-weighted images, respectively, illustrate the fatty component of the distal pectoralis flap (F, outlined by *arrows*) at the oromandibular surgical defect.

reduce postoperative involuntary muscle contraction, as sequela of transected neurovascular bundle with free-flap harvesting, or as a sequela of radiation therapy results in changes appreciated on imaging. The myocutaneous flap may show temporarily swelling and edema in the first few weeks to months of the postoperative period. Over months to years, the myocutaneous flaps undergo muscle atrophy and fat infiltration.[6,8,14] In some instances, the muscles may return to normal appearance after initial swelling, probably reflecting renervation.[15,16]

In the MR imaging assessment of patients with vascularized flaps, the muscle component of the flap and tumor can enhance.[9,17] The preservation of normal striations within the muscle reflects a disease-free status of the flap.[9] Recurrent tumor in the resection bed with a flap reconstruction typically occurs at the margins of the flap where they interface with the surgical bed.[6,8,17,18] In patients with a neopharynx, a new focal luminal soft tissue thickening and narrowing at the surgical margin between the flap and the native mucosa, focal thickening of the wall of the neopharynx, or the formation of a fistula may indicate tumor recurrence (**Fig. 7**).[8,17] A recurrence typically enhances and is best delineated on postcontrast T1-weighted images using fat saturation.[19]

Inflammation and infection associated with a fistulous tract may be indistinguishable from

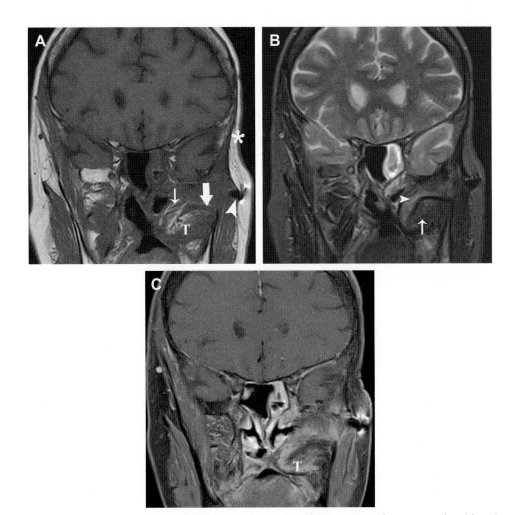

Fig. 3. A 61-year-old woman has 6-month follow-up MR imaging after resection of recurrent adenoid cystic carcinoma involving the left nasopharynx and infratemporal fossa with reconstruction using a rotated temporalis myofascial flap. (*A*) Coronal T1-weighted image shows the temporalis flap in the infratemporal fossa (T) that is isointense to other neck muscles with characteristic muscle striations (*thin arrow*) and fatty components. Susceptibility from the surgical clip marks the zygomatic arch osteostomy (*arrowhead*), and the tendinous insertion to the coronoid process (*thick arrow*). Note the concavity of the donor site at left temporal fossa (*asterisk*). (*B*) Coronal fat-suppressed T2-weighted image shows flap hyperintensity superiorly (*arrowhead*) and hypointensity inferiorly (*thin arrow*). (*C*) Gadolinium-enhanced fat-suppressed coronal T1-weighted image shows enhancement of the flap (T).

neoplastic recurrence. Scar is a dynamic tissue and has a spectrum of imaging appearances. Although scar may enhance, chronic fibrotic scar tissue typically is hypointense compared with muscle on T1 and T2 images and over time shows stability and often retraction.[20] Vascularized granulation tissue may be hyperintense on T2-weighted images with avid enhancement and can be misinterpreted as tumor.[6] The volume of a myocutaneous flap and vascularized granulation tissue remains stable or decreases over time, whereas neoplastic tissue continues to grow (see **Fig. 5**; **Fig. 8**). Therefore, any focal mass-like

tissue at the interface of the normal flap and the recipient bed that demonstrates growth should be highly concerning for tumor (**Fig. 9**).[18,21]

VASCULARIZED FLAPS: SITE-SPECIFIC EXAMPLES
Anterior Skull Base

The primary objective in reconstruction of the anterior cranial base is to provide a water-tight seal between the central nervous system and the sinonasal contents. The secondary objectives are to provide optimal cosmesis, obliterate any

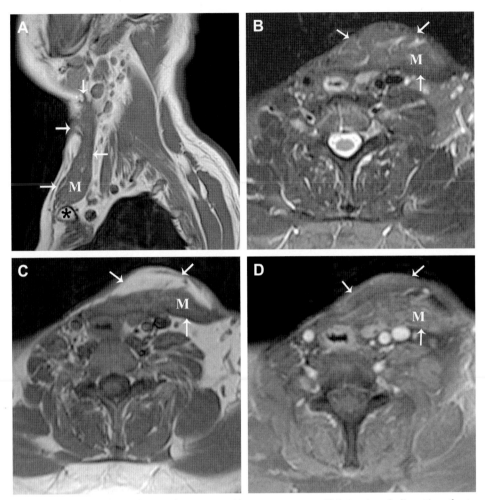

Fig. 4. A 47-year-old man after radiation therapy, total laryngectomy, and bilateral neck dissections for transglottic squamous cell carcinoma and subsequent reconstruction of anterior neck for exposed carotid artery using a left pectoralis flap. Neck MR imaging is performed at 6-month follow-up. (*A*) Sagittal T1-weighted image shows myocutaneous pectoralis flap (outlined by *arrows*) tunneled over the clavicle (*asterisk*) with more bulky muscle component in inferior neck (M). (*B–D*) Axial STIR, unenhanced, and fat-saturated gadolinium-enhanced T1-weighted images, respectively, show the pectoralis flap (outlined by *arrows*) and muscle component (M) with signal intensity and enhancement similar to adjacent muscles.

potential space that may exist, and minimize donor site morbidity.[3] An armamentarium of alloplastic materials is available for reconstruction of small and medium sized defects, whereas vascularized flaps and free-tissue transfers are used for the reconstruction of large surgical defects and reconstructions in an irradiated field.[13] Vascularized bony and alloplastic grafts are rarely necessary for successful skull base reconstruction, which are usually performed with soft tissue flaps.

Anterior skull base defects are reconstructed in a multilayer inlay-onlay fashion to achieve a water-tight cerebrospinal fluid seal. Nonvascularized tissue, such as autologous fascia lata, temporalis fascia, dura, and dermis, can be layered

intracranially in an inlay fashion between the dura and the bone at the edge of the defect. The vascularized tissues including local flaps, myocutaneous pedicled flaps, and free-tissue transfers are layered extracranially in an onlay fashion.

The primary local flap used in reconstruction of small-to-medium endoscopically created anterior skull base defects is mucochondrial-mucoperiosteal nasoseptal flap, which maintains vascular pedicle from the nasoseptal branch of the sphenopalatine artery (**Fig. 10**).[22,23] In open reconstructions of central anterior skull base defects, the pericranial or galeal-pericranial flaps with pedicles from the supratrochlear and supraorbital arteries are readily available in the surgical field

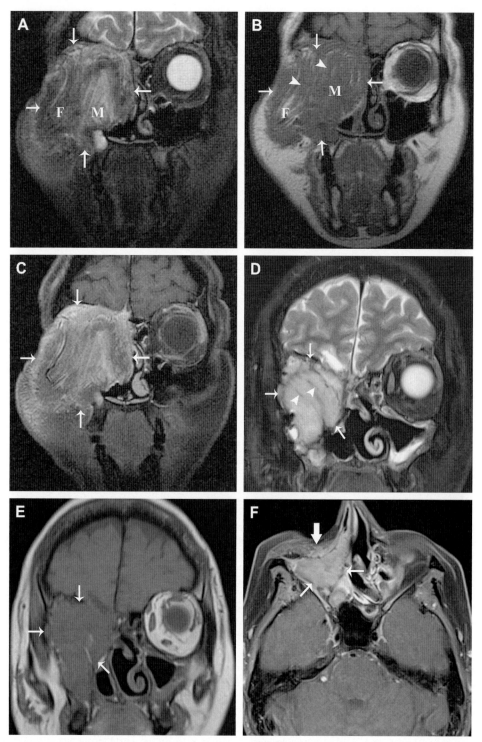

Fig. 5. A 47-year-old woman 3 months after maxillectomy and orbital exenteration for squamous cell carcinoma and reconstruction using a rectus abdominis free flap. (*A–C*) Coronal STIR, unenhanced T1-weighted, and gadolinium-enhanced fat-saturated T1-weighted images, respectively, of the free flap (outlined by *thin arrows*) show the small fatty component (F) and large muscle component (M) with characteristic striations (*arrowheads*), best depicted on T1-weighted imaging (*B*). The flap shows heterogenous T2 hyperintensity and enhancement. (*D–F*) Coronal fat-saturated T2-weighted, unenhanced T1-weighted, and axial gadolinium-enhanced fat-saturated T1-weighted images, respectively, performed at 6-month follow-up show increased T2 hyperintensity and enhancement of the muscular flap (outlined by *arrows*), which maintains striations (*arrowheads*). Note the reduction in volume of the flap (*thick arrow*) best appreciated on axial image (*F*).

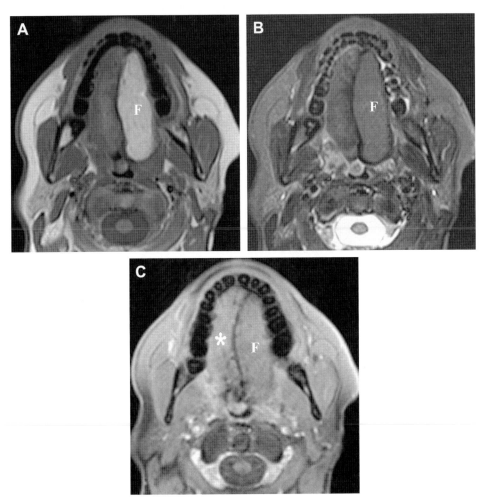

Fig. 6. A 47-year-old man status-post left hemiglossectomy and reconstruction using RFF. (*A*, *B*) Axial T1-weighted and fat-saturated T2-weighted images show fasciocutaneous flap with a large fatty component (F) filling the left hemiglossectomy defect. There is expected bulbous protrusion of the graft into the oropharyngeal lumen. (*C*) Axial fat-saturated gadolinium-enhanced T1-weighted image shows no avid enhancement of the fatty flap compared with the residual tongue (*asterisk*).

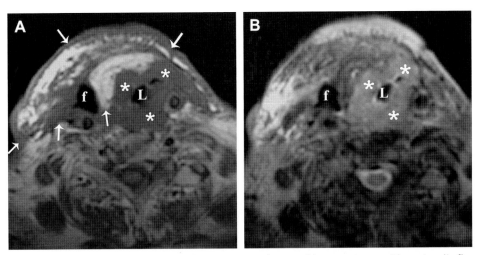

Fig. 7. A 77-year-old man with recurrent carcinoma 1 year after total laryngectomy with pectoralis flap reconstruction. Axial T1-weighted (*A*) and T2-weighted with fat saturation (*B*) images show predominantly fatty right pectoralis flap (outlined by *arrows*) covering the anterior neopharynx. Recurrent tumor (*asterisks*) circumferentially encases the neopharynx. Note the lumen of the neopharynx (L) and air-containing pharyngocutaneous fistula (f) heralding the recurrence.

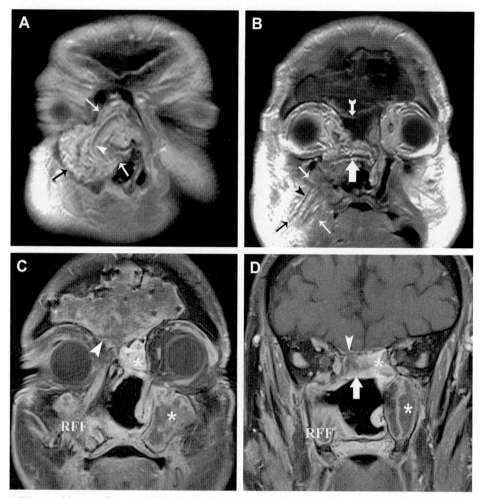

Fig. 8. A 55-year-old man after maxillectomy and anterior skull base (ASB) resection with reconstruction using RFF and pericranial flaps. (*A, B*) Gadolinium-enhanced coronal T1-weighted images without fat saturation performed on postoperative Day 1 show RFF myocutaneous flap (outlined by *thin arrows*) with T1-hyperintense fat and isointense striated muscle fibers (*arrowhead*) filling the maxillectomy defect and nasal side of the ASB reconstruction (*thick arrow*). The pericranial flap shows linear to no enhancement (*bow arrow*). (*C, D*) Gadolinium-enhanced coronal T1-weighted images with fat saturation performed 2 years later show volume loss of the enhancing RFF with cranial retraction at ASB (*arrow*) and sheet-like linear enhancement of the pericranial flap (*arrowhead*). Note normal-enhancing sinonasal mucosa (*asterisks*).

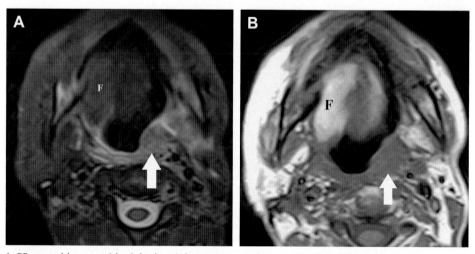

Fig. 9. A 55-year-old man with right hemiglossectomy and reconstruction using RFF 15 years ago. Axial T1-weighted (*A*) and T2 STIR (*B*) images show the largely fat-containing fasciocutaneous flap (F) for reconstruction of right hemiglossectomy. A new primary tumor of the left palatine tonsil is identified (*arrow*).

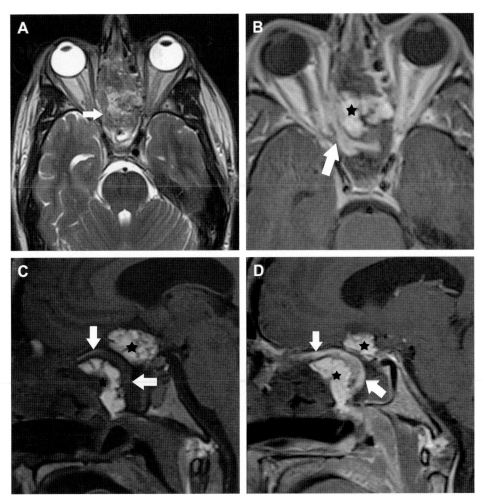

Fig. 10. A 41-year-old man 1 day after resection of a 3-cm meningioma of the planum sphenoidale/tuberculum-sella with reconstruction of the skull base using a nasoseptal flap. Axial T2-weighted (*A*) and gadolinium-enhanced T1-weighted (*B*) images show the enhancing nasoseptal flap isointense to brain on T2-weighted imaging (*arrow*). Sagittal unenhanced T1-weighted (*C*) and enhanced T1-weighted (*D*) images show the multi-layer reconstruction with enhancing C-shaped nasoseptal flap (*arrows*) covering sphenoidectomy defect. Intra-dural and endonasal fat packing (*stars*).

(see **Fig. 8**).[24] For open reconstruction of the lateral skull base defects, the temporoparietal fascia based off the STA or temporalis muscle flap based off the anterior and posterior deep temporal arteries are routinely used (see **Fig. 3**). Free-tissue transfers are reserved for large anterior skull base defects or when a local flap is not available.[25] The free flap pedicle (RFF, rectus abdominis, ALT) can be reanastomosed to STA or facial vessels through a temporal burr hole or craniotomy (**Fig. 11**).

The complex imaging appearance of anterior skull base reconstructions reflects the intricacy of surgical defects and the armamentarium of reconstructive technique and tissues used. The nasoseptal flaps show T1 and T2 isointensity,

variable enhancement, and variable flap thicknesses (range, 2.5–6 mm; mean, 4.4 mm) on immediate postoperative scans and a typical C-shaped configuration at the sphenosellar defect (see **Fig. 10**).[26] The MR imaging features of the used fascial, fasciocutaneous, and myocutaneous flaps reflect the composition of the flaps, as discussed previously, and the pericranial flap shows a thin linear enhancement at the skull base (see **Figs. 3, 8**, and **11**).[10]

Orbit and Midface

The goals of midface reconstruction are to provide support for the orbital contents, to maintain orbital form, to obliterate the defect in cases of orbital

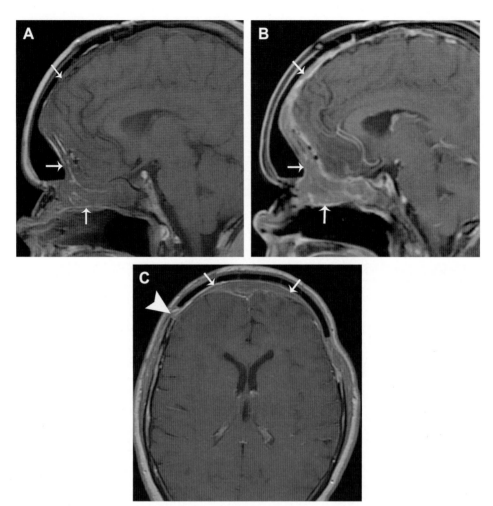

Fig. 11. A 40-year-old man with large frontal scalp sarcoma involving the calvarium and anterior skull base treated with chemoradiation and salvage resection with reconstruction using an ALT flap performed 3 months ago. (*A*) Sagittal unenhanced T1-weighted image shows striated muscular component of the myocutaneous flap (*arrows*) covering the frontal and anterior skull base defect, separating the sinonasal cavity from the intracranial compartment. (*B, C*) Sagittal and axial gadolinium-enhanced T1-weighted images, respectively, show the enhancing flap (*arrows*) and the right temporal burr hole (*arrowhead*) where the vascular pedicle of the flap exits to be anastomosed with superficial temporal artery.

exentoration, and to provide contour and projection to the malar region.[3,27,28] The midface defect is divided into bony and soft tissue components to optimize the choice of flap. The soft tissue defect is often the dominant component of midface reconstructions and dictates the flap choice. The large defect after an orbital exenteration with maxillectomy typically requires a bulky soft tissue flap, such as ALT, rectus abdominis, and latissimus dorsi. In orbital-sparing maxillectomies or in isolated orbital exenterations the less bulky RFF is used (see **Figs. 1, 5,** and **8**). Bony reconstruction of the orbital floor in maxillectomy can be accomplished with osteocutaneous RFF. The RFF pedicle is routinely tunneled through the cheek to reach the facial vessels at the mandibular border.[13] The longer

length of the vascular pedicles with rectus abdominis and latissimus dorsi flaps are advantageous to reach the far cervical vessels for reanastomosis.

Hard Palate and Maxilla

The goals of maxillary reconstruction are to isolate the oral cavity from the nasal cavity, to provide a scaffold for support of dental reconstruction, to obliterate defects, and to restore facial contour. Reconstructive options depend greatly on the type of defects and the availability of reconstructive tissues and individual patient to achieve these goals with the least comorbidity.[27,28]

Palatal obturators and alloplast prostheses may be appropriate for small defects.[29] If used alone for larger defects or after radiotherapy, the cavity may fail to retain the prosthesis or to provide the support necessary for good function. Patient dissatisfaction frequently results from the cumbersome obturator, ongoing maintenance, inadequate oronasal seal, and poor residual dentition. Obturators are removed for MR imaging to limit image degradation from artifact.

The limitations and issues of reconstruction using obturators have led to the expansion of vascularized soft tissue reconstruction for palate defects. Depending on the defect, aesthetic and functional restoration may be achieved with soft tissue alone, a combination of soft tissue and nonvascularized bone graft, or a composite osteofasciocutaneous flap with vascularized bone. The temporalis flap is limited by the length of the vascular pedicle for adequate reach to the surgical defect, its small soft tissue bulk, and the lack of a bone component.[27] Free-tissue transfers (RFF, rectus abdominis, ALT with or without bone component) offer versatile options of tissue choice, volume and contour, no constraints of vascular pedicle length, and tissue orientation (**Fig. 12**).

Oral Cavity and Oropharynx Reconstruction

The site-specific defects after surgery for oral cavity and oropharyngeal cancer dictate the reconstructive procedure intended to prevent wound breakdown and fistula formation; to match the shape, tissue type, and volume of the surgical defect; and to maximize functional outcome.[4] The

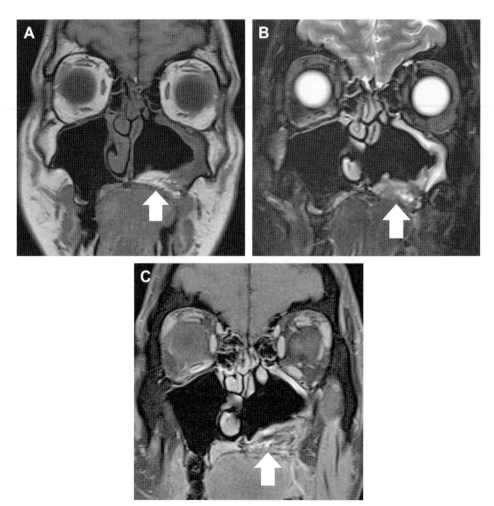

Fig. 12. A 44-year-old man 1 year status-post partial left palatectomy for minor salivary mucoepidermoid carcinoma. Reconstruction was performed using an RFF. Coronal T1-weighted image (A) shows the predominantly fatty content of the fasciocutaneous flap (*arrow*) of the left palate reconstruction. Coronal fat-saturated T2-weighted (B) and gadolinium-enhanced T1-weighted (C) images show heterogenous T2 signal intensity and mild enhancement of the flap (*arrow*).

tongue base propels food to the esophageal inlet while exerting pressure on the soft palate to seal the nasopharyngeal inlet during swallowing. The goal of reconstruction after partial glossectomies and base of tongue resections is a nonbulky RFF or small ALT flap so that the native residual tongue can move and conduct its normal functions (see **Fig. 6**). The more extensive defects involving the tongue base and adjacent tonsil or lateral pharyngeal wall require restoration of tongue base bulk and the complex functional valve of the oropharyngeal and nasopharyngeal soft tissues. The RFF is the most commonly used fasciocutaneous free flap for partial glossectomy and oropharyngeal reconstruction (see **Fig. 6**; **Fig. 13**). Its small-to-medium soft tissue bulk is ideal for partial glossectomies, comprising up to 70% of the tongue volume. Its thin and pliable skin paddle can be contoured to reconstruct the complex three-dimensional relationships of the tongue base, tonsillar fossa, soft palate, and posterior floor of the mouth without crowding the airway lumen. Fibular, scapular, or radial forearm osteocutaneous flaps may be used to treat defects of the lateral oropharynx that also involve the mandibular ramus.

Total glossectomies pose a significant challenge regarding functional restoration regardless of the reconstruction methods. Free-flap reconstruction with rectus abdominis and ALT may provide some function for patients with normally functioning lips and a preserved larynx. However, the overall achieved function is that of severe dysarthria with speech that is usually intelligible, and limited swallowing function necessitating permanent gastrostomy placement.

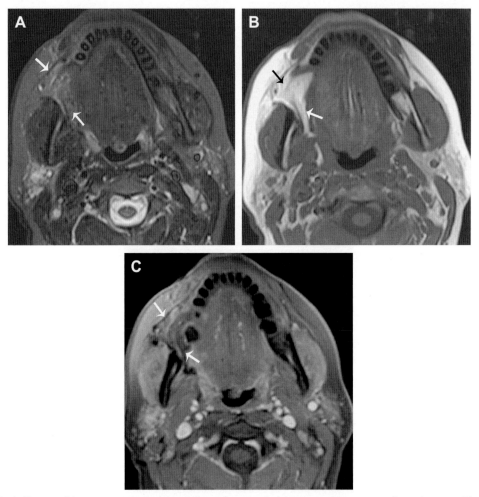

Fig. 13. A 42-year-old woman status-post resection of a retromolar trigone squamous cell carcinoma with reconstruction using RFF 2 years ago. Axial T2 STIR (*A*), unenhanced T1-weighted (*B*), and fat-saturated gadolinium-enhanced T1-weighted (*C*) images show nonenhancing fatty component of fasciocutaneous flap (outlined by *arrows*) filling the right retromolar trigone and marginal mandibulectomy defect.

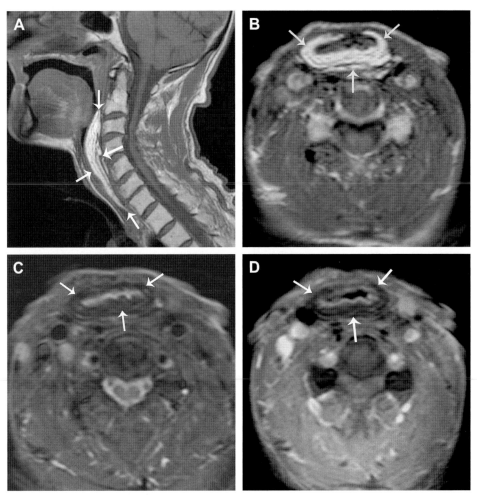

Fig. 14. A 72-year-old man 1 year status-post pharyngolaryngoesophagectomy for laryngeal-hypopharyngeal SCCA with reconstruction using an ALT flap. (*A, B*) Sagittal T1-weighted (*A*) and axial T1-weighted (*B*) images show rolled (tubed) fatty fasciocutaneous flap (outlined by *arrows*) creating the neopharynx. (*C, D*) Axial STIR (*C*) and fat-saturated gadolinium-enhanced T1-weighted (*D*) images show the suppressed (hypointense) nonenhancing fatty component of the flap (*arrows*).

Mandibular Reconstruction

The goals for reconstruction of segmental defects of the mandible are restoration of mandibular continuity; repair of the soft tissue defect; and preservation of mastication, sensation, and dentition. The free-bone graft requires a well-vascularized recipient bed for its survival and a watertight mucosal covering to prevent the graft from bathing in saliva. In an irradiated field where tissue perfusion is compromised and mucosal breakdown is more prone to occur, free-bone grafts are more prone to failure and are rarely used.[30] Therefore, free-tissue transfers are primarily used for segmental defects of all regions. Nonvascularized bone grafts are used for small mandibular defects less than 5 cm in resections

that do not require radiation therapy.[31] For larger bone resections usually associated with large soft tissue defects to treat malignancies that often also require radiation therapy, free-tissue transfers are indicated to reduce the risk of graft failure. Fibular free flaps are the mainstay for mandibular reconstructions. The long segment of fibular bone (approximately 25 cm) with segmental osseous perforators can handle multiple osteotomies without becoming ischemic allowing for contouring that can bridge large defects including those spanning both angles of the mandible. The proximal end of a fibular bone flap can be contoured to fit into the glenoid fossa of the temporomandibular joint as needed. One potential downside to the fibular flap is its associated skin paddle, which is limited in size and flexibility around the bone, but multiple skin paddles can be harvested. In patients with severe peripheral vascular disease, a scapular osteocutaneous free flap may be used. Although the scapula provides less bone length, it provides more skin and is more flexible for large, complex oromandibular wounds. Plate fixation of the mandible uses titanium miniplates or a single microvascular reconstruction plate, both of which result in significant artifact on CT and MR imaging.

Hypopharynx and Laryngeal Reconstruction

The tendency for submucosal spread of hypopharyngeal tumors necessitates wide surgical margins; thus, primary closure with a functional lumen is usually not possible. If insufficient mucosa remains, pedicled or free-tissue transfer flaps may be used for reconstruction to avoid postoperative stenosis. Three types of hypopharyngeal defects are managed by reconstructive surgeons: (1) circumferential pharyngeal defects, (2) noncircumferential defects with some native sensate mucosa remaining, and (3) the more extensive pharyngoesophageal defect. Hypopharyngeal defects are partial losses that cannot be closed primarily, or circumferential losses that require cylindrical reconstruction. These reconstructions are targeted to achieve the best functional outcome while minimizing the risk of complications. Free-flap reconstructions of pharyngolaryngoesophageal defects are frequently used.[7] Laryngectomies with partial pharyngectomies or laryngectomies performed in a previously irradiated patient are best reconstructed with an RFF or pectoralis major myocutaneous flap (see **Fig. 4**). A complete laryngopharyngectomy is most commonly reconstructed with tubed free flaps (RFF, ALT) or the naturally tubed jejunal free flap (**Fig. 14**).[3,32] The jejunum flap has become less favorable because of poorer swallowing and speech function due to mucous formation, higher donor site morbidity, and longer hospital stays.[4,7] The gastro-omental free flap is gaining popularity in the setting of prior chemoradiation where it is thought potentially to decrease fistula rates.[33]

SUMMARY

As technologic advancements, surgical techniques, and multidisciplinary treatment of head and neck cancer continue to evolve, imaging of the treated neck is encountered increasingly in everyday radiologic practices. An understanding of the flaps commonly used to reconstruct surgical beds is paramount to accurate image interpretation. The skill to be able to distinguish between healthy normal flaps and recurrent neoplasm is essential to patient care, especially because many recurrences in reconstructed necks are not detected by clinical examination. Basic knowledge of the surgical techniques and principle of head and neck reconstruction is essential to simplify the complex imaging appearance of these reconstructions. MR imaging provides superior soft tissue resolution, enabling one to recognize the fatty and striated muscular components of a myocutaneous flap, whether pedicled-rotated flap or free flap in free-tissue transfer, and to avoid misinterpretation of flaps for enhancing neoplasm.

REFERENCES

1. Howlader N, Noone AM, Krapcho M, et al. SEER Cancer Statistics Review, 1975-2008. Bethesda, MD: National Cancer Institute. Available at: http://seer.cancer.gov/csr/1975_2008/. based on November 2010 SEER data submission, posted to the SEER web site, 2011. Accessed January, 2012.
2. Turner JH, Reh DD. Incidence and survival in patients with sinonasal cancer: a historical analysis of population-based data. Head Neck 2012;34(6): 877–85.
3. Rosenthal E, Couch M, Farwell DG, et al. Current concepts in microvascular reconstruction. Otolaryngol Head Neck Surg 2007;136:519–24.
4. Smith RB, Sniezek JC, Weed DT, et al. Utilization of free tissue transfer in head and neck surgery. Otolaryngol Head Neck Surg 2007;137:182–91.
5. Schneider DS, Wu V, Wax MK. Indications for pedicled pectoralis major flap in a free tissue transfer practice. Head Neck 2011. DOI:10.1002/hed.21868. Published online Nov 2011.
6. Som PM, Urken ML, Biller HF, et al. Imaging the postoperative neck. Radiology 1993;187:593–603.
7. Murray DJ, Novak CB, Neligan PC. Fasciocutaneous free flaps in pharyngolaryngooesophageal reconstruction: a critical review of the literature. J Plast Reconstr Aesthet Surg 2008;61:1148–56.
8. Wester DJ, Whiteman ML, Singer S, et al. Imaging of the postoperative neck with emphasis on surgical flaps and their complications. AJR Am J Roentgenol 1995;164:989–93.
9. Chong J, Chan LL, Langstein HN, et al. MR imaging of the muscular component of myocutaneous flaps in the head and neck. AJNR Am J Neuroradiol 2001;22:170–4.
10. Naidich MJ, Weissman JL. Reconstructive myofascial skull-base flaps: normal appearance on CT and MR imaging studies. AJR Am J Roentgenol 1996;167:611–4.
11. Bergey DA, Braun TW. The posterior zygomatic arch osteotomy to facilitate temporalis flap placement. J Oral Maxillofac Surg 1994;52(4):426–7.

12. Vartanian JG, Carvalho AL, Carvalho SM, et al. Pectoralis major and other myofascial/myocutaneous flaps in head and neck cancer reconstruction: experience with 437 cases at a single institution. Head Neck 2004;26(12):1018–23.

13. Schmalbach CE, Webb DE, Weitzel EK. Anterior skull base reconstruction: a review of current technique. Curr Opin Otolaryngol Head Neck Surg 2010;18:238–43.

14. Bendszus M, Koltzenburg M, Wessig C, et al. Sequential MR imaging of denervated muscle: experimental study. Am J Neuroradiol 2002;23: 1427–31.

15. Kikuchi Y, Nakamura T, Takayama S, et al. MR imaging in the diagnosis of denervated and reinnervated skeletal muscles: experimental study in rats. Radiology 2003;229(3):861–7.

16. Ylä-Kotola TM, Kauhanen MS, Koskinen SK, et al. Magnetic resonance imaging of microneurovascular free muscle flaps in facial reanimation. Br J Plast Surg 2005;58:22–7.

17. Hudgins PA. Flap reconstruction in the head and neck: expected appearance, complications, and recurrent disease. Eur J Radiol 2002;44:130–8.

18. Hudgins PA, Burson JG, Gussack GS, et al. CT and MR appearance of recurrent malignant head and neck neoplasms after resection and flap reconstruction. AJNR Am J Neuroradiol 1994;15:1689–94.

19. Tomura N, Watanabe O, Hirano Y, et al. MR imaging of recurrent head and neck tumours following flap reconstructive surgery. Clin Radiol 2002;57(2): 109–13.

20. Glazer HS, Lee JK, Levitt RG, et al. Radiation fibrosis: differentiation from recurrent tumor by MR imaging. Radiology 1985;156(3):721–6.

21. Makimoto Y, Yamamoto S, Takano H, et al. Imaging findings of radiation induced sarcoma of the head and neck. Br J Radiol 2007;80:790–7.

22. Hadad G, Bassagasteguy L, Carrau RL, et al. A novel reconstructive technique after endoscopic expanded endonasal approaches: vascular pedicle nasoseptal flap. Laryngoscope 2006;116:1882–6.

23. Kassam A, Thomas A, Carrau R, et al. Endoscopic reconstruction of the skull base using a pedicled nasoseptal flap. Neurosurgery 2008;63(ONS Suppl 1): ONS44–52.

24. Smith JE, Ducic Y. The versatile extended pericranial flap for closure of skull base defects. Otolaryngol Head Neck Surg 2004;130:704–11.

25. Weber SM, Kim JH, Wax MK. Role of free tissue transfer in skull base reconstruction. Otolaryngol Head Neck Surg 2007;136:914–9.

26. Kang MD, Escott E, Thomas AJ, et al. The MR imaging appearance of the vascular pedicle nasoseptal flap. Am J Neuroradiol 2009;30:781–6.

27. O'Connell DA, Futran ND. Reconstruction of the midface and maxilla. Curr Opin Otolaryngol Head Neck Surg 2010;18:304–10.

28. Shrime MG, Gilbert RW. Reconstruction of the midface and maxilla. Facial Plast Surg Clin North Am 2009;17:211–23.

29. Moreno MA, Skoracki RJ, Hanna EY, et al. Microvascular free flap reconstruction versus palatal obturation for maxillectomy defect. Head Neck 2010;32: 860–8.

30. Hurvitz KA, Kobayashi M, Evans GRD. Current options in head and neck reconstruction. Plast Reconstr Surg 2006;118:122e.

31. Miles BA, Goldstein DP, Gilbert RW, et al. Mandible reconstruction. Curr Opin Otolaryngol Head Neck Surg 2010;18:317–22.

32. Disa JJ, Pusic AL, Hidalgo DA, et al. Microvascular reconstruction of the hypopharynx: defect classification, treatment algorithm, and functional outcome based on 165 consecutive cases. Plast Reconstr Surg 2003;111:652.

33. Patel RS, Gilbert RW. Utility of the gastro-omental free flap in head and neck reconstruction. Curr Opin Otolaryngol Head Neck Surg 2009;17(4): 258–62.

Evaluation of the Sellar and Parasellar Regions

Brian M. Chin, MD, MBA[a],*, Richard R. Orlandi, MD[b],
Richard H. Wiggins III, MD[c]

KEYWORDS

- Sellar • Pituitary • Suprasellar • Parasellar • Cavernous sinus

KEY POINTS

- Anatomic localization is essential in the creation of a differential diagnosis of a sellar or parasellar region mass.
- Dedicated magnetic resonance imaging protocols (eg, pituitary, skull base, or sinus) are important for complete characterization, and computed tomography should be considered as a complementary modality to evaluate anatomic variants, calcification, or intraosseous extension.
- Certain diagnoses are dependent on the imaged patient population or clinical presentation; this knowledge further facilitates the provision of a limited, expert differential.

INTRODUCTION

The sellar and parasellar regions are anatomically and pathologically complex areas. Expert knowledge of the anatomy and diseases is important to provide focused differentials and guide patient management. Inflammatory/granulomatous, infectious, neoplastic, and vascular diseases can involve these regions, arising from the pituitary gland, infundibular stalk, hypothalamus, cranial nerves, vascular structures, leptomeninges, or skull base. Abnormalities may be detected incidentally on imaging or when imaged patients present with pituitary dysfunction, vision changes, or cranial nerve III, IV, V, or VI palsies.

ANATOMY
Sellar Region

The sellar region encompasses the sella turcica and the pituitary gland. The parasellar region includes the structures and spaces bordering the sella turcica, namely the cavernous sinuses, suprasellar cistern, hypothalamus, and ventral inferior third ventricle.

The sella turcica (Turkish saddle) is a concave depression in the sphenoid bone. Its ventral borders are the tuberculum sellae and anterior clinoid processes and its dorsal borders are the dorsum sellae and the posterior clinoid processes. The roof of the sella consists of a thin dural covering: the diaphragma sellae.

Within the sella turcica, the pituitary gland consists of the ventral adenohypophysis and the dorsal neurohypophysis. The adenohypophysis is formed by ascending ectodermal cells of the Rathke pouch and consists of the pars distalis, pars intermedia, and pars tuberalis. The adenohypophysis primarily secretes regulatory hormones, such as growth, adrenocorticotropic, prolactin, follicle-stimulating, luteinizing, and thyroid-stimulating hormones.

In contrast, the neurohypophysis is formed as an extension or evagination of neural ectoderm from the floor of the third ventricle (diencephalon).

[a] Department of Radiology, University of Utah, 30 North 1900 East #1A071, Salt Lake City, UT 84132-2140, USA;
[b] Department of Otolaryngology, Head and Neck Surgery, University of Utah, 30 North 1900 East #1A071, Salt Lake City, UT, USA; [c] Department of Radiology, Otolaryngology, Head and Neck Surgery, and BioMedical Informatics, University of Utah, 30 North 1900 East #1A071, Salt Lake City, UT, USA
* Corresponding author.
E-mail address: brian.chin@hsc.utah.edu

Magn Reson Imaging Clin N Am 20 (2012) 515–543
doi:10.1016/j.mric.2012.05.007

The neurohypophysis consists of par nervosa and infundibulum, the latter inserting into the median eminence of the hypothalamus. The infundibulum extends from the hypothalamus through the diaphragma sellae to the pituitary gland. The neurohypophysis primarily consists of axon terminals that secrete hormones formed in the hypothalamus (antidiuretic hormone [vasopressin] and oxytocin) into the blood (**Fig. 1**A, B).

The size of the pituitary gland depends on the age and gender of the imaged patient. Before puberty the gland is small, measuring 6 mm or less in greatest height. During puberty, the pituitary can enlarge up to 10 mm, and in pregnant or postpartum women, it can measure up to 12 mm. In adulthood, the pituitary is otherwise normally 8 mm or less.[1]

Parasellar Region

The parasellar region is a general term that traditionally encompasses the cavernous sinuses and the suprasellar cistern structures. The basisphenoid and the sphenoid sinus are occasionally included as well.

The cavernous sinuses are multilobulated, trabeculated, venous channels lateral to the sella turcica and sphenoid sinus. Cranial nerves III, IV, V1, and V2 lie within the lateral dural wall, whereas cranial nerve VI lies within the cavernous sinus. It also contains the cavernous segment of the internal carotid artery (ICA) (**Fig. 2**A, B).

The suprasellar cistern contains the optic chiasm/nerves, anterior third ventricle, hypothalamus, and tuber cinereum. The anterior margin of the hypothalamus is the lamina terminalis and its posterior margin is imprecise, demarcated as a vertical plane extending from the mammillary bodies to the posterior commissure. Located along the ventral lateral aspect of the third ventricle, the caudal extent is formed by the infundibular stalk, tuber cinereum, and mammillary bodies.

There are two cerebrospinal fluid (CSF)-containing extensions of the third ventricle: the optic nerve recess, which is ventral to the optic chiasm, and the more dorsal infundibular recess, which extends caudally into the superior infundibulum. Located in the tuberal region of the hypothalamus and ventral to the mammillary bodies, the tuber cinereum is a lamina of gray matter. Part of the limbic system, the mammillary bodies are paired globular structures along the floor of the hypothalamus that connect with the hippocampi via the fornices.

Understanding the anatomy is crucial in attempting to localize a process to the: (1) sellar, (2) suprasellar (including infundibulum), or (3) parasellar compartments. Such localization limits the differential possibilities, and when combined with imaging characteristics, clinical history, and patient age, enables the provision of a limited, clinically relevant differential.

Key Point

Understanding the complex anatomy is essential for differential creation.

Imaging Overview

Computed tomography (CT) and magnetic resonance (MR) imaging are complementary modalities for evaluating the sellar and parasellar

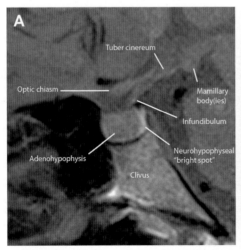
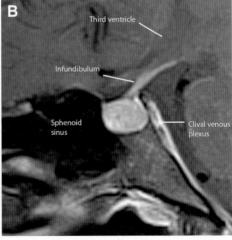

Fig. 1. Anatomy. (*A*) Sagittal precontrast, fat-saturated T1WI image through the midline sella turcica shows the normal T1 shortening in the neurohypophysis. (*B*) Postcontrast T1WI image shows the normal enhancement of the pituitary gland, infundibulum, and tuber cinereum region caused by the lack of a blood-brain barrier.

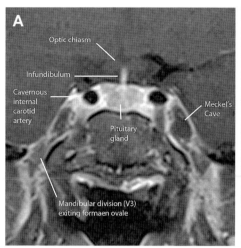
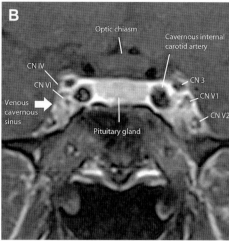

Fig. 2. (*A*, *B*) Anatomy. Coronal postcontrast, fat-saturated T1WI images through the sella turcica show the gland relative to the parasellar cavernous sinuses and suprasellar optic chiasm. The pituitary gland enhances less strongly than the cavernous sinus venous blood.

regions. With rapid acquisition and multiplanar capabilities, CT can characterize and provide a differential for most processes. Specifically, CT is helpful in determining if a process is primarily osseous in origin or is a result of secondary involvement of the skull base. In addition, it readily identifies calcifications, whether vascular, dystrophic, or tumor matrix in origin.

With its high spatial resolution and multiplanar capabilities, MR imaging is superior in determining if a process originates from the sellar, suprasellar cistern structures, cavernous sinus, or skull base as well as characterizing its regional spread. With its various sequences, MR imaging can determine if a mass is solid, cystic, hemorrhagic, or fatty, which narrows the differential depending on the location.

When evaluating a sellar or parasellar process, it is important to use an MR imaging protocol (eg, pituitary or skull base) with the appropriate field of view, slice thickness, and sequences for complete characterization. Pending the indication (eg, microadenoma detection), dynamic postcontrast pituitary imaging should be obtained as well.[2]

It is important to recognize normal MR imaging characteristics of the sellar and parasellar regions. In adults, the adenohypophysis is isointense to the pons on sagittal imaging.[1] The neurohypophysis is usually T1 hyperintense because of vasopressin neurosecretory granules.[3] T1 hyperintense signal of the neurohypophysis is seen in up to 90% of healthy patients,[4] yet if there is growth or endocrine abnormalities, follow-up imaging is important to exclude a developing infiltrative or neoplastic

process. Given the lack of a blood-brain barrier, the infundibulum and pituitary gland enhance homogeneously and rapidly, slightly hypointense to the adjacent venous cavernous sinus.

Dynamic imaging rapidly acquires coronal images through the entire pituitary gland repeatedly during contrast administration. In a normal hypophysis, the contrast first accumulates in the cavernous sinuses, followed by the infundibulum and adjacent superior medial aspect of the hypophysis. The remainder of the adenohypophysis then enhances in a centrifugal fashion.

IMAGING ANALYSIS

Because more than 30 entities/processes can involve this region, this article focuses on the entities most commonly seen in general practice (macroadenoma, microadenoma, hypothalamic-chiasmatic glioma, meningioma, and metastases) as well as less common entities, such as Rathke's cleft cyst (RCC), (epi)dermoid, craniopharyngioma, and hypothalamic hamartoma. Although vascular, inflammatory, infectious, and granulomatous processes can uncommonly involve this region, they are not addressed in this article.

When evaluating sellar diseases, it is important to first localize the process to the sellar, parasellar, or suprasellar compartment and have a systematic approach toward analysis (**Box 1**). With knowledge of the common and uncommon processes in that region, the patient's age and presentation, and the imaging features of the process, one can provide a limited, expert differential (**Table 1**).

ADENOMA

Although rarely ectopic in the nasopharynx, sinonasal region, or skull base, adenomas are the most common intrasellar disease. Based on autopsy and imaging studies, unsuspected pituitary adenoma prevalence ranges from 14% to 22.5% in the general population.[5] By definition, a microadenoma is less than 10 mm, and a macroadenoma is 10 mm or more in its greatest dimension.

Adenomas are either functional or nonfunctional. A functional tumor is named for the hormone it produces. A prolactinoma is the most common adenoma, presenting with amenorrhea-galactorrhea (women) or gynecomastia-hypogonadism-impotence (men). An adrenocorticotropic-producing

Box 1
Approach to analysis of sellar, parasellar, and suprasellar processes.

- What is the patient's age, past medical history, and presenting signs and symptoms?
- Is the center of the mass sellar, suprasellar, or parasellar in location?
- If it involves the sella turcica, is the pituitary gland normal, enlarged, or displaced?
- Is the mass solid, cystic, or mixed in signal characteristics or attenuation?
- Is calcification or hemorrhage present on the CT or gradient echo sequences?
- Does the mass enhance and to what degree?
- What is the enhancement pattern (homogeneous, heterogeneous, rim, solid, dural)?
- Does the mass restrict on diffusion sequences?
- Is there involvement of the surrounding structures (cavernous sinus, skull base, optic chiasm)?
- Is there vascular encasement, narrowing, or occlusion?
- Are there features to suggest a vascular origin (pulsation, flow void, rim calcifications)?
- Are there anatomic variants relevant to the surgical approach?

adenoma presents with Cushing syndrome; a thyroid-stimulating hormone secreting adenoma, hyperthyroidism/thyrotoxicosis; and a growth hormone–producing adenoma, gigantism in children, and acromegaly in adults.

A nonfunctioning adenoma is the second most common intrasellar disease after prolactinoma. It may be asymptomatic until it develops suprasellar and parasellar extension. With superior extension into the suprasellar cistern, optic chiasm impingement may present with loss of temporal vision. With lateral compression or invasion of the cavernous sinuses, patients may experience cranial neuropathy. In rare instances, a patient may acutely present with apoplexy (see later discussion), potentially requiring emergency treatment.

MR is the primary modality used to evaluate both endocrine-active and nonfunctional pituitary adenomas, although multidetector-row contrasted CT has been used as well.[6] The goal of the MR examination is to localize the origin of the adenoma, its extension in relation to the various surrounding structures, and to exclude any alternative diagnosis. CT is obtained either when there is a contraindication to MR imaging or as a complementary modality to evaluate anatomic variant, calcification, or intraosseous involvement.

Macroadenoma

MR imaging is the primary imaging modality for characterization of macroadenomas. Specifically, MR imaging is important to evaluate potential suprasellar extension and mass effect on the optic chiasm, lateral infiltration of the cavernous sinus, and inferior invasion of the clivus or sphenoid sinus.

On MR imaging, the most helpful imaging feature is a mass that cannot be separated from the pituitary gland on the sagittal T1-weighted image (WI) sequence. As it grows, the adenoma enlarges the sella turcica and with suprasellar extension, often has a figure-of-eight or snowman-like appearance in the coronal plane with constriction of the waist caused by the diaphragma sellae (**Fig. 3**). Uncommonly, it mimics an aggressive skull base process (termed an invasive

Table 1
Common and uncommon diseases of the sellar and parasellar compartments

	Sellar[a]	Parasellar[b]
Common	Pituitary hyperplasia Pituitary microadenoma Empty sella	Hypothalamic-chiasmatic glioma Meningioma Craniopharyngioma Schwannoma (cavernous sinus) Metastases (skull base)
Uncommon	Pituitary macroadenoma RCC Craniopharyngioma	Germinoma Langerhans cell histiocytosis Lymphoma Dermoid/epidermoid Tuber cinereum hamartoma Arachnoid cyst Aneurysm Neurosarcoid Neurocysticercosis Carotid-cavernous fistula Cavernous sinus thrombosis
Rare	Arachnoid cyst Apoplexy Aneurysm Lymphocytic hypophysitis Meningioma Metastasis (gland/stalk) Lymphoma	Chordoma Pilomyxoid astrocytoma Leukemia RCC Lymphocytic hypophysitis Pseudotumor Pituicytoma

[a] Includes sella processes extending into the suprasellar region.
[b] Includes processes originating in the cavernous sinuses, suprasellar cistern structures, and the basisphenoid.

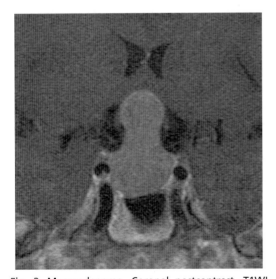

Fig. 3. Macroadenoma. Coronal postcontrast, T1WI image shows a homogeneously enhancing mass that enlarges the sella turcica and extends into the suprasellar cistern, compressing the optic chiasm. It has a figure-of-eight or snowmanlike appearance because of constriction of the waist of the mass by the diaphragma sellae.

macroadenoma) caused by caudal growth into the basisphenoid bone.[7] Up to 8.2% of macroadenomas can have clival invasion.[8] An invasive macroadenoma can be either functional or nonfunctional. As a result, if the pituitary gland is not visualized, consider obtaining endocrine laboratory values before surgical biopsy of a clival mass.

A macroadenoma is usually isointense to gray matter on T1-weighted imaging (T1WI) and T2-weighted imaging (T2WI) sequences,[4] although it is often heterogeneous in signal because of internal hemorrhage, cystic changes, or necrosis.[9,10] There is mild to moderate enhancement. Infrequently, smooth dural enhancement can be present.[11,12] It is important not to erroneously assume a mass is a meningioma if there is dural enhancement, particularly if the pituitary gland cannot be identified and the sella turcica is enlarged.

Best characterized on MR imaging, it is important to attempt to localize normal residual pituitary tissue and evaluate mass effect on the optic nerves and cavernous sinus invasion. On dynamic imaging, nonadenomatous pituitary tissue enhances before the adenoma and is usually displaced superior or posterior to the mass.[9] Mass effect on the optic chiasm is best visualized on coronal T2WI imaging.

Cavernous sinus invasion often limits complete surgical tumor resection, and up to 21% of macroadenomas can have invasion.[13] One study found features that support invasion included: 75% or greater encasement of the cavernous ICA; obliteration of the carotid sulcus venous compartment (the space between the ICA and the carotid sulcus of the sphenoid bone); or crossing of the lateral intercarotid line by the tumor.[14] Another study found that invasion is highly likely with: 45% or greater encasement of the ICA; lack of visualization of 3 or more cavernous sinus venous compartments; or involvement of the lateral venous compartment.[15]

There is unambiguous invasion when the adenoma encircles the cavernous ICA, although this rarely results in luminal narrowing. Cavernous sinus invasion is highly unlikely with: interposition of the normal pituitary gland between the adenoma and the cavernous sinus; an intact medial venous compartment; lack of crossing the medial intercarotid line; and 25% or less encasement of the cavernous ICA (**Fig. 4**A, C).[15]

Key Point

Cavernous sinus invasion affects whether the tumor is likely to be completely resected versus debulked with surveillance imaging or coexistent radiotherapy.

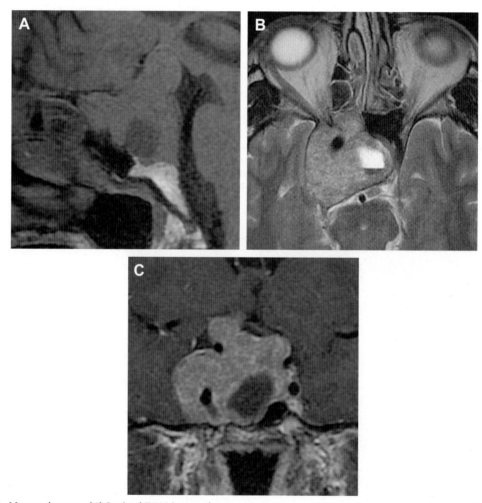

Fig. 4. Macroadenoma. (*A*) Sagittal T1WI image shows an isointense and hypointense sellar and suprasellar mass that invades/erodes the clivus and exerts mass effect on the optic chiasm. (*B*) Axial T2WI image shows a predominantly isointense solid mass with a central, hyperintense cystic/necrotic region with a fluid-fluid level. Hemorrhage and necrosis may be asymptomatic and are not synonymous with the hemorrhagic subtype of pituitary apoplexy. (*C*) Coronal T1WI postcontrast image shows invasion of the right cavernous sinus with encasement of the ICA and abutment of the left ICA without definite cavernous sinus invasion. Note the different enhancing characteristics of the macroadenoma and the left lateral cavernous sinus.

On CT, a macroadenoma appears as an iso-dense to gray matter, noncalcified, solid mass that at least moderately enhances.[4] As a macroadenoma outgrows its blood supply, it becomes heterogeneous in attenuation as a result of necrosis or hemorrhage. Up to 20% of adenomas have hemorrhage, although it is often asymptomatic (**Fig. 5A, B**).[9]

A functional macroadenoma undergoes a trial of medical treatment (eg, dopamine agonist, somatostatin). Surgical therapy is used if medical treatment is inadequate or the tumor is nonfunctional and symptomatic. The most common approach is transsphenoidal resection with fat or surgical packing material. If there is residual disease, patients may also undergo postoperative radiotherapy.[16]

Differential Diagnosis

Pseudoenlargement Pseudoenlargement or physiologic hypertrophy may be misdiagnosed as a macroadenoma. Pseudoenlargement occurs when a shallow sella turcica causes the pituitary to appear enlarged. Physiologic hypertrophy refers to a nonneoplastic increase in size because of puberty, pregnancy/postpartum state, or rarely, end-organ failure (eg, hypothyroidism).[17] In physiologic hypertrophy, the gland increases symmetrically in size and has homogeneous enhancement. Age, gender, and endocrine status must be accounted for to differentiate hypertrophy from a macroadenoma, because an adenoma is uncommonly found in children (**Fig. 6**).[18]

> **Key Point**
>
> Pituitary enlargement may be caused by puberty or pregnancy/postpartum state.

Meningioma A meningioma of the diaphragma sellae or tuberculum sellae can be difficult to differentiate from a macroadenoma if the pituitary gland is not visible. Although uncommon, an intrasellar meningioma can mimic a macroadenoma and compress/obscure the pituitary gland.[19] Although dural enhancement can occasionally be seen with a macroadenoma, the dural thickening with a meningioma is more extensive. Findings that support a meningioma are the visualization of a normal pituitary gland, CSF clefts separating the mass from the gland, and hyperostosis of adjacent bone.

Metastasis A hematogenous metastasis to the pituitary gland is uncommon but can mimic a macroadenoma. Additional enhancing foci within the calvarium, skull base, or intracranial structures support a pituitary metastasis. Often patients have known metastatic disease (**Fig. 7**).

Craniopharyngioma A craniopharyngioma is usually not in the differential with a macroadenoma given differential patient populations. The more common adamantinomatous subtype occurs in children with associated cystic components and calcification. The less common papillary subtype occurs in adults and is predominantly solid, similar to a macroadenoma; however, the pituitary gland can invariably be seen separate from the mass.

Aneurysm An aneurysm from the cavernous, clinoid, ophthalmic, or anterior communication artery complex can uncommonly protrude into the sella, potentially mimicking an adenoma if the normal pituitary gland cannot be visualized.[20] Aneurysms are usually off-midline, partially calcified (particularly the rim) on CT and have a flow-void ± mural thrombus on MR imaging. Even a completely thrombosed aneurysm should not expand the sella turcica or follow the imaging characteristics of a macroadenoma. A cerebral angiogram or CT angiogram should be obtained if there is suspicion of an aneurysm (**Fig. 8A, B**).

> **Key Point**
>
> If there is concern for a suprasellar or intrasellar aneurysm mimicking a macroadenoma on MR imaging, obtain a CT angiogram or cerebral angiogram.

Microadenoma

A patient with a microadenoma usually presents with an endocrine abnormality, which prompts imaging evaluation. Rarely, a microadenoma can be found in ectopic locations, including the cavernous sinus, sphenoid sinus, and clivus,[21] although most commonly it is an oval, round mass within the adenohypophysis.

MR imaging is the best modality for microadenoma detection and localization. Depending on the subtype of tumor and the published series, a microadenoma has a range of appearances on T1WI and T2WI sequences[9] and is best visualized in the coronal plane. It is usually isointense or hypointense on T1WI[22,23] and hypointense or isointense on T2WI sequences.[22] A growth hormone–secreting microadenoma is usually T2WI hypointense. In contrast, a microprolactinoma is often T2WI hyperintense.[9]

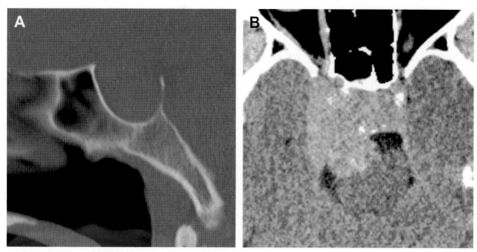

Fig. 5. Macroadenoma. (*A*) Sagittal nonenhanced CT in bone window shows smooth enlargement of the sella turcica, suggestive of an underlying mass or long-standing CSF pulsations/increased CSF pressure. (*B*) Axial nonenhanced CT in soft tissue window (in a different patient) shows an isodense and hyperdense mass expanding sella turcica, invading the right cavernous sinus, and exerting mass effect on the midbrain.

A thyroid-stimulating hormone secreting microadenoma has been described with T2WI hyperintense signal as well (**Fig. 9**A, B).[24]

Dynamic enhanced pituitary imaging has improved sensitivity for microadenoma detection compared with conventional postcontrast imaging.[2,25] A microadenoma characteristically

shows delayed and decreased enhancement relative to the surrounding gland.[23] A normal MR imaging scan does not exclude a microadenoma[26] because it may be very small, obscured by the avidly enhancing pituitary gland (high gadolinium dose), or if the imaging window is too large.[9] Some studies have recommended lower doses of contrast with dynamic imaging to better detect a microadenoma.[22] Postcontrast imaging 30 to 40 minutes after injection may also be helpful for detection.[9]

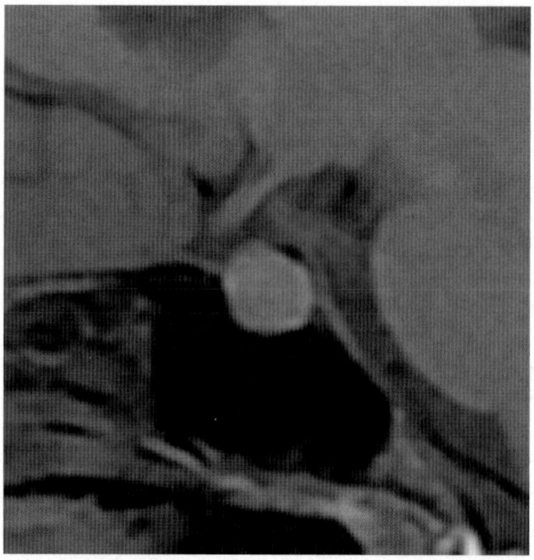

> **Key Point**
>
> Dynamic pituitary MR imaging improves sensitivity of microadenoma detection.

Indirect signs of an underlying mass, such as asymmetric convexity of the diaphragma sellae, asymmetry of the sellar floor, or infundibulum deviation, are neither sensitive nor specific and may be found in normal patients.[27] An infundibulum can be deviated toward a microadenoma.[10]

Although MR imaging is more sensitive for detection,[26] it is important to review the CT appearance of a microadenoma because a patient may have a contraindication to MR imaging. On noncontrast scans, a microadenoma can be hypointense and isodense to the gland.[28,29] Similar to MR imaging, thin-section dynamic imaging is helpful for detection, particularly for the

Fig. 6. Physiologic hypertrophy. Sagittal T1WI image in a 30-year-old pregnant patient shows physiologic enlargement of the pituitary gland, measuring 11 mm. The patient had been referred from an external imaging center for a potential macroadenoma, yet she was asymptomatic with normal laboratory values for her partum state.

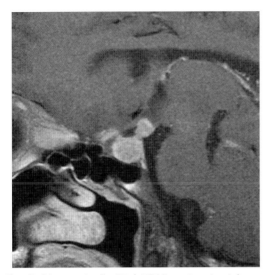

Fig. 7. Metastasis. Sagittal T1WI postcontrast image shows abnormal enlargement of the pituitary gland and the infundibulum. The structures normally enhance but are enlarged. The patient had a history of breast cancer and had metastatic breast cancer with restaging.

precontrast isointense mass. Classically, the microadenoma has decreased and delayed enhancement compared with the surrounding normal enhancing pituitary gland.[30] Uncommonly, the microadenoma can have early enhancement relative to the gland.[31] A microadenoma may be obscured if it is very small or there is extensive dental artifact.

Depending on the subtype of microadenoma, patients undergo medical treatment or transsphenoidal microsurgical resection.[16] Surgery may be performed based on laboratory analysis even if a microadenoma is not seen on MR imaging.

Differential Diagnosis

Nonneoplastic cysts, such as a small intrasellar RCC or pars intermedia cyst, can mimic a nonenhancing, cystic microadenoma. In addition, the insertion of the sphenoid osseous septum may mimic a nonenhancing microadenoma.[32]

APOPLEXY

Clinically symptomatic pituitary apoplexy refers to a specific acute clinical presentation of headache, nausea, visual deficits, altered mental status, ophthalmoplegia, or endocrine deficiencies caused by acute hemorrhagic or ischemic/necrotic pituitary infarction.[33,34] The potential resultant hypopituitarism may be life-threatening. The term subclinical pituitary apoplexy should not be confused with this entity; it is a term used in the literature to refer to asymptomatic pituitary ischemia or hemorrhage found on imaging or pathology specimens.[35]

Although incidences vary depending on the series, apoplexy most commonly occurs in a pre-existing macroadenoma,[36] which can be either functional or nonfunctional.[37] Apoplexy can also occur in an RCC,[38] microadenoma,[39] or even a normal pituitary gland.[33] It can also rarely occur after initiation of bromocriptine or cabergoline for a prolactin-secreting adenoma.[40]

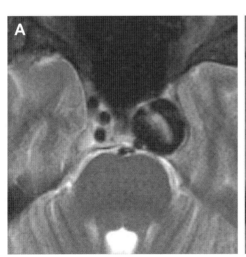
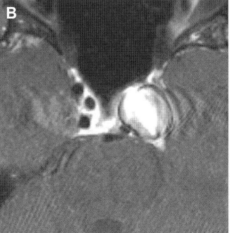

Fig. 8. Cavernous ICA aneurysm. (*A*) Axial fat-saturated T2WI image shows a left parasellar (cavernous sinus) mass with a rim of hypointense signal and central hyperintense signal. (*B*) Axial T1WI fat-saturated, postcontrast imaging shows enhancement and the characteristic pulsation artifact (in the phase encoding direction) from the partially thrombosed, yet patent aneurysm.

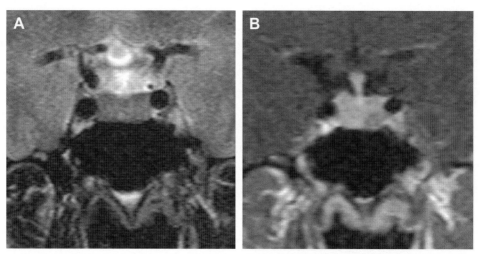

Fig. 9. Prolactin-producing microadenoma. (*A*) Coronal fat-saturated, T2WI image through the sella turcica shows a normal-sized and normal-signal pituitary gland. (*B*) Coronal T1WI postcontrast image shows a subcentimeter area of hypointensity in the left lateral pituitary gland that showed delayed enhancement on dynamic imaging.

Controversy exists regarding the role and timing of surgery compared with medical management. Although some retrospective series recommend conservative support, surgical decompression may be warranted if the patient is unstable or has progressive visual deficits.[37,41] Patients may also need long-term hormone replacement.[42]

CT is not sensitive for pituitary apoplexy detection.[43] CT features depend on the subtype of apoplexy (hemorrhagic or ischemic/necrotic) as well as timing of imaging relative to symptoms. The sella may appear normal, show an isodense/hypodense sellar mass,[44,45] or show a hyperdense mass as a result of hemorrhage.[46,47]

If imaging is obtained days or weeks after symptom onset, it is difficult to differentiate between necrosis, remote hemorrhage, or bland infarction.[48] Although most case reports or series do not include postcontrast imaging, there can be nonenhancement[49,50] or inhomogeneous heterogeneous enhancement,[51] often attributed to an underlying adenoma. Sphenoid sinus mucosal thickening is also a frequent finding with apoplexy, possibly an indirect marker of poor neurologic presentation or outcome.[52]

If apoplexy is suspected, MR imaging is superior in characterization of the pituitary and surrounding structures. It is important to evaluate for mass effect on the optic chiasm or involvement of the cavernous sinus. The T1WI and T2WI features depend on the subtype of apoplexy as well as the timing of imaging (ie, hemoglobin state of oxygenation). As a result, various imaging appearances have been described in the literature. There

can be heterogeneous T1WI and T2WI signal, including T1WI and T2WI hyperintense or hypointense signal characteristics. Enhancement is variable, including rim, homogeneous central, and inhomogeneous global patterns.[53] The adjacent dura uncommonly enhances, and apoplexy should not be mistaken for a diaphragma sellae or tuberculum sellae meningioma (**Fig. 10**A, C).[53,54]

A fluid-fluid level may be present and is pathognomonic for hemorrhage, although it is not pathognomonic for apoplexy.[53,55,56] A coronal or axial gradient echo sequence may also be useful to confirm the presence of hemorrhage.[57]

Key Point

Apoplexy can be life-threatening because of endocrine abnormalities. If suspected, MR imaging should be obtained to screen for an underlying mass and evaluate mass effect or invasion of surrounding structures. Imaging must be correlated with clinical presentation to appropriately diagnose apoplexy.

Differential Diagnosis

Macroadenoma

A macroadenoma can have a clinically silent or mildly symptomatic (eg, headache) hemorrhage. The presence of hemorrhage is not synonymous with the hemorrhagic subtype of pituitary apoplexy. Acutely symptomatic apoplexy has a distinct clinical presentation.

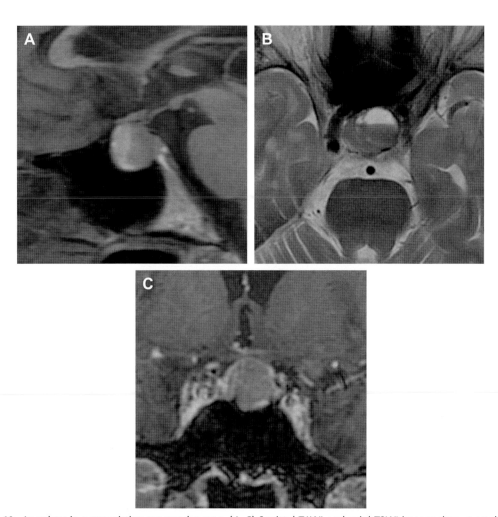

Fig. 10. Apoplexy in a preexisting macroadenoma. (*A*, *B*) Sagittal T1WI and axial T2WI images show a predominantly sellar mass with hyperintense and hypointense signal and a fluid-fluid level. The mass abuts the optic chiasm superiorly. (*C*) On coronal T1WI postcontrast imaging, the mass predominantly has nonenhancement with small peripheral areas of nodular enhancement. Enhancement can be variable in apoplexy, including rim, homogeneous central, and inhomogeneous global patterns, depending on the presence of an underlying mass (eg, macroadenoma) and the type of apoplexy.

RCC

An RCC can have T1WI hyperintense signal similar to subacute hemorrhage seen with the hemorrhagic subtype of apoplexy. However, an RCC is often either an incidental finding or the symptoms are subacute or chronic in origin, which helps to differentiate it from acutely symptomatic apoplexy.

RCC

Arising from Rathke pouch remnants, an RCC is a congenital, nonneoplastic benign cyst. An RCC most commonly involves both the sellar and suprasellar compartments, although it can be solely sellar or rarely solely suprasellar in location.[33,58] An RCC is commonly an incidental discovery on imaging or autopsy, although up to 3% to 9% of symptomatic sellar lesions are caused by RCCs.[33,58] A symptomatic RCC can present with headache, visual disturbances, or endocrine disorders from mass effect on surrounding structures.[33] Rarely, an RCC can present with apoplexy caused by intracystic hemorrhage.[38]

If asymptomatic, an RCC may undergo surveillance imaging. Symptomatic patients undergo surgical drainage or resection. Debate continues regarding complete excision versus partial removal, weighing the risks of recurrence against postoperative morbidity.[59,60] Postoperative surveillance imaging is important because 10% to 14% of RCCs can reaccumulate.[33,58]

Imaging features of an RCC vary among published series.[33,58] On CT, an RCC is an oval, dumbbell-shaped, or multilobular, well-circumscribed mass that is most commonly hypointense, although it can be hyperintense in attenuation as well.[4] There is no internal enhancement, although up to 50% of cases can have rim enhancement, either because of the displaced pituitary gland or the cyst wall.[33] Approximately 5% can have faint rim calcification (Fig. 11A).[33]

MR imaging features of an RCC are variable, depending on its contents (eg, protein, cholesterol, hemorrhage). On T1WI images, an RCC can be hyperintense (38%–40%), hypointense (24%–40%), or isointense (17%–36%). On T2WI images, most are hyperintense (71%–75%).[33,58] On thin-section imaging, an intracystic nodule, composed of protein and cellular debris, is seen in up to 70% of RCCs. The nodule does not enhance and can have T1WI isointense, hyperintense, or hypointense and T2WI isointense or hypointense signal depending on the published series. Similar to CT, an RCC can uncommonly have rim enhancement, as a result of a displaced pituitary gland or pericystic inflammation (see Fig. 11B, C).[33,58]

Key Point

An RCC can have various imaging appearances, particularly on a T1WI sequence. A nonenhancing, intracystic nodule is a helpful discriminator.

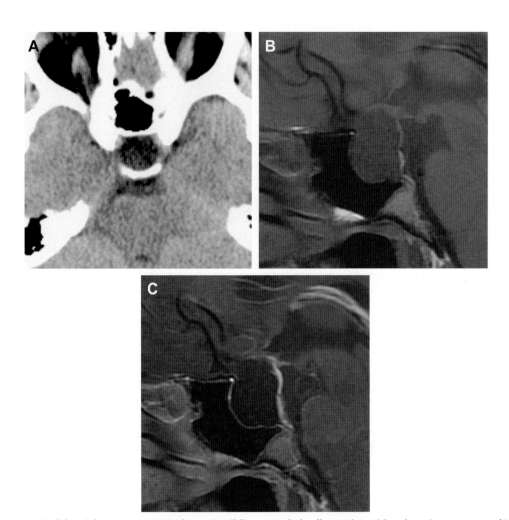

Fig. 11. RCC. (A) Axial noncontrast CT shows a mildly expanded sella turcica with a hypointense mass. (B, C) Sagittal T1WI precontrast and postcontrast images show a predominantly sellar with suprasellar extension mass, which follows CSF signal (T2WI signal not shown) and exerts mass effect on the optic chiasm. There is rim enhancement, attributed to wall inflammation or displaced pituitary tissue.

Differential Diagnosis

Adenoma

Although a macroadenoma may be cystic/necrotic, it enhances more extensively than an RCC and has more heterogeneous signal. A cystic, nonenhancing microadenoma may be difficult to differentiate from a small, sellar RCC. Endocrine laboratory values may be helpful, although RCC can present with endocrine abnormalities as well.

Craniopharyngioma

The adamantinomatous subtype can be cystic and present as a sellar/suprasellar mass similar to an RCC. However, in contrast to an RCC, it usually has nodular or rim enhancement and associated calcifications. If a craniopharyngioma is extensively cystic without calcification or solid enhancing components, it can be mistaken for an RCC.

Nonneoplastic cysts

An arachnoid cyst is uncommon in this location and follows CSF attenuation or signal on all sequences. An epidermoid is rare in this location and follows CSF attenuation or MR imaging signal except for fluid-attenuated inversion recovery (FLAIR) and diffusion-weighted sequences. A dermoid is often suprasellar or parasellar in location and not intrasellar; in addition, it follows fat signal on MR imaging.

MENINGIOMA

After adenoma, a meningioma is the second most common sellar and parasellar region tumor.[61] Five percent to 10% of meningiomas occur in the sellar and parasellar region.[4] A meningioma can originate from the tuberculum sellae, diaphragma sellae, sphenoid wing, cavernous sinus dura, or planum sphenoidale.

Depending on its size and location, a meningioma may be an incidental finding or present with headache, visual deterioration, cranial neuropathy, seizures, and even pituitary dysfunction. If small and asymptomatic, a meningioma may be followed with serial imaging. Depending on extent, treatment includes surgery or radiation therapy.[62–64]

On CT, a meningioma presents as a solid, extra-axial hyperdense mass, with or without areas of cystic degeneration/necrosis.[4] Although not always present, associated CT findings include tumor calcification, hyperostosis, and posterior ethmoid or sphenoid sinus enlargement (pneumosinus dilatans).[65,66] A meningioma may have homogeneous or heterogeneous enhancement.

On MR imaging, most meningiomas are T1WI and T2WI isointense to gray matter. Heterogeneous T2WI signal may be present as a result of calcium (hypointense), cystic changes (hyperintense), or hemorrhage (variable). Given its vascularity, there is avid postcontrast enhancement. Supportive imaging features for a meningioma include hyperostosis, a thickened, enhancing dural tail, and encasement, narrowing, and potential occlusion of the cavernous or supraclinoid segments of the ICA (**Fig. 12**A, B; **Fig. 13**A, D).[61,65,67]

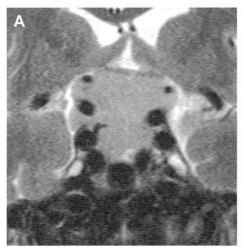
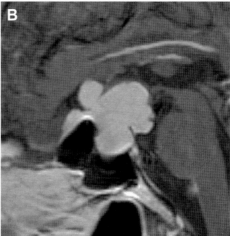

Fig. 12. Diaphragma sellae meningioma. (*A*) Coronal fat-saturated T2WI image shows a predominantly suprasellar, homogeneously T2 isointense mass that partially encases the right supraclinoid ICA. (*B*) Sagittal T1WI postcontrast imaging shows homogeneous enhancement, mild enlargement of the sella turcica (relative to the size of the mass), and a ventral dural tail. The center of the mass as well as its imaging features help to differentiate it from a macroadenoma, even although a normal pituitary gland is not well seen.

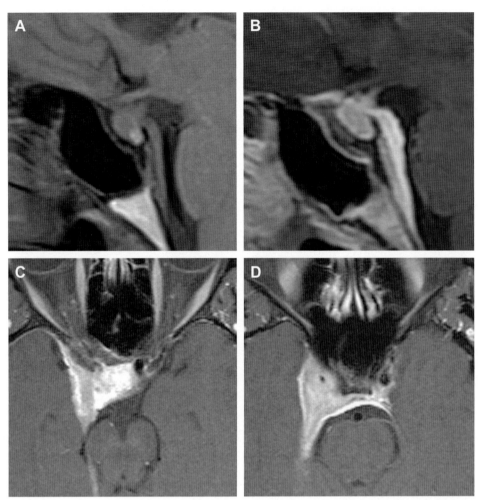

Fig. 13. Cavernous sinus meningioma. (*A*) Sagittal T1WI image shows a normal-sized sella turcica with preservation of the neurohypophyseal bright spot. (*B*) On sagittal T1 postcontrast imaging, there is abnormal thickening and enhancement of the retroclival dura. (*C, D*) On axial T1WI postcontrast imaging, there is an extra-axial, dural-based mass infiltrating the right cavernous sinus and narrowing the ICA. Note the hyperostosis of the right anterior clinoid process.

Key Point

When evaluating a suspected meningioma, look for supportive imaging features (eg, hyperostosis, dural enhancement). It is important to evaluate for potential cavernous/supraclinoid ICA encasement or narrowing.

Differential Diagnosis

Macroadenoma

A macroadenoma may be confused with a meningioma if the macroadenoma has a dural tail, although this is infrequently seen.[11,12] Features that support a meningioma instead of a macroadenoma include identification of a normal-sized

pituitary gland, intense and homogeneous contrast enhancement, a predominantly suprasellar location, and mild enlargement of the sella turcica relative to the size of the tumor.[68] It is important to differentiate these entities because different surgical approaches (craniotomy vs transsphenoidal resection) may be used.

CRANIOPHARYNGIOMA

A craniopharyngioma is a tumor that arises from squamous epithelial remnants of the Rathke pouch. Although it can present in adults, a craniopharyngioma is more common in children and is the most common nonglial tumor in children.[69] The peak incidences of presentation occur between ages 5 and 14 years and less frequently, ages 40 to 74 years.[70,71] Presentation depends on size and location and can include headache, nausea, vomiting, visual changes, hypothalamic or pituitary abnormalities, and hydrocephalus.

The tumor primarily occurs in the infundibular region, although it can arise anywhere along the path of the craniopharyngeal duct, including the nasopharynx, sinonasal region, sphenoid bone, and third ventricle.[72] Although series may differ in overall distribution, more than 90% of craniopharyngiomas have a suprasellar component, either purely suprasellar or sellar/suprasellar in origin. A craniopharyngioma uncommonly arises solely within the sella turcica and rarely within the third ventricle.[65,73]

Although transitional or mixed lesions have been described, there are 2 major histologic subtypes of craniopharyngioma (adamantinomatous and papillary) that vary in clinical and imaging presentation.[72] The adamantinomatous subtype is the most common and predominantly presents in younger patients as a multiloculated, cystic, solid, calcified mass. In contrast, the papillary subtype almost exclusively presents in adults as a predominantly solid, less commonly calcified mass.

Debate continues regarding treatment algorithms. Treatment has traditionally consisted of attempted gross total resection. Adjuvant radiotherapy is often administered, particularly with incomplete resection or recurrent disease.[73,74] However, other studies have suggested that subtotal resection with adjuvant radiotherapy may be more appropriate to minimize morbidity from aggressive resections.[75] Even with gross total resection, long-term surveillance imaging is important given potential recurrence.

CT and MR imaging can be heterogeneous depending on the consistency of the tumor. On CT, the adamantinomatous subtype appears as an isodense to hypodense, multiloculated, sellar/suprasellar mass with predominantly cystic or solid and cystic components. There is often nodular or thin-rim calcification of the cystic components as well as heterogeneous enhancement. In contrast, the papillary subtype is more commonly solid or solid with small cystic components, isodense in attenuation, noncalcified, and with homogeneous enhancement (**Fig. 14**A, B).[72]

Because the cysts contain cholesterol, protein, and hemorrhage, the MR imaging appearance can be variable.[76] Fluid signal is hyperintense to CSF on T1WI sequences and mixed or hyperintense in T2WI signal. Fluid-fluid levels may be present.[76] The solid components are isointense to hypointense on T1WI sequences and inhomogeneously T2WI hyperintense. There is heterogeneous enhancement of both the solid components and cystic walls. Calcification may appear as T1WI/T2WI hypointense foci or gradient echo blooming (**Fig. 15**A, D).[65,72,73]

Key Point

A craniopharyngioma is the most common nonglial tumor in children. The most common presentation is a predominantly suprasellar mass with solid and cystic components, calcification, and enhancement.

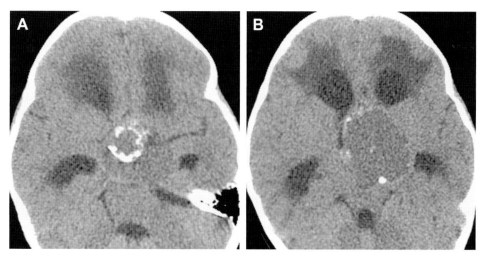

Fig. 14. Adamantinomatous craniopharyngioma. (*A, B*) Axial noncontrast CT shows a large predominantly hypodense suprasellar mass with peripheral calcification. Note the resultant obstructive hydrocephalus with transependymal flow caused by mass effect on the third ventricle/foramen of Monro.

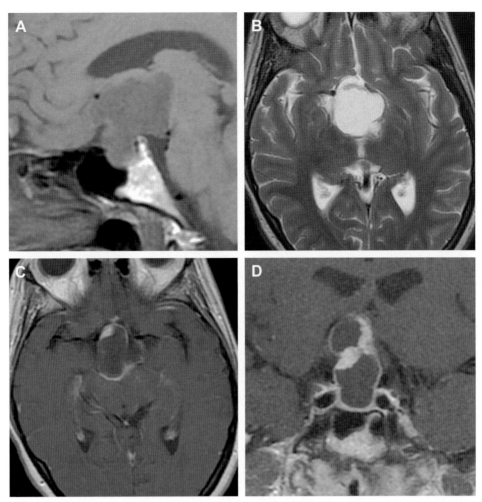

Fig. 15. Adamantinomatous craniopharyngioma (different patient). (*A, B*) Sagittal T1WI and axial T2WI images show a slightly hyperintense to CSF, predominantly suprasellar, cystic mass. There is a smaller intrasellar component. (*C, D*) Axial and coronal T1WI postcontrast imaging shows peripheral, nodular enhancement.

Differential Diagnosis

RCC

Although cystic, an RCC is more homogeneous in appearance compared with the cystic adamantinomatous subtype, and an RCC uncommonly is calcified. A craniopharyngioma has nodular or cystic rim enhancement, in contrast to an RCC, which is nonenhancing or has thin rim enhancement because of inflammation or surrounding pituitary tissue.

Other nonneoplastic cysts

An arachnoid cyst follows CSF attenuation or signal on all sequences and does not calcify. An epidermoid follows CSF attenuation or MR imaging signal except for lack of nullification of CSF signal on FLAIR sequence. In addition, an epidermoid has restricted diffusion on diffusion-weighted imaging and no enhancement or minimal

peripheral enhancement. Although a suprasellar dermoid can have T1WI hyperintense signal as well as calcification, it uncommonly enhances and follows fat signal.

Hypothalamic-chiasmatic glioma

A hypothalamic-chiasmatic glioma (eg, astrocytoma) does occur in children, but in contrast to the adamantinomatous subtype, it is usually a predominantly solid, enhancing mass, without associated calcification. T1WI hyperintense signal is more commonly seen within a craniopharyngioma. The papillary subtype presents in an older patient population and has a more heterogeneous imaging appearance.

EPIDERMOID CYST

An epidermoid is a rare developmental inclusion cyst consisting of ectodermal epithelial elements.

It can occur primarily in the suprasellar or parasellar location or as a result of extension from the prepontine cistern, sylvian fissure, or cerebellopontine angle. The mass is irregular and lobulated and can insinuate and surround neurovascular structures.

An epidermoid can be asymptomatic or, depending on location, can cause seizures, hemifacial spasm, trigeminal neuralgia, gait disturbances, vertigo, or other symptoms. Rarely, an epidermoid cyst can undergo malignant transformation.[77] Although total excision is desirable, surgeons may perform subtotal resection if there is risk of cranial nerve or ischemic deficits with resection.[78]

On CT, the mass is hypodense, often similar to CSF attenuation, without enhancement. Dystrophic calcification is uncommonly present.[79,80] On MR imaging, an epidermoid cyst is classically iso-intense or slightly hyperintense to CSF signal on T1WI and T2WI sequences, with failure of CSF signal nullification on FLAIR sequence. Although hyperintense on a diffusion-weighted imaging sequence, it is often isointense or slightly hyperintense to parenchyma on the apparent diffusion coefficient map.[63,80,81] There is no enhancement or minimal peripheral enhancement.[80] Despite these classic features, there are small series and case reports of epidermoids that have atypical imaging features, such as high attenuation on CT or T1WI/T2WI heterogeneous mixed signal (**Fig. 16**A, C).[81,82]

> **Key Point**
>
> FLAIR or diffusion sequences differentiate an epidermoid from an arachnoid cyst.

Differential Diagnosis

Nonneoplastic cysts
An arachnoid cyst is isodense to CSF on CT and has nulled CSF signal on a FLAIR sequence. Whereas a dermoid can be hypodense on CT, it is differentiated by fat signal on MR imaging. Post-inflammatory cysts (eg, neurocysticercosis) commonly localize to the cisterns. Although these features are not always present, imaging findings that support neurocysticercosis include other sites of infection (eg, parenchyma, ventricles), the presence of a scolex, and rim enhancement.

DERMOID CYST

A dermoid cyst is a congenital inclusion cyst of ectodermal elements (eg, hair, sebaceous/sweat glands, cholesterol crystals) that is most commonly found in the parasellar and suprasellar or other midline locations.[3] Uncommonly, a dermoid can rupture into the subarachnoid space, potentially causing aseptic meningitis, seizures, hydrocephalus, vasospasm, cerebral ischemia, and focal neurologic deficits.[83] Asymptomatic patients with dermoid rupture have also been described.[84] Complete surgical resection is the mainstay of treatment. However, given adherence to surrounding neurovascular structures, subtotal resection may be appropriate to minimize surgical morbidity.[83]

On CT, a dermoid cyst is a nonenhancing, well-circumscribed, hypodense mass. It uncommonly has associated calcification of its capsular rim.[83,84] On MR imaging, a dermoid cyst has predominantly T1WI hyperintense (fat) signal[83] although it may have associated T1WI hypointense signal components as well.[84] T2WI signal is heterogeneous, ranging from hypointense to hyperintense.[84] There is usually minimal to no enhancement of the mass. T1WI hyperintense foci within the subarachnoid space or fat-fluid levels in the lateral ventricles are pathognomonic for a ruptured dermoid (**Fig. 17**; **Fig. 18**A, B).[83]

> **Key Point**
>
> Fat signal within the subarachnoid spaces or ventricles is pathognomonic for a ruptured dermoid. A ruptured dermoid can present with seizures, focal neurologic deficits, or ischemia.

Differential Diagnosis

Craniopharyngioma
A craniopharyngioma can present as a suprasellar mass with T1WI hyperintense features caused by cholesterol, protein, and hemorrhage. However, in contrast to a dermoid, it does not follow fat signal on the fat suppression sequences, usually has associated solid and cystic components, and enhances.

Lipoma
A lipoma is commonly found in the interhemispheric fissure or quadrigeminal/superior cerebellar cistern regions, although it does occur in the suprasellar/interpeduncular regions as well. A lipoma has a more homogeneous appearance on CT and MR imaging compared with an unruptured dermoid. Both can have associated calcifications (**Fig. 19**A, B).

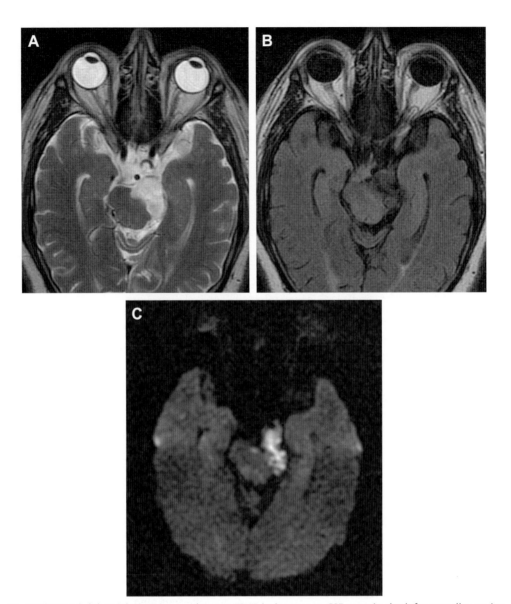

Fig. 16. Epidermoid. (*A*) Axial T2WI image shows a T2WI isointense to CSF mass in the left parasellar region exerting mass effect on the ventral-lateral midbrain. (*B, C*) Axial FLAIR and diffusion show lack of CSF signal nullification and hyperintense diffusion signal. These features differentiate an epidermoid from an arachnoid cyst.

HYPOTHALAMIC (TUBER CINEREUM) HAMARTOMA

A hypothalamic hamartoma is a rare, congenital malformation consisting of hyperplastic neural tissue/heterotopic gray matter that originates from the mammillary bodies, tuber cinereum, or hypothalamus itself.[85] A patient can present with central precocious puberty or gelastic epilepsy. The seizures are often difficult to medically manage, contributing to cognitive and behavior deterioration. Treatment includes medical treatment or excision.[86] Radiotherapy has also been used to treat small or postoperative residual hamartoma.[87]

On imaging, the hamartoma presents as either a pedunculated mass protruding into the interpeduncular cistern or a sessile/intrahypothalamic mass protruding medially into the third ventricle. A hamartoma can range from a few millimeters to centimeters in size.

On CT, it is a well-circumscribed, round, nonenhancing, isodense to gray matter mass. On MR imaging it has T1WI isointense and T2WI isointense to slightly hyperintense signal compared with gray matter and does not enhance.[88] T2WI hyperintense signal characteristics are associated with increased glial contents in the malformations.[89] The

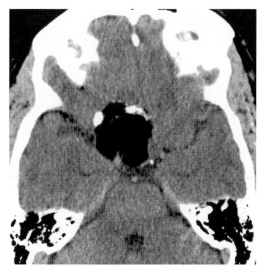

Fig. 17. Dermoid. Nonenhanced CT shows a large hypodense, partially calcified suprasellar mass. Region of interest values ranged from −22 to −40 Hounsfield units (*not shown*).

clinical presentation and MR imaging features differentiate a hypothalamic hamartoma from other pediatric suprasellar masses, such as a craniopharyngioma, germinoma, or glioma (eg, pilocytic astrocytoma) (**Fig. 20**A, C).

Key Point

If there is a history of precocious puberty or gelastic epilepsy in a child, thin-slice, multiplanar MR imaging of the hypothalamus is important to evaluate for an underlying hypothalamic hamartoma.

HYPOTHALAMIC-CHIASMATIC GLIOMA

An astrocytoma is the most common pediatric central nervous system tumor.[69,90] An astrocytoma localizing to the optic pathway or hypothalamic region is typically a low-grade tumor, most commonly a pilocytic astrocytoma. An optic pathway glioma is commonly seen associated with neurofibromatosis type 1, although this association is not always present.[91]

Depending on patient age, location, size, and symptoms, hypothalamic-chiasmatic tumors may undergo surveillance imaging. Case reports of spontaneous regression support surveillance imaging in asymptomatic patients.[92] If patients become symptomatic, chemotherapy often is the initial treatment although surgical resection may be needed for obstructive symptoms. Radiotherapy can be used as well, but given potential long-term morbidity in children, is typically reserved for more advanced cases.[91,93,94] Leptomeningeal spread is rare, but both synchronous and metachronous presentation of CSF spread has been described.[95] Surveillance imaging is recommended, particularly if there is subtotal resection.

Although CT can be used for hypothalamic-chiasmatic astrocytoma evaluation, MR imaging is superior in showing the intracranial extent and relationship to the surrounding structures. On CT, the hypothalamic-chiasmatic astrocytoma mass is hypointense or isointense with enhancement.[96,97]

On MR imaging, a hypothalamic-chiasmatic astrocytoma has classically T2WI hyperintense and T1WI hypointense to isointense signal and mild to avid enhancement.[90] There is usually

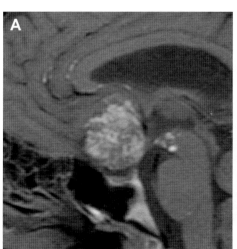

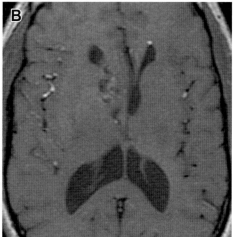

Fig. 18. Dermoid (same case as Fig. 17). (*A*) Sagittal T1WI image shows a hyperintense suprasellar mass as well as scattered T1WI hyperintense foci in the interpeduncular cistern and pericallosal subarachnoid spaces. (*B*) Axial T1WI image shows foci of fat signal in the sylvian fissures, left frontal horn, and right foramen of Monro region caused by the rupture dermoid.

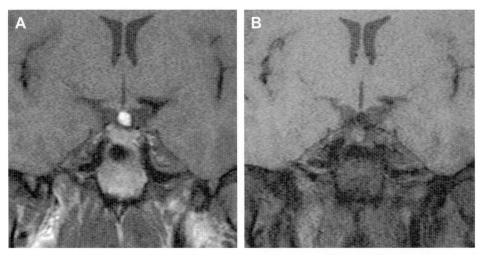

Fig. 19. Lipoma. Coronal T1WI and T1WI with fat-saturation images show a lipoma adjacent to the infundibulum. Note the homogeneous fat suppression seen with a lipoma.

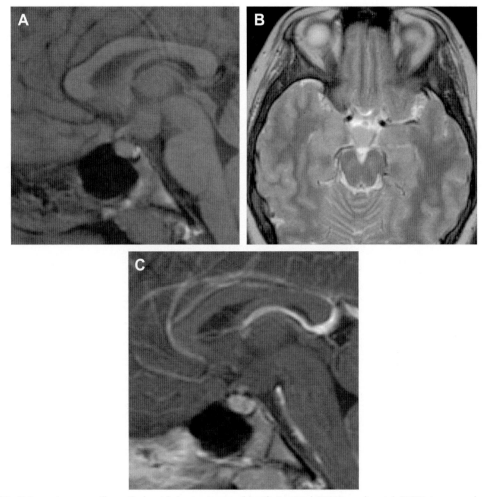

Fig. 20. Tuber cinereum (hypothalamic) hamartoma. (*A*, *B*) Sagittal T1WI and axial T2WI images show an isointense to gray matter, pedunculated mass in the tuber cinereum region. (*C*) Sagittal T1WI postcontrast image shows no enhancement.

complete absence or mild T2WI hyperintense signal in the surrounding brain. Rarely, a pilocytic astrocytoma in this location can have more aggressive imaging features, such as central necrosis or infiltrating margins.[98] In addition, its enhancement pattern may change over time; this does not indicate malignant degeneration if the tumor is otherwise stable in size (**Fig. 21**A, C).[99]

In recent years, a pilomyxoid variant of astrocytoma has been described in the hypothalamic-chiasmatic region as well as other locations. A pilomyxoid astrocytoma has different histologic features and a worse prognosis given the increased tendency for local recurrence and leptomeningeal spread. Although some studies have suggested an increased incidence of central necrosis, peritumoral infiltration, and nonenhancing solid components, there are no reliable imaging features to differentiate a pilomyxoid astrocytoma from a pilocytic astrocytoma.[100–102]

> **Key Point**
>
> A hypothalamic-chiasmatic glioma can be seen in children and adults and has an increased incidence in syndromes such as neurofibromatosis type 1. It is important to characterize the extent (eg, orbital extension) as well as complications (eg, hydrocephalus) to guide management.

Differential Diagnosis

Craniopharyngioma

A craniopharyngioma can also occur in children and should be differentiated from a hypothalamic-chiasmatic glioma given different treatment

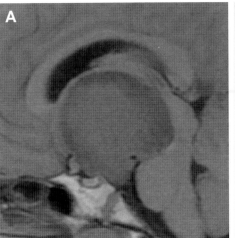
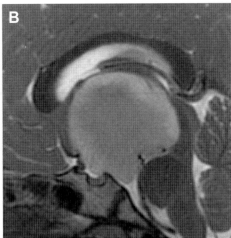
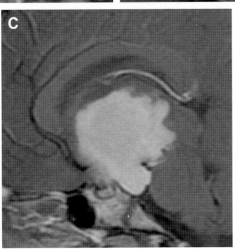

Fig. 21. Hypothalamic pilocytic astrocytoma. (*A*) Sagittal T1WI image shows a large mixed isointense and hypointense suprasellar mass. Given size, it is difficult to differentiate its origin from the hypothalamus or optic pathway/chiasm. Note that the sella is normal in size. (*B*) Sagittal T2WI image shows predominant hyperintense signal. (*C*) Sagittal T1WI postcontrast image shows avid, solid enhancement. There is no evidence of leptomeningeal spread.

approaches. Multiplanar MR imaging can usually determine if the mass originates from the optic chiasm/hypothalamus or exerts mass effect on them. Such differentiation may be difficult when the mass is large or imaging is limited by motion. In contrast to the hypothalamic-chiasmatic glioma presenting in a child, a craniopharyngioma is usually multiloculated, solid, cystic, and partially calcified. In addition, T1WI hyperintense signal is more commonly seen within a craniopharyngioma compared with a glioma.

Germinoma

A germinoma can present in a young patient as a solid, avidly enhancing hypothalamic/infundibular mass. Clinically, a patient more commonly presents with hypothalamic-pituitary axis dysfunction (eg, diabetes insipidus), when compared with the clinical presentation of a glioma. Imaging features supporting a suprasellar germinoma include the simultaneous presentation of a pineal region mass (bifocal disease), leptomeningeal dissemination, and restricted diffusion caused by cellularity of the tumor. Although they may be within the normal range, abnormal tumor markers from the blood and CSF support germinoma (**Fig. 22**A, B).

Langerhans cell histiocytosis

Although Langerhans cell histiocytosis can have multiple presentations, its most common central nervous system presentation is an infiltrative, enhancing mass involving the infundibulum. Clinically, it presents in a very young patient with new-onset hypothalamic dysfunction. Supportive

imaging features include additional sites of disease (eg, calvarium, mastoid), although synchronous disease may not be present.

CHORDOMA

A chordoma is a rare, slow-growing, locally aggressive tumor arising from persistent notochord rests, most commonly localizing to the sacrococcygeal, mobile spine, and clival regions. In the skull base, it most often originates in the midline from the spheno-occipital synchondrosis. Less commonly it is found in the sellar area, paranasal sinuses, nasopharynx, or intradurally.[103] It can be large at diagnosis, extending into the sphenoid sinus, sellar/parasellar region, temporal bone, posterior skull base (jugular foramen, occipital condyles), and nasopharyngeal/parapharyngeal spaces. Clinical presentation often includes a cranial neuropathy[104,105] as well as other nonspecific symptoms, such as headache.

CT and MR imaging are complementary in pretreatment evaluation. MR imaging better characterizes involvement of central and posterior skull base neurovascular structures (eg, carotids, cavernous sinuses, foramina), whereas CT better detects cortical destruction and any associated calcifications. CT or MR angiography is helpful when evaluating for cavernous sinus, ICA, or vertebral-basilar involvement because it may alter surgical approach.[104]

On CT, the classic appearance is a midline, expansile, soft tissue mass with lytic destruction of the clivus and surrounding structures.[103,106] Small

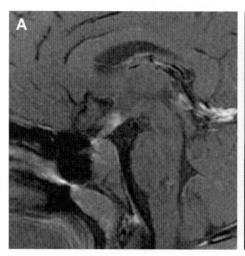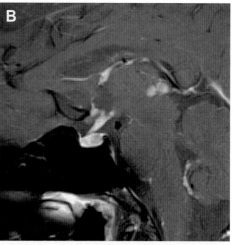

Fig. 22. Germinoma. (*A*) Sagittal T1WI fat-saturated, postcontrast image shows abnormal enlargement of the infundibulum. The patient presented with diabetes insipidus and had no neurohypophyseal T1WI bright spot on precontrast imaging. (*B*) Sagittal T1WI fat-saturated, postcontrast image shows bifocal germinoma with abnormal masslike enhancement of the pineal gland, infundibulum, and ventral third ventricle recesses.

osseous fragments/trabeculae may be present from either destroyed bone or intratumoral calcifications. Given associated necrosis and hemorrhage, there is heterogeneous, marked enhancement (**Fig. 23**A, B).

On MR imaging, the mass has predominantly intermediate to hypointense T1WI signal and T2WI hyperintense signal.[103,106] There may be small T1WI hyperintense and T2WI hypointense foci caused by mucoid and hemorrhage. Entrapped bone spicules as well as septa within the tumor can have T2WI hypointense signal as well. The tumor has heterogeneous, strong enhancement. Occasionally, it has a honeycomb pattern[107] with peripheral enhancement of lobules or septa and more central nonenhancement. Although mass effect on the pons (the thumb sign) has been described on sagittal MR imaging, it is not always present (see **Fig. 23**C, E).

The optimum treatment algorithm is surgical resection with supplemental radiotherapy.[105] Surgical strategies vary because of a surgeon's preference and the tumor extent, and a patient may undergo multiple surgeries to maximize initial tumor resection because it positively correlates with outcome.[104,105] As a result, it is important on immediate postoperative imaging to identify residual disease to guide reoperation or adjuvant therapy options. Total en-bloc resection is difficult to obtain, and although research continues regarding the efficacy of radiotherapy, most patients receive adjuvant therapy.[105] Local recurrence is common,[104] with treatment regimens including reoperation, reirradiation, or chemotherapy.

> **Key Point**
>
> A chordoma is a locally aggressive tumor with outcomes correlated with resection. It is important to obtain CT and MR imaging for staging and closely evaluate postoperative imaging for residual disease.

Differential Diagnosis

Invasive macroadenoma
An invasive macroadenoma can mimic a chordoma by caudal invasion/destruction of the basisphenoid bone. If a normal pituitary gland cannot be visualized, consider endocrine evaluation before surgical biopsy. Other features that may support a macroadenoma include lack of prepontine cistern extension and exclusive involvement of the sphenoid bone.[107]

Metastasis
A metastasis should remain in the differential, even if there is no history of malignancy. Detecting an additional osseous or intracranial lesion supports metastasis.

Other primary osseous malignancy
Other osseous malignancies, such as a plasmacytoma or lymphoma, are less common but remain in the differential. In contrast to a chordoma, a plasmacytoma generally presents with isointense to hyperintense T1WI and isointense to hypointense T2WI signal, the latter attributed to the cellularity and nucleocytoplasmic ratio.[108]

METASTASIS

A metastasis can involve the infundibulum or pituitary gland and mimic a primary sellar process, such as an adenoma. The most common metastatic tumors to the pituitary gland are breast and lung cancer.[109] Both the anterior and posterior gland can be affected, with some series supporting posterior gland and infundibulum preferential involvement, given a direct arterial supply (see **Fig. 7**).[109]

Although most metastases are clinically silent based on autopsy studies, patients can present with diabetes insipidus, anterior endocrine abnormalities, ophthalmoplegia from cavernous sinus invasion, and visual defects caused by suprasellar extension.[109,110]

> **Key Point**
>
> A metastasis should be considered in the differential for an enhancing sella or suprasellar mass, particularly if there is a history of breast or lung malignancy.

Differential Diagnosis

Macroadenoma
There are no specific differentiating imaging features between a macroadenoma and a pituitary metastasis. A dumbbell-shaped sellar/suprasellar mass with a wide waist at the level of the diaphragma sellae supports a slow-growing macroadenoma over a metastasis, which usually has a narrow waist.[111] However, the clinical history is more helpful in differentiation. A patient with a short duration of signs and symptoms, new-onset diabetes insipidus or ophthalmoplegia, or a quickly growing sellar mass supports a metastasis over a macroadenoma.[111] In addition, a metastasis uncommonly presents with hormonal excess.

OPERATIVE PLANNING

Preoperative imaging is obtained both for characterization and stereotactic localization. For

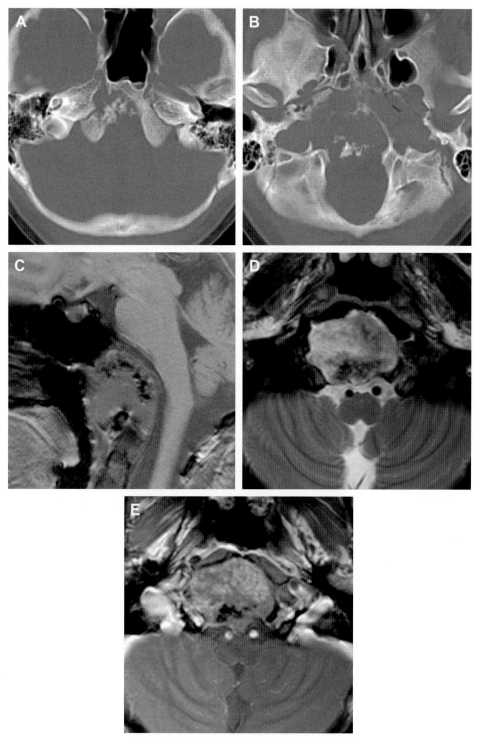

Fig. 23. Chondroid chordoma (a variant of chordoma). (*A, B*) Axial noncontrast CT shows a lytic lesion involving the clivus with associated osseous spicules/matrix. (*C, D*) Sagittal T1WI and axial T2WI images show a predominantly isointense T1 and hyperintense T2 mass with hypointense areas corresponding to the osseous spicules/matrix on the CT. Note the characteristic T2 hyperintense signal and midline location for chordoma. (*E*) Axial T1WI postcontrast image shows heterogeneous enhancement.

characterization, it is important to obtain multiplanar, thin-section imaging because the extent of disease (eg, cavernous sinus, central skull base foramina involvement) may alter the surgical approach. Fat suppression on postcontrasted MR imaging is particularly important when a process involves the skull base. Preoperative CT or MR angiography should be obtained if there is vascular displacement or encasement.

Depending on the size, primary location, and suspected disease of a sellar or parasellar mass, multiple surgical approaches may be taken. For a sellar mass, sublabial transsphenoidal surgery and the more recently developed transnasal endoscopic surgery are used.[112] Subfrontal craniotomy and other techniques may be used when the disease has a large suprasellar component. Knowledge of the surgical approach and potential anatomic variants that may affect outcomes is important. For example, it is important to assess for medially positioned internal carotid arteries within the sella turcica or dehiscence of the sphenoid bone around the arteries, given the increased risk of arterial injury from a transsphenoidal approach.

POSTOPERATIVE IMAGING EVALUATION

Postoperative imaging is important to obtain a baseline for subsequent comparison and to evaluate for complications, such as CSF leak and vascular or optic nerve injury. Depending on the suspected complication, tailored sequences are important, such as coronal T2WI images to evaluate the optic nerves or thin-section CT to look for an osseous defect as the source of the CSF leak. If a patient has new-onset hypothalamic-pituitary dysfunction, look for loss of neurohypophysis T1WI hyperintense signal, stalk transection, or other injury.

Postoperative imaging is particularly important because it may be difficult to differentiate residual tumor and fibrosis on imaging obtained months after surgery.[113] Postoperative hemorrhage, hemostatic agents, and packing material are often intermixed, causing heterogeneous T1WI and T2WI signal on MR imaging. Because fat packing is routinely used to prevent or treat a CSF leak, it is important to have fat-saturated postcontrast imaging in at least 1 plane.[114,115]

SUMMARY

The sellar and parasellar regions are anatomically and pathologically complex areas. In daily practice, adenomas, meningiomas, or aneurysms are the most common diseases. However, with more than 30 different potential entities localizing to this region, knowledge of the anatomy and diseases in addition to clinical information is essential for expert imaging differential diagnosis and management guidance.

REFERENCES

1. Elster AD. Modern imaging of the pituitary. Radiology 1993;187:1–14.
2. Friedman TC, Zuckerbraun E, Lee ML, et al. Dynamic pituitary MRI has high sensitivity and specificity for the diagnosis of mild Cushing's syndrome and should be part of the initial workup. Horm Metab Res 2007;39:451–6.
3. Bonneville F, Cattin F, Marsot-Dupuch K, et al. T1 signal hyperintensity in the sellar region: spectrum of findings. Radiographics 2006;26:93–113.
4. Pisaneschi M, Kapoor G. Imaging the sella and parasellar region. Neuroimaging Clin North Am 2005;15:203–19.
5. Daly AF, Tichomirowa MA, Beckers A. The epidemiology and genetics of pituitary adenomas. Best Pract Res Clin Endocrinol Metab 2009;23:543–54.
6. Miki Y, Kanagaki M, Takahashi JA, et al. Evaluation of pituitary macroadenomas with multidetector-row CT (MDCT): comparison with MR imaging. Neuroradiology 2007;49:327–33.
7. Zhao B, Wei YK, Li GL, et al. Extended transsphenoidal approach for pituitary adenomas invading the anterior cranial base, cavernous sinus, and clivus: a single-center experience with 126 consecutive cases. J Neurosurg 2010;112:108–17.
8. Chen X, Dai J, Ai L, et al. Clival invasion on multidetector CT in 390 pituitary macroadenomas: correlation with sex, subtype and rates of operative complication and recurrence. AJNR Am J Neuroradiol 2011;32:785–9.
9. Bonneville JF, Bonneville F, Cattin F. Magnetic resonance imaging of pituitary adenomas. Eur Radiol 2005;15:543–8.
10. Rumboldt Z. Pituitary adenomas. Top Magn Reson Imaging 2005;16:277–88.
11. Rokni-Yazdi H, Sotoudeh H. Prevalence of "dural tail sign" in patients with different intracranial pathologies. Eur J Radiol 2006;60:42–5.
12. Cattin F, Bonneville F, Andrea I, et al. Dural enhancement in pituitary macroadenomas. Neuroradiology 2000;42:505–8.
13. Hofstetter CP, Shin BJ, Mubita L, et al. Endoscopic endonasal transsphenoidal surgery for functional pituitary adenomas. Neurosurg Focus 2011;30:E10.
14. Cottier JP, Destrieux C, Brunereau L, et al. Cavernous sinus invasion by pituitary adenoma: MR imaging. Radiology 2000;215:463–9.
15. Vieira JO Jr, Cukiert A, Liberman B. Evaluation of magnetic resonance imaging criteria for cavernous

sinus invasion in patients with pituitary adenomas: logistic regression analysis and correlation with surgical findings. Surg Neurol 2006;65:130–5 [discussion: 5].

16. Chanson P, Salenave S. Diagnosis and treatment of pituitary adenomas. Minerva Endocrinol 2004;29: 241–75.

17. Simsek E, Simsek T, Savas-Erdeve S, et al. Pituitary hyperplasia mimicking pituitary macroadenoma in two adolescent patients with long-standing primary hypothyroidism: case reports and review of literature. Turk J Pediatr 2009;51:624–30.

18. Pandey P, Ojha BK, Mahapatra AK. Pediatric pituitary adenoma: a series of 42 patients. J Clin Neurosci 2005;12:124–7.

19. Matsumoto S, Hayase M, Imamura H, et al. A case of intrasellar meningioma mimicking pituitary adenoma. No Shinkei Geka 2001;29:551–7 [in Japanese].

20. Hanak BW, Zada G, Nayar VV, et al. Cerebral aneurysms with intrasellar extension: a systematic review of clinical, anatomical, and treatment characteristics. J Neurosurg 2012;116:164–78.

21. Pluta RM, Nieman L, Doppman JL, et al. Extrapituitary parasellar microadenoma in Cushing's disease. J Clin Endocrinol Metab 1999;84:2912–23.

22. Portocarrero-Ortiz L, Bonifacio-Delgadillo D, Sotomayor-Gonzalez A, et al. A modified protocol using half-dose gadolinium in dynamic 3-Tesla magnetic resonance imaging for detection of ACTH-secreting pituitary tumors. Pituitary 2010;13:230–5.

23. Rennert J, Doerfler A. Imaging of sellar and parasellar lesions. Clin Neurol Neurosurg 2007;109:111–24.

24. Usui T, Izawa S, Sano T, et al. Clinical and molecular features of a TSH-secreting pituitary microadenoma. Pituitary 2005;8:127–34.

25. Xing B, Deng K, Ren ZY, et al. Magnetic resonance imaging characteristics and surgical results of adrenocorticotropin-secreting pituitary adenomas. Chin Med Sci J 2008;23:44–8.

26. Ciric I, Zhao JC, Du H, et al. Transsphenoidal surgery for Cushing disease: experience with 136 patients. Neurosurgery 2012;70:70–80 [discussion: 1].

27. Hall WA, Luciano MG, Doppman JL, et al. Pituitary magnetic resonance imaging in normal human volunteers: occult adenomas in the general population. Ann Intern Med 1994;120:817–20.

28. Wu W, Thuomas KA. Pituitary microadenoma. MR appearance and correlation with CT. Acta Radiol 1995;36:529–35.

29. Hemminghytt S, Kalkhoff RK, Daniels DL, et al. Computed tomographic study of hormone-secreting microadenomas. Radiology 1983;146:65–9.

30. Abe T, Izumiyama H, Fujisawa I. Evaluation of pituitary adenomas by multidirectional multislice dynamic CT. Acta Radiol 2002;43:556–9.

31. Bonneville JF, Cattin F, Gorczyca W, et al. Pituitary microadenomas: early enhancement with dynamic CT–implications of arterial blood supply and potential importance. Radiology 1993;187:857–61.

32. D'Ercole M, Della Pepa GM, Carrozza C, et al. Two diagnostic pitfalls mimicking a prolactin-secreting microadenoma. J Clin Endocrinol Metab 2010;95:5171.

33. Kim E. Symptomatic Rathke's cleft cyst: clinical features and surgical outcomes. World Neurosurg 2011. [Epub ahead of print].

34. Semple PL, Webb MK, de Villiers JC, et al. Pituitary apoplexy. Neurosurgery 2005;56:65–72 [discussion: 3].

35. Liu ZH, Chang CN, Pai PC, et al. Clinical features and surgical outcome of clinical and subclinical pituitary apoplexy. J Clin Neurosci 2010;17:694–9.

36. Moller-Goede DL, Brandle M, Landau K, et al. Pituitary apoplexy: re-evaluation of risk factors for bleeding into pituitary adenomas and impact on outcome. Eur J Endocrinol 2011;164:37–43.

37. Leyer C, Castinetti F, Morange I, et al. A conservative management is preferable in milder forms of pituitary tumor apoplexy. J Endocrinol Invest 2011;34:502–9.

38. Chaiban JT, Abdelmannan D, Cohen M, et al. Rathke's cleft cyst apoplexy: a newly characterized distinct clinical entity. J Neurosurg 2011;114: 318–24.

39. Randall BR, Couldwell WT. Apoplexy in pituitary microadenomas. Acta Neurochir (Wien) 2010;152:1737–40.

40. Singh P, Singh M, Cugati G, et al. Bromocriptine or cabergoline induced pituitary apoplexy: rare but life-threatening catastrophe. J Hum Reprod Sci 2011;4:59.

41. Seuk JW, Kim CH, Yang MS, et al. Visual outcome after transsphenoidal surgery in patients with pituitary apoplexy. J Korean Neurosurg Soc 2011;49: 339–44.

42. Ranabir S, Baruah MP. Pituitary apoplexy. Indian J Endocrinol Metab 2011;15(Suppl 3):S188–96.

43. Sibal L, Ball SG, Connolly V, et al. Pituitary apoplexy: a review of clinical presentation, management and outcome in 45 cases. Pituitary 2004;7:157–63.

44. Gruber A, Clayton J, Kumar S, et al. Pituitary apoplexy: retrospective review of 30 patients–is surgical intervention always necessary? Br J Neurosurg 2006;20:379–85.

45. Ostrov SG, Quencer RM, Hoffman JC, et al. Hemorrhage within pituitary adenomas: how often associated with pituitary apoplexy syndrome? AJR Am J Roentgenol 1989;153:153–60.

46. Harris SM, Cannon JE, Carroll PV, et al. Pituitary apoplexy: two very different presentations with one unifying diagnosis. JRSM Short Rep 2010;1:53.

47. Haboubi H, Azam I, Edavalath M, et al. Apoplexy in a corticotrophin-secreting pituitary macroadenoma: a case report and review of the literature. QJM 2010;103:607–9.

48. Nawar RN, AbdelMannan D, Selman WR, et al. Pituitary tumor apoplexy: a review. J Intensive Care Med 2008;23:75–90.

49. Perotti V, Dexter M. Post-partum pituitary apoplexy with bilateral third nerve palsy and bilateral carotid occlusion. J Clin Neurosci 2010;17:1328–30.

50. Thurtell MJ, Besser M, Halmagyi GM. Pituitary apoplexy causing isolated blindness after cardiac bypass surgery. Arch Ophthalmol 2008;126:576–8.

51. Das NK, Behari S, Banerji D. Pituitary apoplexy associated with acute cerebral infarct. J Clin Neurosci 2008;15:1418–20.

52. Liu JK, Couldwell WT. Pituitary apoplexy in the magnetic resonance imaging era: clinical significance of sphenoid sinus mucosal thickening. J Neurosurg 2006;104:892–8.

53. Piotin M, Tampieri D, Rufenacht DA, et al. The various MRI patterns of pituitary apoplexy. Eur Radiol 1999;9:918–23.

54. Koenigsberg RA, Patil K. Pituitary apoplexy associated with dural (tail) enhancement. AJR Am J Roentgenol 1994;163:227–8.

55. Ginath S, Golan A. Images in clinical medicine. Gestational pituitary-tumor apoplexy. N Engl J Med 2010;363:e10.

56. Yang BP, Yang CW, Mindea SA, et al. Pituitary apoplexy. Pediatr Radiol 2005;35:830–1.

57. Tosaka M, Sato N, Hirato J, et al. Assessment of hemorrhage in pituitary macroadenoma by T2*-weighted gradient-echo MR imaging. AJNR Am J Neuroradiol 2007;28:2023–9.

58. Zhong W, You C, Jiang S, et al. Symptomatic Rathke's cleft cyst. J Clin Neurosci 2012;19:501–8.

59. Post KD. Rathke's cleft cysts: unanswered questions. World Neurosurg 2012. [Epub ahead of print].

60. Higgins DM, Van Gompel JJ, Nippoldt TB, et al. Symptomatic Rathke's cleft cysts: extent of resection and surgical complications. Neurosurg Focus 2011;31:E2.

61. Johnsen DE, Woodruff WW, Allen IS, et al. MR imaging of the sellar and juxtasellar regions. Radiographics 1991;11:727–58.

62. Chandler WF, Barkan AL. Treatment of pituitary tumors: a surgical perspective. Endocrinol Metab Clin North Am 2008;37:51–66, viii.

63. Hakyemez B, Aksoy U, Yildiz H, et al. Intracranial epidermoid cysts: diffusion-weighted, FLAIR and conventional MR findings. Eur J Radiol 2005;54:214–20.

64. Alexiou GA, Gogou P, Markoula S, et al. Management of meningiomas. Clin Neurol Neurosurg 2010;112:177–82.

65. Rao VJ, James RA, Mitra D. Imaging characteristics of common suprasellar lesions with emphasis on MRI findings. Clin Radiol 2008;63:939–47.

66. Kizana E, Lee R, Young N, et al. A review of the radiological features of intracranial meningiomas. Australas Radiol 1996;40:454–62.

67. Hirsch WL, Sekhar LN, Lanzino G, et al. Meningiomas involving the cavernous sinus: value of imaging for predicting surgical complications. AJR Am J Roentgenol 1993;160:1083–8.

68. Cappabianca P, Cirillo S, Alfieri A, et al. Pituitary macroadenoma and diaphragma sellae meningioma: differential diagnosis on MRI. Neuroradiology 1999;41:22–6.

69. Pinho RS, Andreoni S, Silva NS, et al. Pediatric central nervous system tumors: a single-center experience from 1989 to 2009. J Pediatr Hematol Oncol 2011;33:605–9.

70. Nielsen EH, Feldt-Rasmussen U, Poulsgaard L, et al. Incidence of craniopharyngioma in Denmark (n = 189) and estimated world incidence of craniopharyngioma in children and adults. J Neurooncol 2011;104:755–63.

71. Bunin GR, Surawicz TS, Witman PA, et al. The descriptive epidemiology of craniopharyngioma. J Neurosurg 1998;89:547–51.

72. Zada G, Lin N, Ojerholm E, et al. Craniopharyngioma and other cystic epithelial lesions of the sellar region: a review of clinical, imaging, and histopathological relationships. Neurosurg Focus 2010;28:E4.

73. Karavitaki N, Wass JA. Non-adenomatous pituitary tumours. Best Pract Res Clin Endocrinol Metab 2009;23:651–65.

74. Hofmann BM, Hollig A, Strauss C, et al. Results after treatment of craniopharyngiomas: further experiences with 73 patients since 1997. J Neurosurg 2012;116:373–84.

75. Schoenfeld A, Pekmezci M, Barnes MJ, et al. The superiority of conservative resection and adjuvant radiation for craniopharyngiomas. J Neurooncol 2012;108(1):133–9.

76. Huang BY, Castillo M. Nonadenomatous tumors of the pituitary and sella turcica. Top Magn Reson Imaging 2005;16:289–99.

77. Hao S, Tang J, Wu Z, et al. Natural malignant transformation of an intracranial epidermoid cyst. J Formos Med Assoc 2010;109:390–6.

78. Schiefer TK, Link MJ. Epidermoids of the cerebellopontine angle: a 20-year experience. Surg Neurol 2008;70:584–90 [discussion: 90].

79. Praveen KS, Devi BI. Calcified epidermoid cyst of the anterior interhemispheric fissure. Br J Neurosurg 2009;23:90–1.

80. Aribandi M, Wilson NJ. CT and MR imaging features of intracerebral epidermoid–a rare lesion. Br J Radiol 2008;81:e97–9.

81. Hu XY, Hu CH, Fang XM, et al. Intraparenchymal epidermoid cysts in the brain: diagnostic value of MR diffusion-weighted imaging. Clin Radiol 2008;63:813–8.

82. Bohara M, Yonezawa H, Hanaya R, et al. Posterior fossa epidermoid cysts presenting with unusual

radiological appearances–two case reports. Neurol Med Chir (Tokyo) 2011;51:85–8.

83. Liu JK, Gottfried ON, Salzman KL, et al. Ruptured intracranial dermoid cysts: clinical, radiographic, and surgical features. Neurosurgery 2008;62:377–84 [discussion: 84].

84. Orakcioglu B, Halatsch ME, Fortunati M, et al. Intracranial dermoid cysts: variations of radiological and clinical features. Acta Neurochir (Wien) 2008; 150:1227–34 [discussion: 34].

85. Coons SW, Rekate HL, Prenger EC, et al. The histopathology of hypothalamic hamartomas: study of 57 cases. J Neuropathol Exp Neurol 2007;66:131–41.

86. Wait SD, Abla AA, Killory BD, et al. Surgical approaches to hypothalamic hamartomas. Neurosurg Focus 2011;30:E2.

87. Mathieu D, Deacon C, Pinard CA, et al. Gamma Knife surgery for hypothalamic hamartomas causing refractory epilepsy: preliminary results from a prospective observational study. J Neurosurg 2010;113(Suppl):215–21.

88. Qiu XM, Wang H, Wei F, et al. Magnetic resonance imaging findings of hypothalamic hamartoma correlated with clinical features. Neurosciences (Riyadh) 2010;15:209–10.

89. Amstutz DR, Coons SW, Kerrigan JF, et al. Hypothalamic hamartomas: correlation of MR imaging and spectroscopic findings with tumor glial content. AJNR Am J Neuroradiol 2006;27:794–8.

90. Koeller KK, Rushing EJ. From the archives of the AFIP: pilocytic astrocytoma: radiologic-pathologic correlation. Radiographics 2004;24:1693–708.

91. Segal L, Darvish-Zargar M, Dilenge ME, et al. Optic pathway gliomas in patients with neurofibromatosis type 1: follow-up of 44 patients. J AAPOS 2010;14:155–8.

92. Rozen WM, Joseph S, Lo PA. Spontaneous regression of low-grade gliomas in pediatric patients without neurofibromatosis. Pediatr Neurosurg 2008;44:324–8.

93. Akiyama H, Nakamizo S, Kawamura A, et al. Management of chiasmatic-hypothalamic gliomas in children: report of nine pediatric cases. No Shinkei Geka 2007;35:1079–85 [in Japanese].

94. Sawamura Y, Kamada K, Kamoshima Y, et al. Role of surgery for optic pathway/hypothalamic astrocytomas in children. Neuro Oncol 2008;10:725–33.

95. Mazloom A, Hodges JC, Teh BS, et al. Outcome of patients with pilocytic astrocytoma and leptomeningeal dissemination. Int J Radiat Oncol Biol Phys 2012. [Epub ahead of print].

96. Valdueza JM, Lohmann F, Dammann O, et al. Analysis of 20 primarily surgically treated chiasmatic/hypothalamic pilocytic astrocytomas. Acta Neurochir (Wien) 1994;126:44–50.

97. Nitta T, Sato K. A clinicopathological study of 16 cases with optico-hypothalamic glioma. No Shinkei Geka 1995;23:217–22 [in Japanese].

98. Kumar AJ, Leeds NE, Kumar VA, et al. Magnetic resonance imaging features of pilocytic astrocytoma of the brain mimicking high-grade gliomas. J Comput Assist Tomogr 2010;34:601–11.

99. Gaudino S, Quaglio FR, Schiarelli C, et al. Spontaneous modifications of contrast enhancement in childhood non-cerebellar pilocytic astrocytomas. Neuroradiology 2012. [Epub ahead of print].

100. Lee IH, Kim JH, Suh YL, et al. Imaging characteristics of pilomyxoid astrocytomas in comparison with pilocytic astrocytomas. Eur J Radiol 2011;79:311–6.

101. Komakula ST, Fenton LZ, Kleinschmidt-DeMasters BK, et al. Pilomyxoid astrocytoma: neuroimaging with clinicopathologic correlates in 4 cases followed over time. J Pediatr Hematol Oncol 2007;29:465–70.

102. Komotar RJ, Zacharia BE, Sughrue ME, et al. Magnetic resonance imaging characteristics of pilomyxoid astrocytoma. Neurol Res 2008;30:945–51.

103. Erdem E, Angtuaco EC, Van Hemert R, et al. Comprehensive review of intracranial chordoma. Radiographics 2003;23:995–1009.

104. Sen C, Triana AI, Berglind N, et al. Clival chordomas: clinical management, results, and complications in 71 patients. J Neurosurg 2010;113:1059–71.

105. Walcott BP, Nahed BV, Mohyeldin A, et al. Chordoma: current concepts, management, and future directions. Lancet Oncol 2012;13:e69–76.

106. Gehanne C, Delpierre I, Damry N, et al. Skull base chordoma: CT and MRI features. JBR-BTR 2005;88:325–7.

107. Doucet V, Peretti-Viton P, Figarella-Branger D, et al. MRI of intracranial chordomas. Extent of tumour and contrast enhancement: criteria for differential diagnosis. Neuroradiology 1997;39:571–6.

108. Cerase A, Tarantino A, Gozzetti A, et al. Intracranial involvement in plasmacytomas and multiple myeloma: a pictorial essay. Neuroradiology 2008;50:665–74.

109. Fassett DR, Couldwell WT. Metastases to the pituitary gland. Neurosurg Focus 2004;16:E8.

110. Mao JF, Zhang JL, Nie M, et al. Diabetes insipidus as the first symptom caused by lung cancer metastasis to the pituitary glands: clinical presentations, diagnosis, and management. J Postgrad Med 2011;57:302–6.

111. Dutta P, Bhansali A, Shah VN, et al. Pituitary metastasis as a presenting manifestation of silent systemic malignancy: a retrospective analysis of four cases. Indian J Endocrinol Metab 2011; 15(Suppl 3):S242–5.

112. Neal JG, Patel SJ, Kulbersh JS, et al. Comparison of techniques for transsphenoidal pituitary surgery. Am J Rhinol 2007;21:203–6.

113. Yoon PH, Kim DI, Jeon P, et al. Pituitary adenomas: early postoperative MR imaging after transsphenoidal resection. AJNR Am J Neuroradiol 2001;22:1097–104.

114. Shiley SG, Limonadi F, Delashaw JB, et al. Incidence, etiology, and management of cerebrospinal fluid leaks following trans-sphenoidal surgery. Laryngoscope 2003;113:1283–8.

115. Tamasauskas A, Sinkunas K, Draf W, et al. Management of cerebrospinal fluid leak after surgical removal of pituitary adenomas. Medicina (Kaunas) 2008;44:302–7.

Applications of Magnetic Resonance Imaging in Adult Temporal Bone Disorders

Suyash Mohan, MD, PDCC[a],*, Ellen Hoeffner, MD[b],
Douglas C. Bigelow, MD[c], Laurie A. Loevner, MD[a]

KEYWORDS

- MR imaging • Adult temporal bone • Cholesteatoma • Vestibulocochlear schwannoma
- Aberrant ICA • Petrous apicitis

KEY POINTS

- Magnetic resonance imaging is the primary imaging modality for evaluation of the nonosseous components of the adult temporal bone.
- Both temporal bones are always imaged to compare sides and the brain/skull base included so that intracranial extension can be evaluated.
- Middle ear congenital cholesteatoma presents as a nodular soft tissue mass, without osseous erosions or involvement of Prussak space, and with normal pars flaccida.
- A non–echo planar (EP) diffusion-weighted (DW) imaging sequence should be preferred rather than an EP DW imaging sequence because it is less sensitive to susceptibility artifacts and is therefore able to show cholesteatomas as small as 2 mm.
- In early stages of necrotizing external otitis, nonspecific soft tissue swelling is present in the external auditory canal with erosion at the petrotympanic fissure and obliteration of the retrocondylar fat pad.

INTRODUCTION

Temporal bone imaging is challenging because the normal anatomy includes many small but clinically important structures, and a significant abnormality in this area may be less than 1 mm in size. With isotropic sections, bone algorithm, and three-dimensional (3D) reconstructions, computed tomography (CT) has been the mainstay for evaluating the temporal bone since its inception in the early 1970s,[1,2] whereas magnetic resonance (MR) imaging is the primary imaging modality for evaluation of the nonosseous components including major blood vessels, fluid spaces (cerebrospinal fluid [CSF], endolymph, perilymph), nerves, muscle, cartilage, brain, salivary glands, and fat.[3–10] MR imaging has superior soft tissue resolution, multiplanar capability, does not use ionizing radiation, and is the most effective technique for the evaluation of these structures and their disorders.[11–16] Both of these techniques are complimentary, and it often becomes necessary to use both CT and MR imaging for satisfactory tissue characterization and identification of disorders or confident exclusion of abnormalities. This article reviews current clinical applications of MR imaging

[a] Department of Radiology, Division of Neuroradiology, University of Pennsylvania School of Medicine, 3400 Spruce Street, Philadelphia, PA 19104, USA; [b] Department of Radiology, Division of Neuroradiology, University of Michigan Health System, 1500 East Medical Center Drive, Ann Arbor, Michigan 48109-0030, USA; [c] Department of Otorhinolaryngology: Head and Neck Surgery, University of Pennsylvania School of Medicine, Philadelphia, PA 19104, USA
* Corresponding author.
E-mail address: drsuyash@gmail.com

mri.theclinics.com

techniques appropriate for diagnosing adult temporal bone disorders, and presents appropriate examples.

TECHNIQUE

MR imaging of the temporal bone is typically performed using a dedicated multichannel head coil and a high field strength MR imaging system. The signal/noise ratio can be improved approximately 3 to 5 times compared with that of a routine head coil by using dedicated phased-array surface coils specifically designed for temporal bone imaging.[17,18] The disadvantage of using these coils is that the images are not homogeneous in signal intensity, the coils are more cumbersome for the technologist to position, and are not routinely used at the authors' institutions. Both temporal bones are always imaged to compare sides and the brain/skull base included, so that intracranial extension of a disease process can be evaluated. To address these specific goals, 4 basic MR imaging techniques are used: whole-brain imaging, high-resolution T2/fluid space imaging, precontrast-enhanced and postcontrast-enhanced high-resolution T1-weighted imaging, and vascular (MR angiography) imaging.

Routine Brain Survey

An MR imaging protocol of the temporal bone should start with a brain examination using a T2-weighted, or fluid-attenuated inversion recovery (FLAIR) and whole-brain postgadolinium T1-weighted sequence to exclude associated brain pathologic processes. For example, a patient who presents with symptoms of dizziness could have disorders that result from brainstem demyelination, ischemia, or a neoplasm. Diffusion-weighted (DW) imaging should be added, which helps in differentiation between congenital or acquired cholesteatoma and epidermoid cysts.

High-Resolution T2-Weighted Imaging

Fluid-sensitive high-resolution images are noncontrast enhanced and show the CSF and endolymphatic spaces as regions of high signal intensity. The cisternal cranial nerves can be visualized without contrast using this technique because the nerves are surrounded by fluid of higher signal intensity. Fluid in the otic capsule structures is best visualized using this technique, making it possible to evaluate cochlear or vestibular disorders. This technique has also been used as for screening to rule out vestibular schwannomas.[19]

A heavily T2-weighted sequence, usually a submillimetric 3D turbo spin echo (TSE)/fast spin echo (FSE) T2-weighted sequence, is performed to evaluate the fluid content and signal intensity characteristics in the membranous labyrinth. Postprocessing of the image data can create any specific projection or surface desired. Steady-state T2-weighted gradient echo images using constructive interference techniques also have excellent quality and are not marred by increased magnetic susceptibility artifacts because of their short echo times.[20–22]

High-Resolution Precontrast-Enhanced and Postcontrast-Enhanced T1-Weighted Images

T1-weighted sequences are performed before and after intravenous administration of gadolinium: a 1-mm (or even submillimeter) axial 3D T1-weighted gradient echo sequence or a thin-slice (2 mm or less) axial and coronal spin echo (SE) T1-weighted sequence can be used. Fat saturation techniques can be applied in 1 direction after contrast administration. This sequence is ideal for identification of subtle changes, like those seen with labyrinthitis/vestibulitis or small vestibular tumors.

T1-weighted gradient echo images can be acquired by using a moderate recovery time (30–50 milliseconds) and flip angle (30°–50°) and by spoiling (destroying residual transverse magnetization). Spoiling is needed to eliminate T2 contrast components from the acquired signal, thus yielding T1-weighted images similar to routine spin echo images but can also show the vessels to advantage.[19] Caution must be exercised, because high signal of vessels may be mistaken for enhancement in a tumor. Routine spin echo T1-weighted images can be used, but the resolution is significantly lower. The lack of any high signal within the canal on this sequence is a reliable indicator that no eighth nerve tumor is present. Some radiologists add fat suppression to eliminate potentially confusing high signal from the fat in the petrous apex.

With the increasing use of 3-T magnets, the axial submillimeter 3D T1-weighted gradient echo sequence is likely to become the sequence of choice because it gives the maximum number of slices through the temporal bone.

Acquisition of a noncontrast T1-weighted sequence is of value to help characterize high-signal regions on contrast studies because, without a noncontrast examination, it may be difficult to differentiate fat or subacute hemorrhage.

MR Angiography

In addition, a dedicated MR angiography acquisition may be of value in specific instances, especially in a case of suspected glomus tumor or in the evaluation of a patient with pulsatile tinnitus. Most commonly, noncontrast 3D time-of-flight sequences are used, which generate the best detail. Postprocessing of these volume data sets can be used to create detailed 3D projections in different planes and perspectives. Flow compensation decreases signal from the moving CSF and thereby increases the contrast/noise ratio between the blood vessels and the CSF in MR angiography; therefore, the soft tissue detail may be poor. Although current MR angiography can provide high-quality images, they cannot substitute for traditional catheter angiography in many cases, which remains the gold standard to exclude small dural arteriovenous fistulas.

NORMAL MR IMAGING ANATOMY

Normal anatomic structures of the temporal bone as seen on precontrast-enhanced and postcontrast-enhanced T1-weighted MR imaging are shown in **Fig. 1**. Corresponding anatomy, as seen on thin-section high-resolution T2-weighted images, is shown in **Fig. 2**. Additional relevant anatomy is discussed, along with specific disease processes.

INTERNAL AUDITORY CANAL AND CPA LESIONS
Anatomy

The cerebellopontine angle (CPA) is an inverted triangular-shaped CSF space anterior to the cerebellar hemispheres and lateral to the pons. It extends into the petrous bone as the internal auditory canal (IAC), with its medial aperture being the porus acusticus. Lesions that arise within or involve the IAC can be considered together with lesions affecting the CPA cistern. The fifth cranial nerve traverses the superior aspect of the cistern from the lateral pons to the Meckel cave. The seventh (facial) and eighth (vestibulocochlear) cranial nerves arise from the low CPA cistern at the lateral aspect of the inferior medulla, emerging at the level of the foramen of Luschka. These nerves ascend to the porus acusticus, with the facial nerve slightly anterior and superior to the eighth cranial nerve. Both nerves are intimately related to the anterior inferior cerebellar artery (AICA), and, in two-thirds of patients, the AICA loops into the IAC on at least 1 side.

The IAC is located within the midsubstance of the petrous apex. It runs in the coronal plane in relation to the skull but in an angle of approximately 45° in relation to the long axis of the petrous bone. It houses the vestibulocochlear and facial nerves (cranial nerves VIII and VII, respectively). Within the IAC, the facial nerve is located in the anterior superior portion. The cochlear nerve runs in the anterior inferior portion of the IAC, whereas the superior and the inferior divisions of the vestibular nerve course in the superior posterior and inferior posterior portions of the internal auditory canal, respectively. Within the lateral portion of the IAC, all 4 nerve components can be seen on volumetric, heavily T2-weighted images, whereas only 2 nerves are identified in the medial portion because the vestibulocochlear nerve separates first in the midportion of the internal auditory canal into its 3 components (cochlear, superior vestibular, and inferior vestibular divisions).[23]

Common disorders in this region include various neoplastic and nonneoplastic masses, inflammatory and vascular processes that affect the CPA

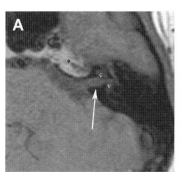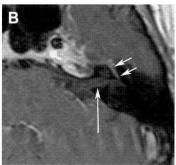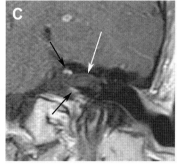

Fig. 1. (*A*) Precontrast 3-mm-thick axial T1-weighted spin echo (SE) image through the left temporal bone obtained on a 1.5-T magnet shows the VII and VIII cranial nerve complex in the internal auditory canal (IAC) (*arrow*). The cochlea (c) and vestibule (v) are seen as areas of intermediate signal. High signal fat is seen in the petrous apex (*asterisk*). (*B*) Postcontrast image through the left IAC with no enhancement of the VII and VIII cranial nerve complex within the IAC (*long arrow*). Normal enhancement of the tympanic segment of the facial nerve is seen (*short arrows*). (*C*) Postcontrast 3-mm-thick direct coronal T1-weighted SE image through the left IAC. There is no enhancement within the IAC (*long white arrow*). High signal fat in the petrous bone adjacent to the left IAC (*short black arrows*) should not be mistaken for enhancement.

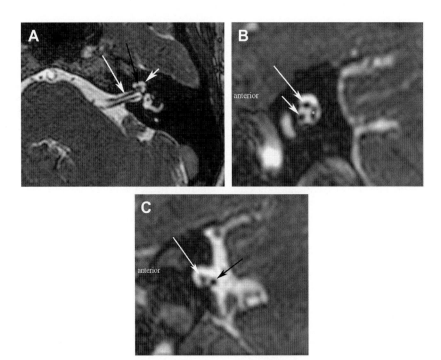

Fig. 2. (A) High-resolution, heavily T2-weighted, fast field echo (FFE) Sensitivity Encoding (SENSE) image through left IAC obtained on a 1.5-T magnet. The cochlear nerve is seen anteriorly in the IAC (*long white arrow*), whereas the inferior vestibular nerve is seen posteriorly. High signal is seen within the inner ear structures, including the cochlea (*short white arrow*) and the vestibule (*asterisk*). The modiolus (*long black arrow*) is seen as an area of low signal with in the cochlea. (B) Sagittal reformatted image through lateral left IAC from the same sequence. The facial (*long arrow*) and cochlear (*short arrow*) nerves are seen anteriorly in the IAC, whereas the still conjoined vestibular nerves (*asterisk*) are posterior. (C) Sagittal reformatted image from the same sequence through medial left IAC shows 2 nerves, anteriorly the facial nerve (*long white arrow*) and posteriorly the vestibulocochlear nerve (*short black arrow*).

and IAC cisterns and the cranial nerves located there. In addition to lesions specific to this region, any intra-axial or extra-axial process that involves subarachnoid/cisternal spaces can also be seen here. These processes typically present because of mass effect on the 5th to 12th cranial nerves, or over the pons or cerebellum, which may result in fourth ventricular obstruction.

Vestibulocochlear Schwannoma

Vestibulocochlear Schwannoma (VCS) is a benign, slowly growing neoplasm that accounts for 70% to 80% of all CPA lesions and approximately one-tenth of all intracranial tumors.[24] These lesions were previously known as acoustic neuromas, and most often arise from the inferior vestibular nerve within the IAC and present with hearing loss or tinnitus.[25] Vestibular symptoms of vertigo and dizziness are less common, which is curious given that most of these tumors arise from the vestibular portion of the nerve. This phenomenon may be caused by a lesser susceptibility of the nerve to the effects of compression or by the central nervous system's greater ability to compensate

for unilateral vestibular denervation.[26] Schwannomas can be entirely intracanalicular or have intracanalicular and cisternal components, resulting in the typical ice-cream-cone appearance (**Fig. 3**). Vestibular schwannomas can, rarely, be purely intracisternal, and these tend to reach a larger size before presenting with mass effect

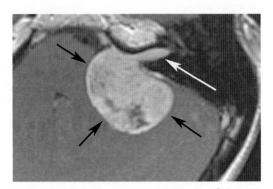

Fig. 3. Typical ice-cream-cone appearance of vestibulocochlear schwannoma with an intracanalicular component (*long white arrow*) and a larger cisternal component (*short black arrows*) that enhances heterogeneously on postcontrast T1-weighted SE image.

on the cerebellar hemispheres and fourth ventricle rather than hearing loss.

Contrast-enhanced MR imaging is considered the first-line imaging technique for VCS evaluation, because of the sensitivity afforded by the intense enhancement that these tumors typically manifest, even in small lesions.[27] High-resolution T2 imaging is a supplemental noncontrast technique that can provide exquisite imaging of the CSF and nerves in the CPA and IAC. On T2 FSE, VCSs appear as nodules or filling defects against the background of bright CSF (**Fig. 4**). This technique allows detection of tumors as small a few millimeters and can provide adjunctive information that is useful in surgical planning, such as identifying from which nerve component the tumor arises, defining the extent of the tumor boundaries, and determining whether there is a CSF cap at the fundus of the IAC. In the proper clinical setting, T2 FSE can serve as an inexpensive screening technique for patients with uncomplicated sensorineural hearing loss (SNHL).[28]

Although small lesions tend to have homogeneous enhancement, larger lesions more frequently have cystic spaces and show heterogeneous enhancement. Those tumors with cystic areas tend to be faster growing and to have a less favorable surgical outcome with regard to integrity of facial nerve function.[29] Hence, when describing these masses, it is important to describe the tumor dimensions in terms of the cisternal component and the component within the IAC. Lateral extent of the tumor within the IAC should be assessed, and particular mention should be made of whether or not the mass extends up to or into the cochlear aperture. If the mass is associated with a cyst, the size of this cyst should also be described.

VCS is associated with neurofibromatosis type 2 (NF-2),[30] and this condition should be suspected when VCS is bilateral or is discovered in a child or young adult. The presence of NF-2 should also heighten the radiologist's awareness of possible associated lesions, including meningiomas and ependymomas.

Malignant degeneration of VCS is rare and is associated with NF-1.[31] Melanotic schwannoma is another malignant variant of VCS that may arise from melanocytes, which share their neural crest origin with Schwann cells.[32]

Treatment options depend to a large extent on tumor size, extension into the IAC, and presence of cystic components, and mainly include observation, microsurgical removal, and stereotactic radiosurgery. Observation is reserved for elderly patients who do not experience mass effect.

Meningioma

Meningiomas are the second most common tumor to arise in the CPA, representing up to 10% to 15% of tumors. These slow-growing masses are well circumscribed, arise from arachnoid meningoepithelial cells, and are epidemiologically and histologically similar to meningiomas that occur elsewhere in the cranial vault. In the CPA, these tumors tend to arise from the dura of the dorsal aspect of the petrous temporal bone. They typically present with hearing loss, tinnitus, and headache, whereas larger tumors may present with cerebellar signs and trigeminal neuropathy.[33] The imaging hallmarks of meningioma include extraaxial dural-based location, intense enhancement, hyperostosis, and calcification on CT, which is seen in up to one-fourth of lesions (**Fig. 5**).[34] Sometimes a meningioma may mimic a VCS both clinically and on imaging. The following imaging features are helpful in their differentiation, despite some overlap (**Table 1**).

Epidermoid and Other Cystic Masses

Epidermoid tumors, also known as congenital cholesteatoma, represent the third most common

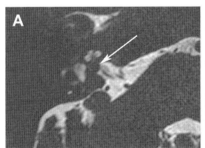 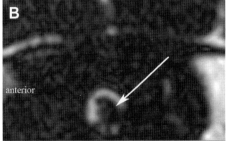

Fig. 4. (*A*) Axial high-resolution TSE T2-weighted image obtained on a 3-T magnet shows a low signal mass in the distal right IAC (*arrow*) outlined by high-signal CSF. (*B*) Sagittal reformatted image from same sequence through the right IAC shows a mass (*arrow*) in the posterior superior aspect of the IAC, compatible with a vestibular schwannoma.

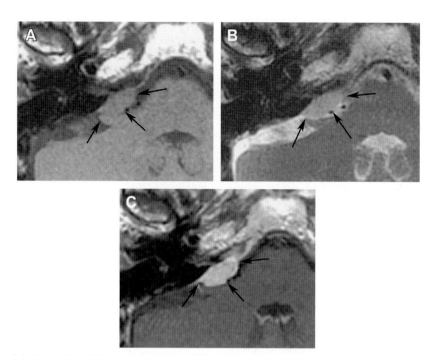

Fig. 5. (*A*) Axial T1-weighted SE image through the right CPA cistern shows a dural-based mass arising from the dorsal aspect of petrous temporal bone (*arrows*) that is isointense to brain. (*B*) On an axial FSE T2-weighted image, the mass (*arrows*) is slightly hyperintense to brain. (*C*) There is homogeneous enhancement (*arrows*) on postcontrast T1-weighted SE image.

masses in this location. They arise from inclusion of ectodermal epithelial tissue during neural tube closure. These masses are lined by stratified keratinized epithelium, and grow from desquamation and accumulation of keratin and cholesterol within the cysts. The gross appearance is glistening and pearly, and this has led to this lesion being called the beautiful tumor.[35] These lobulated malleable masses have a tendency to insinuate between cranial nerves and vessels. Because of this characteristic, they tend to present only when large. Epidermoids present clinically with symptoms similar to schwannomas and meningiomas: tinnitus, hearing loss, or even hemifacial spasm. However, epidermoid tumors are readily distinguished from schwannomas and meningiomas by their imaging appearance. These cysts are nonenhancing on CT and MR imaging, following the density and intensity of CSF on most sequences. The feature that distinguishes these lesions from arachnoid cysts is a relative hyperintensity to CSF on FLAIR imaging and reduced diffusion signal intensity on DW imaging sequences (**Fig. 6**).[36] This characteristic of epidermoid tumors also serves as a useful feature for the detection of any residual tumor on postoperative follow-up examinations.

Table 1
Imaging features of meningiomas and schwannomas

Characteristics	Meningioma	Schwannoma
Signal intensity on T2	Isointense to hyperintense to GM	Hyperintense
Hyperostosis	+	−
Calcification	+	−
Dural tail	+	−
DW imaging/ADC	Lower ADC than schwannomas	Higher ADC than meningiomas
Perfusion-weighted imaging	High rCBV	Low rCBV
MR spectroscopy	Cho, low Cr/NAA and alanine	mI

Abbreviations: ADC, apparent diffusion coefficient; Cho, choline; Cr/NAA, creatine/*N*-acetylaspartate ratio; GM, gray matter; mI, myoinositol; rCBV, regional cerebral blood volume.

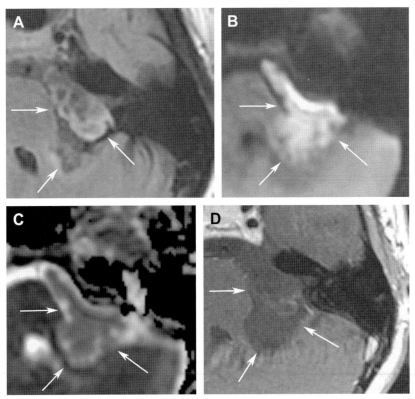

Fig. 6. Left CPA cistern epidermoid. (*A*) Axial FLAIR image shows an extra-axial mass heterogeneously hyperintense to CSF (*arrows*). There is mass effect on adjacent cerebellum and middle cerebellar peduncle. (*B*) The mass is of markedly hyperintense signal is seen on DW imaging (*arrows*). (*C*) On the corresponding apparent diffusion coefficient (ADC) map, the mass is isointense to brain (*arrows*). (*D*) On a T1-weighted SE postcontrast image the mass (*arrows*) is isointense to CSF with minimal heterogeneity and no enhancement.

Malignant transformation of an epidermoid to squamous cell carcinoma is an extremely rare event, characterized by areas of contrast enhancement within the lesion.[37] Unusual appearances of epidermoids have been reported and include the so-called white epidermoids. These epidermoids show reversed signal intensities; that is, hyperintensity on T1-weighted sequences and hypointensity on T2-weighted sequences, attributed to the high proteinaceous content.[38] When the appearance is atypical, MR spectroscopy may aid in diagnosis, because epidermoids have been reported to depict elevated lactate peaks.[39]

Arachnoid cysts (AC) are the major differential diagnosis for a nonenhancing cystic CPA mass. These cysts are simple loculated CSF collections that form as a result of a congenital focal defect or duplication of the arachnoid membrane.[40] ACs can be seen in any location where the arachnoid membrane is found, but some of the more common locations include middle cranial fossa, hemispheric convexities, CPA cisterns, suprasellar cistern, and cisterna magna. DW imaging has proved to be able to distinguish these lesions

and other nonenhancing CPA masses. Because ACs are thin-walled masses containing only CSF, they have no enhancement and show facilitated diffusion. Mass effect on adjacent brain or mild remodeling of adjacent bone are often present (**Fig. 7**). High-resolution T2-weighted sequences can be used to identify the cyst wall, but, in cases in which the cyst wall cannot be shown, differentiation between a simple enlarged CSF space and a small AC becomes difficult.

Dermoid cyst (DC) is similar to EC in that it is the result of a congenital ectodermal inclusion, but it differs in that it includes tissues from all 3 ectodermal layers. DCs may contain fat, hair, teeth, and calcification. DCs may rupture, resulting in a characteristic appearance of scattered fat droplets in the CSF space, and may cause chemical meningitis.

Lipomas are benign hamartomatous lesions that are distinct from DCs. Lipomas are masses of ectopic fat that probably form as a result of fatty maldevelopment of primitive meningeal mesodermal tissues.[41] Intracranial lipomas most commonly are seen at the midline, but can also occur

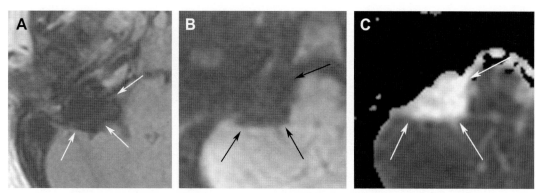

Fig. 7. Right CPA arachnoid cyst. (*A*) Axial FLAIR image shows an extra-axial mass that is isointense to CSF (*arrows*). There is mild mass effect on the cerebellum. (*B*) The mass is also isointense to CSF on the DW imaging (*arrows*). (*C*) On the corresponding ADC map, the mass remains isointense to CSF (*arrows*).

in the CPA region, or within the IAC. Unlike their supratentorial counterparts, posterior fossa lipomas are not usually associated with cerebral malformations. Both DCs and lipomas on MR imaging show characteristic hyperintense fat signal on T1-weighted imaging. Lipomas tend to be smaller and more homogeneous and they do not enhance on contrast administration. Neurovascular structures seem to pass through the lipoma and are usually not displaced.[42] DCs often contain heterogeneous elements, including calcification, which is best appreciated on CT.

Malignant and Inflammatory Meningitides

Any inflammatory or infectious process affecting the dura or leptomeninges can involve the CPA cistern. Differentiating between these entities and metastatic disease (leptomeningeal carcinomatosis) by imaging features alone is difficult (**Fig. 8A**). A clear clinical history is important, but the final diagnosis often requires CSF analysis.

Meningeal disease is evaluated best with fat-suppressed contrast-enhanced MR imaging. Abnormal enhancement may appear as multiple nodular deposits or as focal or diffuse leptomeningeal or pachymeningeal thickening.[43] A solitary meningeal deposit may mimic a meningioma. In the setting of carcinomatous meningitis, abnormal enhancement within IAC is a sensitive imaging marker of leptomeningeal carcinomatosis and the remainder of the craniospinal axis should be examined to evaluate for possible involvement.

INNER EAR LESIONS
Large Endolymphatic Duct and Sac

Large endolymphatic sac anomaly is the most common congenital inner ear anomaly found by imaging and is bilateral in 90% of cases.[44] It is also the most commonly missed cause of congenital deafness. It is a familial lesion with autosomal recessive inheritance. There is an association with Pendred syndrome, which is severe

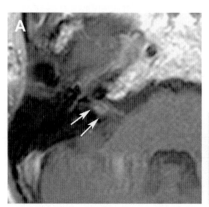

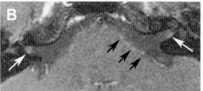

Fig. 8. (*A*) Enhancement and thickening along the intracanalicular portion of right VII and VIII cranial nerve (*arrows*) on postcontrast T1-weighted SE image related to metastatic breast cancer. (*B*) Enhancement within both IACs (*white arrows*) and along the surface of the pons (*black arrows*) on postcontrast T1-weighted SE image related to neurosarcoidosis.

SNHL with thyroid disorder. Patients typically present with progressive, severe SNHL in childhood or early adulthood, often exacerbated by minor trauma.

The hallmark imaging characteristic of large endolymphatic sac anomaly on CT is enlargement of the bony vestibular aqueduct, and a diameter greater than 1.5 mm at a point halfway between the crus communis and the intracranial aperture of the aqueduct, or an opercular measurement of more than 2 mm, are generally considered to be the defining characteristics.[45] On T2 FSE MR imaging, the underlying endolymphatic structure abnormalities are shown readily, consisting of enlargement of the endolymphatic sac and duct (Fig. 9). In some cases, enlargement of the sac is more conspicuous than that of the duct, on T2 FSE MR. The vestibular aqueduct is usually found at the level of the vestibule and lateral semicircular canal, so it is easy to compare the diameter of the sac with the lateral and posterior semicircular canals, which should be larger than the aqueduct.[44] There is no relationship between the size of the endolymphatic sac and the severity of the SNHL. Although the aqueduct is best evaluated with CT, the bright signal intensity on T2 within the sac is best seen on thin T2-weighted images. In more than 75% of cases, there is an associated cochlear dysplasia, with dysmorphic apical turn and modiolar deficiency.[46] High-resolution T2 MR imaging may be able to distinguish more subtle abnormalities of scalar chamber asymmetry with the more anterior scala vestibuli larger than the more posterior scala tympani. Approximately 50% of cases have associated vestibular or semicircular canal anomalies. In patients with sudden hearing loss, studies have shown wider vestibular aqueducts in the affected ear compared with controls.[47] The endolymphatic sac can show enhancement, which may be caused by inflammation of the endolymphatic tissue or venous engorgement.[47] It is hypothesized that a wide vestibular aqueduct may be associated with insufficient maturation of the inner ear.[48] The congenital fragile inner ear may receive abnormal pressure transmission through the vestibular aqueduct.[49]

Labyrinthitis/Labyrinthine Ossificans

Labyrinthitis is a nonspecific inflammation of the membranous labyrinth,[50] with a variety of causes (Box 1), viral infection being most common. It may arise as a complication of meningitis when purulent material reaches the endolymph via CSF. The cochlear aqueduct, which links the subarachnoid space to the basal turn of the tympanic scale, is generally proposed as the most probable conduit of meningogenic labyrinthitis.[51] This might explain why the concentration of bacteria and inflammatory cells is high and the ossification more frequently occurs in the basal turn of scala tympani, and high-frequency hearing loss associated to the basal turn of the cochlea is more pronounced than low-frequency hearing loss associated to the apex of the cochlea. A host of other conditions can lead to labyrinthitis, including otomastoid disease, demyelinating disease, granulomatous disease, and metastatic disease. Meningogenic labyrinthitis typically is bilateral, whereas tympanogenic and traumatic causes are unilateral.

The clinical presentation of labyrinthitis typically includes vertigo, dizziness, and SNHL. Contrast-enhanced MR imaging of the temporal bone is the most sensitive technique for detecting labyrinthine inflammation. Labyrinthitis usually manifests as diffuse mild or moderate enhancement that involves the entire membranous labyrinth, or a portion of the labyrinth.[50] Enhancement may be unilateral or bilateral, and may persist for months after the onset of symptoms. The distinction between labyrinthitis and labyrinthine schwannoma (LS) may be difficult on enhanced MR imaging. On T2 FSE MR imaging, labyrinthitis usually shows

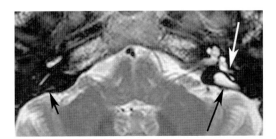

Fig. 9. An enlarged left endolymphatic duct and sac is seen as a tubular area of high signal (*long black arrow*) at the level of the aqueduct on this axial high-resolution TSE T2-weighted image obtained on a 3-T magnet. It is larger in diameter than the lateral semicircular canal (*white arrow*). A normal-sized vestibular aqueduct is seen on the right (*short black arrow*).

Box 1
Etiologic classification of labyrinthitis

- Hematogenic
- Tympanogenic
- Meningogenic
- Traumatic
- After stapedectomy or other inner ear surgery
- Spontaneous

normal or minimal diminished T2 fluid signal in the labyrinth, in contrast with the filling defect seen with LS.

In the chronic phase, labyrinthitis may progress to labyrinthitis ossificans (LO), which begins with fibrosis and progresses to ossification as early as 2 months and causes obliteration of the labyrinth. The clinical presentation of LO is chronic profound hearing loss and loss of vestibular function. The imaging hallmark of LO is osseous obliteration of the labyrinth, which is seen as loss of normal high signal on thin-section T2 FSE images.[52] In the early stages of LO, the membranous labyrinth begins to fill with ill-defined fibrous inflammatory debris. These early changes are more difficult to detect on CT, and T2 FSE is a useful adjunct to CT at this stage. As osseous proliferation continues, portions of the labyrinth become filled in by bone and may progress to complete obliteration in severe cases (**Fig. 10**). In the absence of appropriate clinical history, end-stage LO may be mistaken for congenital labyrinthine hypoplasia.

In cochlear LO, the fluid spaces of the cochlea are affected. In noncochlear LO, the fluid spaces of the semicircular canal or vestibule are affected. On 3D FT-constructive interference steady-state sequences, there is loss of normal fluid signal intensity within the cochlea because of fibrous proliferation of the labyrinth. The modiolus can appear enlarged. The enhancement of membranous labyrinthitis can persist in the ossifying stages of LO.

Intralabyrinthine hemorrhage can occur in patients with history of anticoagulation, sickle cell disease, trauma, leukemia, or other hyperviscosity syndromes. Patients experience acute onset of unilateral SNHL. There is high signal within normally fluid-filled spaces of the labyrinth on T1 MR imaging.

Intralabyrinthine Schwannoma

Intralabyrinthine schwannoma is a benign tumor that arises from Schwann cells with the membranous labyrinth, which results in progressive hearing loss. Before the advent of MR imaging, the diagnosis of LS was not made without surgical exploration of the labyrinth. It is seen as focal enhancement on thin-section fat-suppressed postcontrast T1-weighted imaging, within the membranous labyrinth, with a corresponding filling defect within the perilymph on thin-section T2 FSE imaging (**Fig. 11**). These lesions can be subdivided according to location: intracochlear, vestibulocochlear, transmodiolar, transmacular, and transtotic.[53]

Endolymphatic Sac Tumor

Endolymphatic sac tumor (ELST), also referred to as papillary adenomatous tumor of the temporal bone, is a rare neoplasm that occurs as a locally invasive mass in a retrolabyrinthine location. They are centered in the fovea of the endolymphatic sac in the posterior surface of the petrous temporal bone. Larger lesions (>3 cm) can spread to involve the middle ear, CPA cistern, and/or jugular foramen. The tumor is vascular and predominantly fed by distal branches of the ascending pharyngeal and occipital arteries.[54]

SNHL is seen in virtually all patients. Other symptoms include facial nerve palsy, pulsatile tinnitus, and vertigo. If ELST is bilateral, then von Hippel-Lindau syndrome should be suspected. Hearing loss and ELST are frequently associated with von Hippel-Lindau syndrome and should be considered when screening individuals at risk for von Hippel-Lindau syndrome and when monitoring patients with an established diagnosis of von

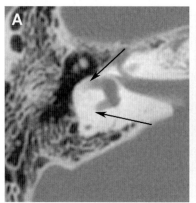
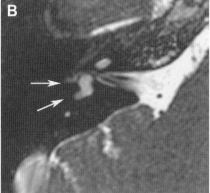

Fig. 10. Postmeningitic noncochlear LO. (*A*) Axial CT image thorough right temporal bone shows dense ossification in the lateral semicircular canal (*arrows*). (*B*) Axial T2-weighted FFE SENSE image through right temporal bone in the same patient shows loss of normal high T2 signal in the lateral semicircular canal (*arrows*).

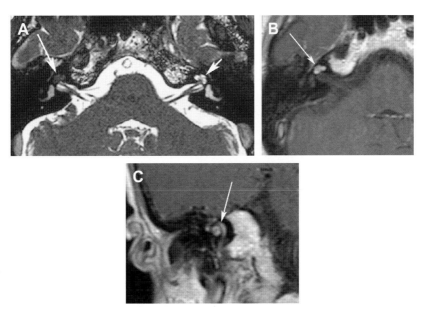

Fig. 11. Intracochlear schwannoma. (*A*) Axial high-resolution TSE T2-weighted image shows a filling defect (*long arrow*) within the middle and apical turns of the right cochlea compared with normal left cochlea (*short arrow*). (*B*) Postcontrast axial T1-weighted SE image shows corresponding intense enhancement (*arrow*). (*C*) Postcontrast coronal T1-weighted image shows enhancement throughout the cochlea including the basal turn (*arrow*).

Hippel-Lindau syndrome. On CT, the lesion shows intratumoral bone spicules, with destructive and aggressive-appearing margins. A thin rim of calcification along the posterior margin of the tumor is common. There are high signal foci within the tumor matrix on T1 MR imaging when the lesion is larger than 3 cm, and along the margin when the lesion is less than 3 cm. Most tumors (80%) have these foci of increased signal intensity.[55] Flow voids can be seen when the tumor is larger than 2 cm. These lesions show heterogeneous enhancement on contrast-enhanced MR imaging (**Fig. 12**).

PETROUS BONE LESIONS

The petrous apex is the most medial portion of the temporal bone that cannot be directly examined on clinical examination; hence, the referring physician has to rely completely on imaging interpretation.

Anatomy

The petrous apex represents the pyramid-shaped medial portion of the temporal bone located between the inner ear structures laterally, petrosphenoid fissure anteriorly, and petrooccipital fissure medially.[56] It is obliquely positioned within the skull base, with the apex anteromedially located and the base posterolaterally located. Its anterosuperior portion forms the floor of the middle cranial fossa, whereas the posterosuperior

portion constitutes the anterior wall of the posterior cranial fossa. The petrous apex is subdivided by the IAC into an anterior portion containing marrow, and a denser posterior portion derived from the otic capsule.[56] In 35% of patients, the petrous apex is pneumatized by infralabyrinthine, anterior, superior, posteromedial, or subarcuate tracts that provide direct pathways for diseases to spread from the mastoid or middle ear cavity to the petrous apex. The petrous apex houses a few important vascular and neuronal channels. The petrous carotid and the IAC are the largest channels, whereas the Dorello, singular, and arcuate canals are smaller and not always visualized.[57] The foramen lacerum is the fibrocartilaginous, medial extension of the bony floor of the petrous carotid canal that is located between the petrous apex, the basiocciput, and the basisphenoid bone. The Dorello canal extends through the medial portion of the petrous apex and contains the abducens nerve (cranial nerve VI). The arcuate canal courses between the crura of the superior semicircular canal within the superior portion of the petrous apex and holds the arcuate artery.

NORMAL ANATOMIC VARIATIONS
Asymmetric Pneumatization

In most patients, the petrous apex is nonpneumatized. Even if pneumatization occurs, it is typically symmetric with no diagnostic concern. Only when the pneumatization is asymmetric is the

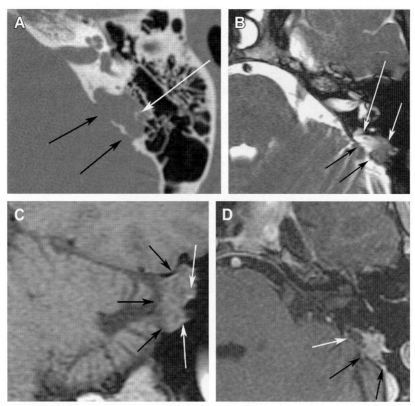

Fig. 12. Endolymphatic sac tumor. (*A*) Axial CT image through the temporal bone shows a destructive process centered in the region of the endolymphatic sac along the posterior surface of the petrous temporal bone (*black arrows*). Intratumoral bone spicules are seen (*white arrow*). (*B*) Axial heavily T2-weighted FIESTA (fast imaging employing steady state acquisition) sequence shows a corresponding destructive lesion (*black arrows*) with a solid component isointense to brain (*short white arrow*) and a medial cystic component (*long white arrow*). (*C*) A coronal precontrast T1-weighted image shows a mass isointense to brain (*black arrows*) with foci of high signal along the periphery (*white arrows*). (*D*) Following contrast administration, there is intense enhancement of the solid component of the mass (*black arrows*) and peripheral enhancement of the cystic component (*white arrow*).

nonpneumatized petrous apex typically misinterpreted as a petrous apex lesion such as cholesteatoma, petrous apicitis, or cholesterol granuloma, especially on MR imaging. The nonpneumatized petrous apex shows variable signal intensity depending on a patient's age. In younger patients, it is of intermediate signal intensity on all sequences and is unlikely to be mistaken for cholesteatoma or fluid-filled or pus-filled petrous apex, which typically shows high signal intensity on T2-weighted images. In contrast, the high T1 signal intensity of the fatty bone marrow within the nonpneumatized petrous apex in older adults may be mistaken for cholesterol granuloma (**Fig. 13**). Lack of mass effect and suppression of the fatty bone marrow on fat-suppressed sequences yields the correct diagnosis. Cholesterol granuloma often shows even higher T1 signal intensity than the surrounding bone marrow or subcutaneous adipose tissues.

Giant Air Cell/Petrous Apex Effusion

A giant air cell is defined as a petrous apex air cell that is more than 1.5 cm in its largest diameter.[58] When air filled, it is typically of no diagnostic concern. When it is fluid filled with preservation of the internal septations without clinical signs of acute infections, it is known as petrous apex effusion.[59] Until recently, such petrous apex effusions were considered to be leave-alone lesions, but more recent publications suggest that it is a true clinical disorder that may present with indolent infections, hearing loss, headache, facial spasm, and positional vertigo in more than half of the involved patients.[59] If the appearance on MR imaging is more complicated, appearing hyperintense both on T2-weighted imaging and T1-weighted imaging, the signal characteristics of benign fluid mimic those of cholesterol granuloma (CG). If there is uncertainty about the diagnosis in this situation, comparison with CT to exclude an

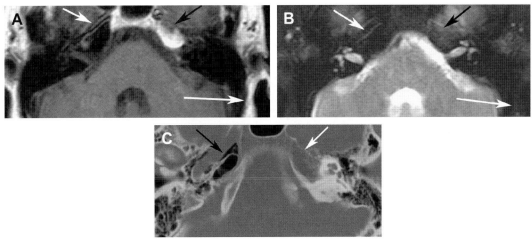

Fig. 13. Asymmetry of the petrous apices. (*A*) The high signal of the marrow fat in the left petrous apex (*black arrow*), similar to subcutaneous fat (*long white arrow*), should not be mistaken for abnormality despite its asymmetry compared with the hypointense right petrous apex (*short white arrow*) on this axial, precontrast, T1-weighted SE image. (*B*) Comparison with an axial fat-suppressed FSE T2-weighted image shows low signal in left petrous apex (*black arrow*), again similar to that of subcutaneous fat (*long white arrow*). The right petrous apex remains hypointense (*short white arrow*). (*C*) Axial CT shows a nonpneumatized left petrous apex containing marrow (*white arrow*). The right petrous apex is pneumatized (*black arrow*), resulting in the hypointense signal on all MR sequences.

expansile lesion and long-term imaging follow-up are prudent to rule out early CG (**Fig. 14**).

ANOMALOUS INTERNAL CAROTID ARTERY

Aberrant internal carotid artery malformation, also called intratympanic ICA, is a rare vascular congenital malformation of the petrous apex that is caused by regression of the cervical internal carotid artery during embryogenesis. It develops from the anastomosis of an enlarged ascending pharyngeal branch (the inferior tympanic artery) and an enlarged derivative of the primitive hyostapedial trunk (the caroticotympanic artery). This uncommon lesion is often asymptomatic, although patients may experience conductive hearing loss or subjective or objective pulsatile tinnitus. In the clinical setting of a vascular retrotympanic mass,

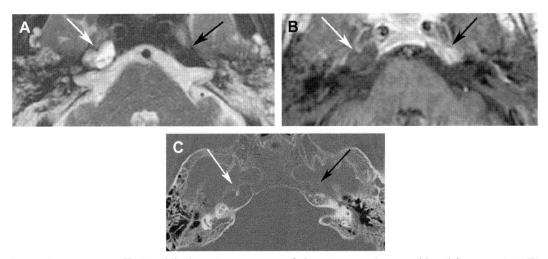

Fig. 14. Petrous apex effusion. (*A*) There is asymmetry of the petrous apices on this axial, noncontrast T1-weighted SE image, with hypointense signal on the right (*white arrow*) and hypointense signal on the left (*black arrow*). (*B*) On the axial FSE T2-weighted image, the right petrous apex is hyperintense (*white arrow*). Signal characteristics are consistent with fluid. The left petrous apex is hypointense (*black arrow*), consistent with fat. (*C*) Axial CT image shows a normal, nonpneumatized left petrous apex (*black arrow*); whereas a right petrous apex air cell is opacified (*white arrow*). There is no bone expansion or destruction.

differentiation of aberrant ICA from surgical lesions, such as paraganglioma, is critical. Intratympanic ICA is recognized most easily on CT, but, in uncertain cases, MR angiography is useful if aberrant ICA is easily recognized by the abnormally lateral and posterior position of the vertical petrous ICA (**Fig. 15**).

CG

The most common location for CG is the middle ear, although classic descriptions often focus on petrous apex. CG was initially recognized as a complication of chronic otomastoid inflammation but the cause is still unknown. According to the most accepted theory, it is caused by inadequate ventilation of the pneumatized petrous apex, which results in negative pressure, reabsorption of air, mucosal edema, and hemorrhage, with local tissue breakdown and cholesterol formation leading to foreign body reaction.[60] A newer theory is based on exposed bone marrow as a result of the aggressive pneumatization of the petrous apex that leads to coaptation of bone marrow and mucosa, eliciting hemorrhage that obstructs the apical outflow tract. This process, in turn, leads to breakdown of the blood and foreign body reaction with subsequent cyst formation and bony

expansion.[61] Regardless of the cause, both theories support 2 important points for the radiologist: (1) accumulation of blood products and cholesterol leading to high signal intensity on T1-weighted and T2-weighted images; and (2) a CG starts out in a pneumatized petrous apex (**Fig. 16**). Because pneumatization of the petrous apex is typically symmetric in distribution, presence of a contralateral highly pneumatized petrous apex supports the diagnosis of CG rather than cholesteatoma.[62]

Because of the depth in location, these granulomas can be large at the time of diagnosis and cause seventh and eighth cranial nerve dysfunction. Their large size also may make distinction from other petrous apex lesions difficult, particularly for petrous apex aneurysm. A related lesion is mucocele of the petrous apex, which develops as a postobstructive sequel to inflammatory insult, similar to that seen in the sinonasal cavities. The petrous apex is an uncommon place for mucocele, but, when large, can present clinically as similar to CG. On MR imaging, petrous apex mucocele typically shows hypointensity on T1-weighted imaging and hyperintensity on T2-weighted imaging, distinguishing mucocele from CG. However, signal on T1-weighted imaging is variable, depending on the protein composition of the fluid contents,

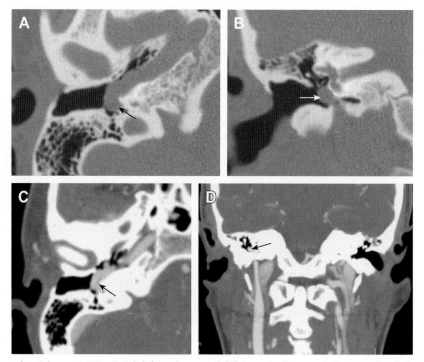

Fig. 15. Anomalous/aberrant ICA. Axial (*A*) and coronal (*B*) images (bone window settings) from CT of the temporal bone depict an internal carotid artery that courses adjacent to the jugular bulb (*black arrow in A*) and, at a higher level, within the hypotympanum (*white arrow in B*); findings confirmed on axial (*C*) and coronal (*D*) CT angiography images (*black arrow*).

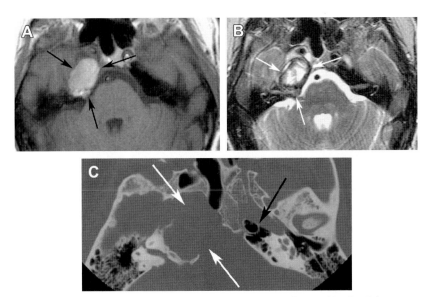

Fig. 16. Petrous apex CG. (*A*) There is an expansile T1 hyperintense mass (*arrows*) in the right petrous apex on this axial, noncontrast T1-weighted image. (*B*) The mass (*arrows*) is also hyperintense centrally on this axial TSE T2-weighted image with a hypointense rim, compatible with hemosiderin from remote hemorrhage. (*C*) Axial CT image shows the expansile nature of this (*white arrows*) and a pneumatized petrous apex on the contralateral side (*black arrow*).

and may appear hyperintense, in which case differentiation from CG becomes more difficult.

PETROUS APICITIS AND OSTEOMYELITIS

Petrous apicitis is a subtype of skull base osteomyelitis that is caused by medial extension of acute otitis media into a pneumatized petrous apex. *Streptococcus pneumoniae*, *Haemophilus influenzae*, and *Staphylococcus aureus* are the most common causative organisms. Patients with petrous apicitis are usually acutely sick with fever and some or all of the symptoms of the Gradenigo triad: ipsilateral cranial nerve VI paralysis, severe facial pain in V1 distribution, and otomastoiditis.[63] In early stages, imaging shows simple opacification or air fluid levels in petrous apex cells with enhancement and evidence of otomastoid disease (**Fig. 17**). As the infection progresses to osteomyelitis, trabecular breakdown and cortical destruction become apparent. Because of the proximity of the petrous apex to the brain, patients who have petrous apicitis are prone to intracranial complications best assesses by MR imaging, which may show involvement of the adjacent cisterns or IAC and possible complications of abscess or venous sinus thrombosis.

Petrous apicitis has traditionally been treated with debridement; however, successful conservative treatment of uncomplicated petrous apicitis has recently been reported. In such cases, gallium single-photon emission CT imaging might be beneficial for evaluating response to therapy.[64]

Petrous Apex Osteomyelitis

Petrous osteomyelitis is caused by direct medial extension of malignant otitis externa or by retrograde spread of thrombophlebitis along the petrous carotid canal venous plexus into the non-pneumatized petrous apex.[56] *Pseudomonas* is the most common causative organism.[65] Patients typically complain of severe, deep ear pain that is out of proportion to the physical findings.[65] MR imaging is superior in determining the extent of the disease by better showing the replacement of the fatty bone marrow by the infectious process and the surrounding soft tissue and intracranial involvement. Nuclear medicine studies such as technetium-99 bone scan and gallium scan are sensitive and used to monitor the response to antibiotic therapy.

MIDDLE EAR AND MASTOID LESIONS

Lesions that affect the middle ear and mastoid include congenital anomalies, congenital and acquired inflammatory conditions, and infectious and neoplastic processes.

CONGENITAL CHOLESTEATOMA

Congenital cholesteatoma is caused by the presence of an ectopic rest of epithelial tissue, and is

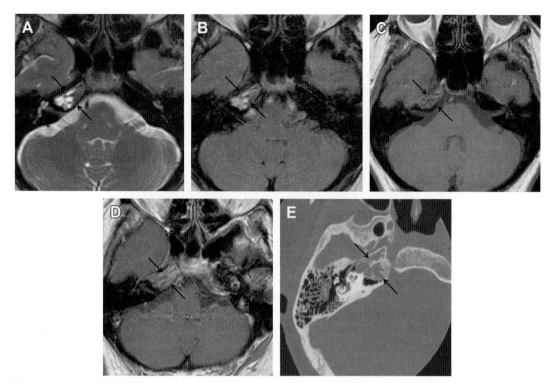

Fig. 17. Petrous apicitis. (*A*) Axial T2-weighted, (*B*) axial FLAIR, and (*C*) precontrast T1-weighted images show opacification of the right petrous air cells (*black arrows*), with diffuse enhancement on the gadolinium-enhanced T1-weighted image (*D*). Although the axial CT image (bone window settings) (*E*) showed no frank osseous destruction, the patient improved significantly on antibiotic treatment.

the third most common tumor of the middle ear. Although classically described in the petrous apex, congenital cholesteatoma is found more commonly in the middle ear and also may occur in the mastoid and external canal. Congenital cholesteatoma should always be included in the differential diagnosis of a lytic lesion in the petrous bone. By definition, congenital cholesteatomas are found behind an intact tympanic membrane with no history of inflammatory middle ear disease. They can be found anywhere in the middle ear cavity but have a propensity to occur anteriorly in the tympanic cavity near the eustachian tube, or near the stapes.[66]

On CT, middle ear congenital cholesteatoma usually presents as a small nodular soft tissue mass, often without any associated ossicular erosion (**Fig. 18**). The Prussak space is not involved, and the scutum is sharply delineated with normal pars flaccid of the tympanic membrane.[66] MR imaging can be used to differentiate these middle ear lesions, because cholesteatomas appear hyperintense on B1000 DW imaging sequences. A non-EPI DW imaging sequence should be preferred rather than an EPI DW imaging sequence because the former sequence is less sensitive to

susceptibility artifacts at the brain-bone interface, and is therefore able to show cholesteatomas as small as 2 mm.[67,68] On T2-weighted MR imaging, a congenital cholesteatoma (and an acquired cholesteatoma) displays a moderate intensity, which is lower than that of inflammatory middle ear changes. On T1-weighted images, a congenital cholesteatoma is hypointense without any contrast enhancement apart from some peripheral enhancement.[68]

ACQUIRED CHOLESTEATOMA

Acquired cholesteatoma (AC) is a complication of chronic otomastoiditis that consists of a collection of keratinaceous debris contained within a sac lined by stratified squamous epithelium. AC arises as a result of disruption of the normal physiologic maintenance of the tympanic squamous epithelium, although some disagreement exists as to the mechanism of AC formation. The most widely accepted theory suggests that posterosuperior retraction pockets form in the tympanic membrane (pars flaccida cholesteatoma) as a result of inflammatory insult, which in turn disrupt the normal migration and turnover of squamous epithelial

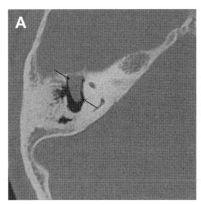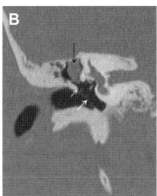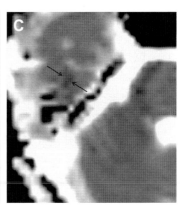

Fig. 18. Congenital cholesteatoma. Axial (*A*) and coronal (*B*) images (bone window settings) from CT of the temporal bone show a nodular soft tissue mass in the epitympanum (*black arrows*), with intact scutum (*small white arrow* in *B*), and tympanic membrane (*long white arrow* in *B*). This mass was hyperintense on B1000 DW imaging sequences (not shown), with low ADC values (*C; black arrows*).

layers. A less frequent variant originates from the lower part of the tympanic membrane (pars tensa cholesteatoma).

Acquired pars flaccida cholesteatoma progressively grows into the Prussak space and starts eroding surrounding structures, such as the scutum, lateral epitympanic wall, and ossicular chain (mainly the head of the malleus and the long process and body of the incus). By definition, acquired cholesteatoma is always associated with tympanic membrane abnormalities and associated infection history of repeated episodes of otitis media. Patients with AC suffer from progressive conductive hearing loss and may experience symptoms of facial nerve and vestibulocochlear dysfunction as osseous erosion progresses to involve adjacent temporal bone structures.

On imaging, the hallmark feature of cholesteatoma is osseous erosion associated with nonenhancing soft tissue mass. Complications of cholesteatoma are the result of erosion into adjacent vital structures and include facial canal dehiscence, labyrinthine fistula (particularly at the lateral superior semicircular canal [SCC]), dehiscence of the tympanic tegmen, and extension into the dural venous sinuses. Evidence of these potential complications should be sought on all studies in which cholesteatoma is suspected. MR imaging signal of ACs is similar to that described for congenital lesions, consisting of hypointensity on T1-weighted imaging, variable hyperintensity on T2-weighted imaging, and mild peripheral enhancement.

Postcontrast T1-weighted MR imaging has been advocated as an effective technique for distinguishing granulation tissue from residual cholesteatoma.[69] Cholesteatomas are avascular and do not enhance following contrast administration, whereas granulation tissue is poorly vascularized and does enhance on delayed images. During the past several years, data have been published advocating DW imaging for evaluation of residual or recurrent cholesteatoma following mastoidectomy (**Fig. 19**). Newer DW imaging techniques with thinner section acquisition and decreased susceptibility artifacts allow detection of small lesions. DW imaging can be useful as the primary imaging technique when visualization is impaired by canal wall up mastoidectomy or cartilaginous reconstruction. The DW imaging technique may be used in place of second-look surgery, sparing patients the morbidity of repeat exploration.

ACUTE OTOMASTOIDITIS

Acute otomastoiditis (AOM) is a common infectious process that stems from upper respiratory infection and usually affects children. Bacterial cause is the rule, with *S pneumoniae* and *H influenzae* accounting for most cases. Tuberculous otitis is uncommon but occurs more often in immunocompromised patients. AOM is readily managed with a course of antibiotics in most patients. The condition becomes complicated when secondary osseous infection develops that involves the ossicles, tympanic cavity, or mastoid. Coalescent mastoiditis, abscess formation, and fistula development are part of the spectrum of untreated disease. In advanced cases, intracranial extension of infection may result in meningitis, cerebritis, empyema, or dural venous thrombosis. In the setting of acute uncomplicated disease, imaging is not necessary; if imaging is done; nonspecific fluid and debris are apparent in the middle ear and mastoid without evidence of bony erosion. In more advanced disease, evidence of

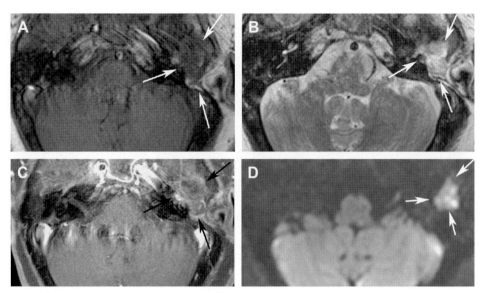

Fig. 19. Recurrent acquired cholesteatoma. (*A*) Axial, noncontrast T1-weighted image shows a mass in the middle ear/mastoid region that is of low signal (*arrows*). (*B*) The mass is hyperintense on the axial T2 SENSE image (*arrows*). (*C*) An axial, fat-saturated, postcontrast T1-weighted image shows only peripheral enhancement (*arrows*). (*D*) The mass is of high signal on axial DW imaging (*arrows*).

osseous destruction is present, with loss of middle ear and mastoid bony landmarks and dehiscence into the inner ear and intracranial compartment. Intracranial complications are best appreciated on contrast-enhanced MR imaging (**Fig. 20**).

PARAGANGLIOMA

Paragangliomas arise from the extra-adrenal neural crest–derived paraganglia, the glomus bodies. These glomus bodies lie along the nerves in the inferior temporal bone along the cochlear promontory in the middle ear, giving rise to the glomus tympanicum (GTP). When a large glomus jugulare extends into the middle ear, the term glomus jugulotympanicum is used. Most of these jugulotympanic tumors arise in association with

the glomus formations of the inferior tympanic branch of the glossopharyngeal nerve (Jacobson nerve) or the mastoid branch of the vagus nerve (Arnold nerve).[70,71] The GTP tumor is the most common neoplasm of the middle ear. The peak age of incidence is during the fifth and sixth decades of life, and there is a clear female predisposition (3:1 ratio).

Patients typically present with pulsatile tinnitus, conductive hearing loss, or inner ear symptoms. Large jugulotympanicum tumors also may present with multiple lower cranial neuropathies. On otologic examination, GTP appears as a bluish-red vascular retrotympanic mass, and becomes difficult to differentiate between a GTP tumor, a glomus jugulotympanicum tumor, and vascular variants (eg, high-riding dehiscent jugular bulb,

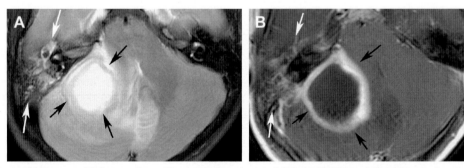

Fig. 20. Acute otomastoiditis complicated by cerebellar abscess. (*A*) Axial TSE T2-weighted image shows scattered opacification of the right middle ear and mastoid air cells (*white arrows*). The abscess cavity can be seen in the adjacent cerebellum (*black arrows*). (*B*) Axial, postcontrast T1-weighted image shows patchy enhancement in the mastoid region (*white arrows*) and peripheral enhancement of the cerebellar abscess (*black arrows*).

aberrant internal carotid artery). Because surgical intervention or biopsy can potentially be hazardous, imaging plays a critical role in accurate diagnosis.

Small GTP tumors are seen as a soft tissue nodule situated anteriorly in the hypotympanum against the cochlear promontory. Larger tumors fill the middle ear, but typically do not cause bone erosion and tend to spare the ossicles. Glomus tumors show intense enhancement on MR imaging because of their vascular nature. MR imaging plays a critical role in defining the extension of GTP intracranially and into the skull base (**Fig. 21**). Unenhanced T1-weighted images show the mass lesion in the jugular fossa with its characteristic salt-and-pepper appearance. The pepper represents the hypointense dots caused by the signal voids of large feeding arteries, whereas the salt is secondary to subacute hemorrhage in the tumor.[70–72] On an unenhanced 3D time-of-flight MR angiography sequence, serpiginous high signal intensities can be found in the tumor, representing the high-velocity flow of the large feeding arteries. In the assessment of paragangliomas, the combination of conventional MR imaging and contrast-enhanced MR angiography is significantly superior to conventional MR imaging sequences alone.[72]

INTRATEMPORAL FACIAL NERVE LESIONS
Anatomy

Imaging plays a critical role in the evaluation of the complex anatomy of the facial nerve. The anatomy of the facial nerve can conceptually be broken down into 3 major segments: intracranial, intratemporal, and extratemporal. The intracranial segment refers to that portion of the nerve that runs from the brainstem to the IAC. The intratemporal segment begins as the nerve enters the IAC, with the first intratemporal segment being the intracanalicular segment, then the labyrinthine segment, which runs from the fundus of the IAC to the geniculate ganglion, or the first/anterior genu. The portion of the facial nerve that runs from the geniculate ganglion to the second genu is termed the tympanic segment, which is the most commonly injured portion of the facial nerve during middle ear/mastoid surgery. The next segment is the mastoid or descending segment, before the nerve exits the temporal bone through to the stylomastoid foramen, as the extratemporal segment. It then enters the parotid gland and splits into 2 major segments at a point termed the pes anserinus. The upper segment is termed the temporozygomatic segment, and the lower segment is termed the cervicofacial segment,

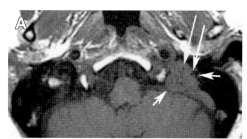
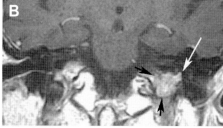
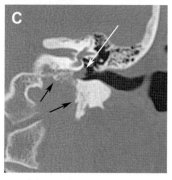

Fig. 21. Glomus jugulotympanicum tumor. (*A*) A soft tissue mass is seen in the jugular foramen (*short arrows*) with signal voids within it (*long arrows*) on this axial, noncontrast T1-weighted image. (*B*) Coronal, postcontrast T1-weighted image shows intense enhancement of the mass (*black arrows*) with a small component extending into the hypotympanum (*white arrow*). (*C*) A direct coronal CT scan through the temporal bone shows the extension into the hypotympanum (*white arrow*) and the expansion of, and permeative bone changes around, the jugular foramen (*black arrows*).

which further splits into 5 major branches: the temporal, zygomatic, buccal, mandibular, and cervical branches.[73] Some disease processes may involve 1 segment, whereas others may involve multiple segments, but only those conditions that affect the intratemporal segment are discussed here. Contrast-enhanced thin-section MR imaging remains the preferred imaging technique for evaluating facial nerve lesions.

INFLAMMATORY DISORDERS OF THE FACIAL NERVE

Bell palsy, the most common cause of facial paralysis, is characterized by an abrupt onset of facial weakness, which peaks by 48 hours. It has been associated with Herpes simplex infection, and is thought to result from inflammatory edema of the facial nerve, with resultant compression of the vascular supply within the tight fallopian canal. The labyrinthine segment resides in the narrowest portion of the canal and hence is most susceptible to ischemia. The diagnosis of Bell palsy is one of exclusion, with imaging reserved only for atypical cases (ie, weakness that persists for a longer period than would be expected in an uncomplicated Bell palsy). Other atypical features include slowly progressive palsy, facial palsy accompanied by spasm, recurrent palsy, bilateral symptoms, unusual degrees of pain, and the presence of multiple cranial neuropathies or other neurologic symptoms.

MR imaging using gadolinium shows enhancement of the inflamed segment, which is most pronounced in the region of the geniculate ganglion at the lateral end of the IAC, but more diffuse enhancement of the intratemporal portion may be seen (**Fig. 22**). Because mild enhancement of the geniculate ganglion and tympanic segment can be normal, comparison with the uninvolved contralateral nerve provides an important internal control.[74] The pattern of enhancement does not correlate with prognosis and may persist for months after resolution of symptoms. The diameter of the nerve is the key difference between Bell palsy and tumors involving the nerve. In Bell palsy, the nerve enhances with little or no enlargement and no focal nodularity. Enlargement of the intratemporal segments of the facial nerve should raise suspicion for a neoplasm. Gadolinium MR imaging scans of patients with facial palsy should include the course of the facial nerve, from its exit from the brain stem to its terminal branches on the face.

Herpes zoster oticus (Ramsay Hunt syndrome [RHS]) is another type of herpetic facial neuritis, resulting from reactivation of latent varicella zoster virus in the geniculate ganglion that is triggered by stress, aging, or immunosuppression. Patients with RHS present with facial palsy and painful vesicles involving the pinna. Involvement of the vestibulocochlear nerve also may result in SNHL, vertigo, tinnitus, and nystagmus. MR imaging shows enhancement of the facial nerve in a manner identical to Bell palsy, along the vestibulocochlear nerve, the labyrinth, and also in the lesions of the external ear.

The facial nerve may also be secondarily involved in inflammatory disorders of the temporal bone.

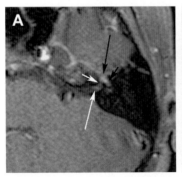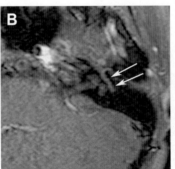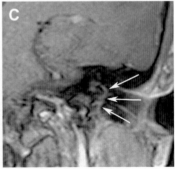

Fig. 22. Presumed Bell palsy in a patient with acute onset of facial nerve paralysis. The patient had an MR imaging examination because of slow resolution of symptoms. (*A*) This fat-saturated, postcontrast, axial T1-weighted SE image through the left temporal bone shows enhancement within the intracanalicular (*long white arrow*), labyrinthine (*short white arrow*) and tympanic (*short black arrow*) segments of the facial nerve as well as the anterior genu (*long black arrow*). (*B*) Slightly inferior image from same sequence shows enhancement throughout the tympanic segment (*arrows*) of the facial nerve. (*C*) Postcontrast, coronal T1-weighted SE image shows enhancement along the mastoid segment (*arrows*) of the facial nerve.

About 5% of patients who have acute otitis media and 1% of patients who have cholesteatoma may present with facial nerve paralysis.

NEOPLASMS OF THE FACIAL NERVE

Neoplasms of the facial nerve usually present with progressive facial paralysis in a pattern not typical of Bell palsy (eg, insidious onset, progression for more than 3 weeks, persistence for longer than 6 months). Two common facial nerve neoplasms, schwannoma and hemangioma, are discussed here. However, the facial nerve can be secondarily involved by tumors of the temporal bone or by perineural spread of malignancy, which is outside the scope of this article.

FACIAL SCHWANNOMA

Facial schwannomas can occur along any segment of the facial nerve, with a predilection for the geniculate ganglion and a tendency to involve multiple segments.[75] Clinical presentation of facial schwannoma depends on tumor location, with facial nerve palsy being a common, but not universal, symptom.[76] Facial schwannomas in the

IAC are more likely to present with SNHL and may be indistinguishable from acoustic schwannoma. Those that affect the geniculate ganglion are clinically silent for long periods of time and are incidentally detected during imaging for unrelated conditions. Tympanic segment schwannomas may show a lobulated growth pattern, project into the middle ear cavity, displace the ossicular chain, and result in conductive hearing loss.

On MR images, they may present as lobulated masses (when in the CPA cistern, IAC, tympanic segment, and parotid space) or segments of fusiform expansion (when in the labyrinthine and mastoid segments) (**Fig. 23**). Tumors arising from the geniculate ganglion may grow along the greater superficial petrosal nerve and project into the middle cranial fossa, occasionally mimicking other extra-axial tumors of the middle fossa, such as a meningioma. Geniculate ganglion schwannomas may resemble hemangiomas, but they produce smooth expansion of the fallopian canal, unlike the rarefied margins encountered with hemangiomas, which may also contain ossific spicules. Facial nerve schwannomas that span the posterior and middle cranial fossae do so by straddling the midportion of the petrous bone, as opposed to

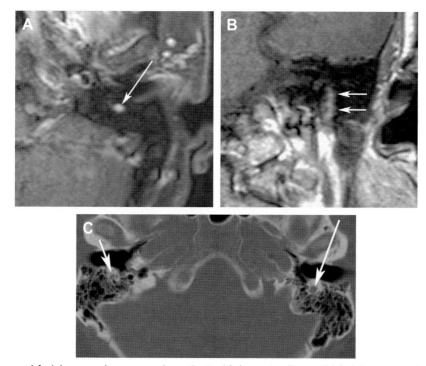

Fig. 23. Presumed facial nerve schwannoma in patient with long-standing, mild facial nerve weakness. (*A*) Fat-saturated, postcontrast axial T1-weighted image through the temporal bone shows enlargement and intense enhancement (*arrow*) of the mastoid segment of the left facial nerve. (*B*) Postcontrast, coronal T1-weighted SE image shows the enlarged, enhancing (*arrows*) mastoid segment of the facial nerve. (*C*) Axial CT image through the temporal bones shows enlargement of the mastoid segment (*long white arrow*) of the left facial nerve canal. The normal-sized mastoid segment of the right facial nerve (*short white arrow*) can be seen for comparison.

trigeminal schwannomas, which are centered the petrous apex. CT best depicts the expansion of the bony facial canal produced by these tumors.

FACIAL NERVE HEMANGIOMA

Facial nerve hemangioma is a benign vascular malformation composed of multiple vascular channels of varying size, with cavernous and capillary subtypes. Hemangiomas present with symptoms of facial palsy and hemifacial spasm, often at an earlier stage than schwannomas, because they invade the nerve rather than simply compressing it. They are most often encountered in the geniculate ganglion, in the fundus of the IAC, and, less often, in the posterior genu. Complete characterization of hemangiomas usually requires CT and contrast MR imaging, with intratumoral bone spicules on CT images the best clue to diagnosis (**Fig. 24**). They also show subtle expansion of the fallopian canal, with rarefaction of the bony margins as opposed to the fusiform expansion of a schwannoma. Because of their vascular nature, these are markedly hyperintense on T2-weighted imaging with intense contrast enhancement. Internal heterogeneity secondary to bony matrix may be evident.

EXTERNAL EAR LESIONS
Inflammatory Lesions of the External Ear

Of the many infectious and inflammatory conditions of the external ear, only necrotizing external otitis is discussed here because of its tendency to spread to the temporal bone and surrounding structures.

Necrotizing external otitis is considered a complication of external otitis, and is a potentially life-threatening disease. It was initially referred to as malignant otitis externa because of its associated high mortality.[77] Being an inflammatory disease rather than a neoplastic process, this term has been replaced by necrotizing external otitis. Necrotizing external otitis is mostly seen in elderly diabetics or immunocompromised patients, with occasional reports in children or in nondiabetic, immunocompetent people. The most common pathogen is *Pseudomonas aeruginosa*, with fungi (mainly *Aspergillus fumigatus*) being the causative agent in nondiabetic patients. The propensity of diabetics to develop necrotizing external otitis is thought to be partly caused by the compromised blood supply in diabetic microangiopathy.[78,79] In addition, the cerumen has a higher pH in diabetic patients, which might impair its bactericidal function.[80] *Pseudomonas* colonizes the ear canal and causes infection of the soft tissues of the external auditory canal (EAC), which then slowly progresses to cellulitis, chondritis, and osteomyelitis. The infection extends through the fissures of Santorini and the tympanomastoid suture to the osseous EAC and subtemporal soft tissues, and spreads along vascular and facial planes to surfaces of the mastoid and petrous portion of the temporal bone, petrous apex, and skull base. In advanced cases, intracranial extension can occur. The diagnosis is suspected in severe and refractory external otitis, which may be associated with neurologic symptoms or cranial nerve deficits.

Imaging evaluation includes multiple modalities. In the early stages, nonspecific soft tissue swelling is present in the EAC with erosion at the petrotympanic fissure and obliteration of the retrocondylar fat pad (**Fig. 25**).[81] The soft tissue involvement extends to the parapharyngeal space, nasopharynx, masticator space, and stylomastoid foramen, and infection eventually spreads to the contralateral side. These soft tissue changes and

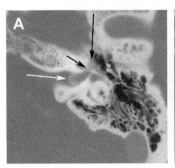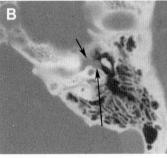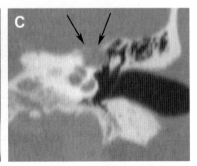

Fig. 24. Presumed facial nerve hemangioma in a patient with slowly progressive facial nerve palsy. (*A*) Axial CT image through the left temporal bone shows mass with bony/ossific spicules within it enlarging the fundus (*long white arrow*), fallopian canal (*short black arrow*), and anterior genu (*long black arrow*) of the left facial nerve canal. (*B*) Slightly superior axial image again shows the involvement of the anterior genu (*short black arrow*) with extension onto the proximal tympanic segment (*long black arrow*) of the facial nerve canal. (*C*) Direct coronal CT image shows the enlarged anterior genu (*arrows*) with small bony/ossific densities in the lesion.

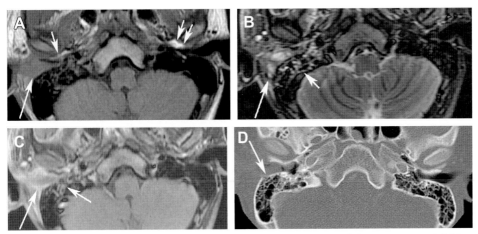

Fig. 25. Otitis externa in a patient with right ear pain and purulent drainage. (*A*) Precontrast, axial T1-weighted image shows soft tissue infiltration into the right EAC (*long white arrow*) with partial obliteration or retrocondylar fat pad (*short white arrow*) compared with normal left side (*double short white arrows*). (*B*) Axial short tau inversion recovery image shows that the soft tissue extending into the EAC is of intermediate to high signal (*long white arrow*). There is scattered right mastoid opacification, concerning for possible extension (*short white arrow*). (*C*) Fat-saturated, postcontrast, axial T1-weighted image shows patchy enhancement of EAC abnormality (*long white arrow*) and within the mastoid region (*short white arrow*). (*D*) Axial CT image shows subtle, focal erosion of mastoid cortex (*arrow*) forming the posterior wall of the EAC.

medullary bone changes are more obvious on MR imaging, with cortical bone erosion best seen on CT. Unlike other inflammatory diseases, necrotizing external otitis shows low signal intensity of soft tissue changes on both T1-weighted and T2-weighted images, reflecting a fibrotic necrotizing process rather than edema. After contrast administration, limited enhancement of the abnormal tissues is seen. Dural enhancement may be present. In cases of intracranial extension or dural sinus thrombosis, signs of meningitis or cerebral abscesses may be visualized. It can be effectively treated with a prolonged course of antibiotics and control of diabetes, with or without surgical debridement.

Neoplasms of the External Ear

Malignant tumors of the EAC are rare. The most frequently encountered primary malignant neoplasms of the EAC are SCC, basal cell carcinoma, adenoid cystic carcinoma, and ceruminous gland carcinoma.[82,83] SCC of the EAC and external ear is usually seen in elderly patients with a prior

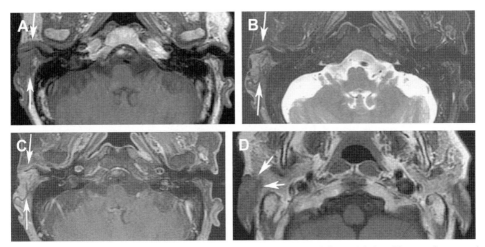

Fig. 26. Squamous cell carcinoma of the right auricle. (*A*) Precontrast, axial T1-weighted image shows an infiltrative soft tissue mass centered posterior to, but extending into, the right EAC (*arrows*) that is of intermediate signal. (*B*) Fat-saturated, axial FSE T2-weighted image shows the mass to be slightly hyperintense (*arrows*). (*C*) Fat-saturated, postcontrast, axial T1-weighted image shows enhancement of the lesion (*arrows*). (*D*) More inferiorly, a precontrast, axial T1-weighted image shows possible infiltration into the parotid gland (*arrows*).

history of chronic external and middle ear infection. The most frequently encountered secondary neoplasms are metastatic lesions in the EAC or parotid adenoid cystic carcinoma directly invading the EAC.[83] Breast carcinoma is the most common hematogenous metastatic lesion to occur within the temporal bone.[83] Malignant melanoma has been reported to arise on the external ear, secondarily invading the EAC.

The purpose of imaging evaluation of these malignancies is to assess the degree of deep extension and regional spread of disease, because the prognosis depends on the local invasion and the extent of the disease.[82] Bony abnormalities are better seen on CT, and MR imaging is useful in determining soft tissue extent and degree of skull base invasion in more advanced lesions. Local spread to the parotid gland or regional lymphatic spread to parotid lymph nodes also are important features of radiologic staging (**Fig. 26**).

GENERALIZED/SYSTEMIC CONDITIONS

Processes that affect osseous structures generically elsewhere in the body also may also affect the temporal bone, with MR imaging being particularly useful in various osseous neoplasms.

BENIGN AND MALIGNANT OSSEOUS NEOPLASM

Both primary and secondary malignancies can involve the temporal bone. Common primary neoplasms include lymphoma and myeloma, with the most common metastatic tumor arising from

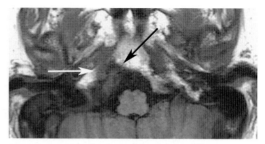

Fig. 27. Prostate cancer metastatic to skull base. Precontrast, axial T1-weighted image shows intermediate signal replacing the normal fatty marrow of the right petrous apex (*white arrow*) and lateral clivus (*black arrow*).

a breast primary (**Fig. 27**). In pediatric patients, additional considerations include histiocytosis and rhabdomyosarcoma. Both giant cell tumor (GCT) and aneurismal bone cyst (ABC) have been described in the temporal bone. GCTs are often large, expansile, variably destructive tumors, whereas ABCs are expansile, multiloculated lesions with fluid levels. Osteoblastoma can occur in the temporal bone and usually is seen in younger patients. Osteosarcoma is rare in the temporal bone and may be seen secondarily in the setting of prior irradiation or Paget disease. Chondrosarcoma has a predilection for the skull base, is typically centered in the petrosphenoid and petrooccipital synchondroses, and frequently extends into the petrous temporal bone (**Fig. 28**). The imaging features of primary and metastatic neoplasms of the temporal bone are generally nonspecific. Both CT and MR imaging are complimentary, with enhanced fat-suppressed MR

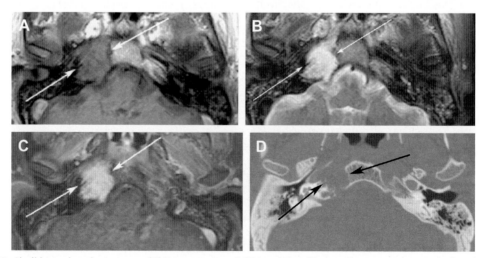

Fig. 28. Skull base chondrosarcoma. (*A*) Precontrast, axial T1-weighted image shows a mass centered in the right petroclival fissure of intermediate signal replacing normal marrow of the petrous apex and lateral clivus (*arrows*). (*B*) The mass (*arrows*) is very hyperintense on an axial TSE T2-weighted image. (*C*) There is intense enhancement of the mass (*arrows*) on a fat-saturated, postcontrast, axial T1-weighted image. (*D*) Axial CT image through the skull base shows a corresponding destructive lesion centered in the petroclival fissure (*arrows*).

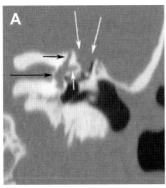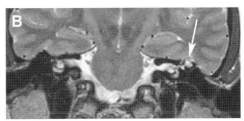

Fig. 29. Meningoencephalocele. (*A*) Coronal reformatted image through the left temporal bone shows a bony defect in the tegmen tympani with soft tissue protruding through it into the epitympanum (*long white arrows*). Portions of the adjacent lateral semicircular canal (*short white arrow*), superior semicircular canal (*short black arrow*) and vestibule (*long black arrow*) are seen. (*B*) Coronal T2-weighted image shows CSF and brain protruding through the small defect (*arrow*).

imaging being slightly better than CT in its ability to show the soft tissue extent of malignant tumors and in assessing the extent of intracranial disease.

SPONTANEOUS MENINGOENCEPHALOCELES AND CSF LEAKS FROM INTRACRANIAL HYPERTENSION

Spontaneous, idiopathic nasal meningoencephaloceles are herniations of arachnoid/dura and CSF through anatomically fragile sites within the skull base. The underlying condition is hypothesized to represent a form of intracranial hypertension that exerts hydrostatic pressure at anatomically weakened sites within the skull base.[84] MR imaging is the ideal imaging method and provides valuable information in detecting brain tissue and meningeal herniation, which is critical for accurate diagnosis and surgical planning. MR imaging should always be performed if there is an osseous defect on CT and complete opacification of an adjacent sinus in the patient with a possible CSF leak, because CT has limited ability in differentiating between obstructed secretions and the possibility of a meningoencephalocele (**Fig. 29**).

SUMMARY

MR imaging has increasing applications in the assessment of temporal bone disorders. It has improved detection and understanding of various disease conditions involving the temporal bone and allows for a precise assessment of most pathologic entities. Moreover, MR imaging is the imaging modality of choice for evaluating retrocochlear lesions, disorders of the membranous labyrinth; evaluation before cochlear implantation;

showing complicated infectious and inflammatory diseases, and showing the location and extension of primary and secondary temporal bone neoplasms. A thorough understanding of the anatomy is important in correctly assessing abnormality.

REFERENCES

1. Jäger L, Bonell H, Liebl M, et al. CT of the normal temporal bone: comparison of multi- and single-detector row CT. Radiology 2005;235:133–41.
2. Casselman JW. Diagnostic imaging in clinical neuro-otology. Curr Opin Neurol 2002;15:23–30.
3. Brogan M, Chakeres D. Computed tomography and magnetic resonance imaging of the normal anatomy of the temporal bone. Semin Ultrasound CT MR 1989;10:178–94.
4. Mafee MF, Charletta D, Kumar A, et al. Large vestibular aqueduct and congenital sensorineural hearing loss. AJNR Am J Neuroradiol 1992;13:805–19.
5. McGhee R, Chakeres DW, Schmalbrock P, et al. The extracranial facial nerve: high resolution three dimensional Fourier transform MR imaging. AJNR Am J Neuroradiol 1993;14:464–72.
6. Schmalbrock P, Brogan M, Chakeres DW, et al. Optimization of submillimeter resolution MR imaging methods for the inner ear. J Magn Reson Imaging 1993;3:451–9.
7. Tien R, Felsberg G. Fast spin echo high resolution MR imaging of the inner ear. AJR Am J Roentgenol 1992;159:395–8.
8. Mark AS, Seltzer S, Harnsberger HR. Sensorineural hearing loss: more than meets the eye? AJNR 1993;13:37–45.
9. Seltzer S, Mark AS. Contrast enhancement of the labyrinth on MR scans in patients with sudden

hearing loss and vertigo: evidence of labyrinthine disease. AJNR Am J Neuroradiol 1991;12:13–6.

10. Weisman JL, Curtin HD, Hirsch BE, et al. High signal from the otic labyrinth on unenhanced MRI. AJNR Am J Neuroradiol 1992;13:1183–7.

11. Niyazov DM, Andrews JC, Strelioff D, et al. Diagnosis of endolymphatic hydrops in vivo with magnetic resonance imaging. Otol Neurotol 2001; 22:813–7.

12. Hegarty JL, Patel S, Fischbein N, et al. The value of enhanced magnetic resonance imaging in the evaluation of endocochlear disease. Laryngoscope 2002;112:8–17.

13. Schick B, Brors D, Koch O, et al. Magnetic resonance imaging in patients with sudden hearing loss, tinnitus and vertigo. Otol Neurotol 2001;22:808–12.

14. Dobben GD, Raofi B, Mafee MF, et al. Otogenic intracranial inflammations: role of magnetic resonance imaging. Top Magn Reson Imaging 2000;11: 76–86.

15. Davidson HC. Imaging evaluation of sensorineural hearing loss. Semin Ultrasound CT MR 2001;22: 229–49.

16. Naidich TP, Mann SS, Som PM. Imaging of the osseous, membranous, and perilymphatic labyrinths. Neuroimaging Clin North Am 2000;10:23–34.

17. Schmalbrock P, Pruski J, Sun L, et al. Phased array RF coils for high-resolution MRI of the inner ear and brain stem. J Comput Assist Tomogr 1995;19(1):8–14.

18. Hayes H, Tsaruda J. Temporal lobes: surface MR coil phased array imaging. Radiology 1993;189: 918–20.

19. Schmalbrock P, Chakeres DW, Monroe JW, et al. Assessment of internal auditory canal tumors: a comparison of contrast-enhanced T1-weighted and steady-state T2-weighted gradient-echo MR imaging. AJNR Am J Neuroradiol 1999;20(7):1207–13.

20. Casselman JW, Kuhweide R, Deimling M, et al. Constructive interference in steady state 3DFT MRI of the inner ear and CP angle. AJNR Am J Neuroradiol 1993;14:47–57.

21. Oehler M, Schmalbrock P, Chakeres DW, et al. Magnetic susceptibility artifacts on high resolution MR of the temporal bone. AJNR Am J Neuroradiol 1995;16:1135–43.

22. Schmalbrock P, Yuan C, Chakeres DW, et al. Methods to achieve very short echo times for volume magnetic resonance angiography. Radiology 1990; 175:861–5.

23. Davidson HC. Imaging of the temporal bone. Neuroimaging Clin North Am 2004;14:721–60.

24. Swartz JD, Harnsberger HR. Imaging of the temporal bone. New York: Thieme Medical; 1998. p. 420.

25. Moffat DA, Ballagh RH. Rare tumours of the cerebellopontine angle. Clin Oncol (R Coll Radiol) 1995;7:28–41.

26. Weissman JL. Hearing loss. Radiology 1996;199: 593–611.

27. Curati WL, Graif M, Kingsley DP, et al. Acoustic neuromas: Gd-DTPA enhancement in MR imaging. Radiology 1986;158:447–51.

28. Allen RW, Harnsberger HR, Shelton C, et al. Low-cost high-resolution fast spin-echo MR of acoustic schwannoma: an alternative to enhanced conventional spin-echo MR? AJNR Am J Neuroradiol 1996;17:1205–10.

29. Fundova P, Charabi S, Tos M, et al. Cystic vestibular schwannoma: surgical outcome. J Laryngol Otol 2000;114:935–9.

30. Lo WW, Solti-Bohman LG. Tumors of the temporal bone and the cerebellopontine angle. In: Som PM, Curtin HD, editors. Head and neck imaging, vol. 2, 3rd edition. St Louis (MO): Mosby-Year Book; 1996. p. 1451.

31. Gruskin P, Carberry JN. Pathology of acoustic tumors. In: House WF, Luetze CM, editors. Acoustic tumors, vol. 1. Baltimore (MD): University Park Press; 1979. p. 85–148.

32. Earls JP, Robles HA, McAdams HP, et al. General case of the day. Malignant melanotic schwannoma of the eighth cranial nerve. Radiographics 1994;14: 1425–7.

33. Gerganov V, Bussarsky V, Romansky K, et al. Cerebellopontine angle meningiomas. Clinical features and surgical treatment. J Neurosurg Sci 2003; 47(3):129–35.

34. Valavanis A, Schubiger O, Hayek J, et al. CT of meningiomas on the posterior surface of the petrous bone. Neuroradiology 1981;22:111–21.

35. Osbom AG. Diagnostic neuroradiology. St Louis (MO): Mosby; 1994. p. 631.

36. Ikushima I, Korogi Y, Hirai T, et al. MR of epidermoids with a variety of pulse sequences. Am J Neuroradiol 1997;18:1359–63.

37. Michael LM II, Moss T, Madhu T. Malignant transformation of posterior fossa epidermoid cyst. Br J Neurosurg 2005;19(6):505–10.

38. Timmer FA, Sluzewski M, Treskes M, et al. Chemical analysis of an epidermoid cyst with unusual CT and MR characteristics. Am J Neuroradiol 1998;19(6): 1111–2.

39. Nguyen JB, Ahktar N, Delgado PN, et al. Magnetic resonance imaging and proton magnetic resonance spectroscopy of intracranial epidermoid tumors. Crit Rev Comput Tomogr 2004;45:389–427.

40. Rock IP, Zimmerman R, Bell WO, et al. Arachnoid cysts of the posterior fossa. Neurosurgery 1986;18: 176–9.

41. Smimiotopoulos JG, Yue NC, Rushing L. Cerebellopontine angle masses: radiologic-pathologic correlation. Radiographics 1993;13:1131–47.

42. Dahlen RT, Johnson CE, Harnsberger HR, et al. CT and MR characteristics of intravestibular lipoma. Am J Neuroradiol 2002;23:1413–7.

43. Sze G. Diseases of the intracranial meninges: MR imaging features. Am J Roentgenol 1993;160:727–33.

44. Harnsberger HR. Endolymphatic sac anomaly. In: Harnsberger HR, et al, editors. Diagnostic imaging head and neck. Amirsys (Diagnostic Imaging (Lippincott)); 2004. I2-108-111.

45. Levenson MJ, Parisier SC, Jacobs M, et al. The large vestibular aqueduct syndrome in children: a review of 12 cases and the description of a new clinical entity. Arch Otolaryngol Head Neck Surg 1989;115:54–8.

46. Naganawa S, Ito T, Iwayama E, et al. MR imaging of the cochlear modiolus: area measurement in healthy subjects and in patients with a large endolymphatic duct and sac. Radiology 1999;213(3):819–23.

47. Sugiura M, Naganawa S, Ishida IM, et al. Vestibular aqueduct in sudden sensorineural hearing loss. J Laryngol Otol 2007;122:887–92.

48. Ishida IM, Sugiura M, Naganawa S, et al. Cochlear modiolus and lateral semicircular canal in sudden deafness. Acta Otolaryngol 2007;127:1–5.

49. Boston M, Halsted M, Meinzen-Derr J, et al. The large vestibular aqueduct: a new definition based on audiologic and computed tomography correlation. Otolaryngol Head Neck Surg 2007;136:972–7.

50. Mark AS, Seltzer S, Nelson-Drake J, et al. Labyrinthine enhancement on gadolinium-enhanced magnetic resonance imaging in sudden deafness and vertigo: correlation with audiologic and electronystagmographic studies. Ann Otol Rhinol Laryngol 1992;101:459–64.

51. Merchant SN, Gopen Q. A human temporal bone study of acute bacterial meningogenic labyrinthitis. Am J Otol 1996;17:375–85.

52. Casselman JW, Kuhweide R, Ampe W, et al. Pathology of the membranous labyrinth: comparison of T1- and T2-weighted and gadolinium-enhanced spin echo and 3DFT-CISS imaging. AJNR Am J Neuroradiol 1993;14:59–69.

53. Fitzgerald DC, Grundfast KM, Hecht DA, et al. Intralabyrinthine schwannomas. Am J Otol 1999;20(3):381–5.

54. Baltacioglu F, Ekinci G, Türe U, et al. MR imaging, CT and angiography features of endolymphatic sac tumors: report of two cases. Neuroradiology 2002;44(1):91–6.

55. Harnsberger HR. Endolymphatic sac tumor. In: Harnsberger HR, et al, editors. Diagnostic imaging head and neck. Amirsys (Diagnostic Imaging (Lippincott)); 2004. I2-126-129.

56. Connor SE, Leung R, Natas S. Imaging of the petrous apex: a pictorial review. Br J Radiol 2008;81(965): 427–35.

57. Koesling S, Kunkel P, Schul T. Vascular anomalies, sutures and small canals of the temporal bone on axial CT. Eur J Radiol 2005;54(3):335–43.

58. Dubois PJ, Roub LW. Giant air cells of the petrous apex: tomographic features. Radiology 1978;129(1):103–9.

59. Arriaga MA. Petrous apex effusion: a clinical disorder. Laryngoscope 2006;116(8):1349–56.

60. Farrior B, Kampsen E, Farrior JB. The positive pressure of cholesterol granuloma idiopathic blue eardrum: differential diagnosis. Laryngoscope 1981;91(8):1286–96.

61. Jackler RK, Cho M. A new theory to explain the genesis of petrous apex cholesterol granuloma. Otol Neurotol 2003;24(1):96–106.

62. Jackler RK, Parker DA. Radiographic differential diagnosis of petrous apex lesions. Am J Otol 1992; 13(6):561–74.

63. Motamed M, Kalan A. Gardenigo's syndrome. Postgrad Med J 2000;76:559–60.

64. Lee YH, Lee NJ, Kim JH, et al. CT, MRI and gallium SPECT in the diagnosis and treatment of petrous apicitis presenting as multiple cranial neuropathies. Br J Radiol 2005;78:948–51.

65. Lee S, Hooper R, Fuller A, et al. Otogenic cranial base osteomyelitis: a proposed prognosis-based system for disease classification. Otol Neurotol 2008;29(5):666–72.

66. Magliulo G. Petrous bone cholesteatoma: clinical longitudinal study. Eur Arch Otorhinolaryngol 2007; 264:115–20.

67. Vercruysse JP, De Foer B, Pouillon M, et al. The value of diffusion-weighted MR imaging in the diagnosis of primary acquired and residual cholesteatoma: a surgical verified study of 100 patients. Eur Radiol 2006;16:1461–7.

68. De Foer B, Vercruysse JP, Bernaerts A. The value of single-shot turbo spin-echo diffusion-weighted MR imaging in the detection of middle ear cholesteatoma. Neuroradiology 2007;49:841–8.

69. Williams MT, Ayache D, Alberti C, et al. Detection of post-operative residual cholesteatoma with delayed contrast-enhanced MR imaging: initial findings. Eur Radiol 2003;13:169–74.

70. Rao AB, Koeller KK, Adair CF. From the archives of the AFIP. Paragangliomas of the head and neck: radiologic-pathologic correlation. Radiographics 1999;19:1605–32.

71. Caldemeyer KS, Mathews VP, Azzarelli B, et al. The jugular foramen: a review of anatomy, masses, and imaging characteristics. Radiographics 1997;17: 1123–39.

72. Neves F, Huwart L, Jourdan G, et al. Head and neck paragangliomas: value of contrast-enhanced 3D MR angiography. Am J Neuroradiol 2008;29: 883–9.

73. Curtin H, Sanelli P, Som P. Temporal bone: embryology and anatomy. In: Som PM, Curtin HD, editors. Head and neck imaging. 4th edition. St Louis (MO): Mosby; 2003. p. 1057–92.

74. Gebarski SS, Telian SA, Niparko JK. Enhancement along the normal facial nerve in the facial canal: MR imaging and anatomic correlation. Radiology 1992;183(2):391–4.

75. Latack JT, Gabrielsen TO, Knake JE, et al. Facial nerve neuromas: radiologic evaluation. Radiology 1983;149:731–9.

76. Dort JC, Fisch U. Facial nerve schwannoma. Skull Base Surg 1991;1:51–7.

77. Chandler JR. Malignant external otitis. Laryngoscope 1968;78:1257–94.

78. Sreepada GS, Kwartler JA. Skull base osteomyelitis secondary to malignant otitis externa. Curr Opin Otolaryngol Head Neck Surg 2003;11(5):316–23.

79. Slattery WH, Brackmann DE. Skull base osteomyelitis: malignant external otitis. Otolaryngol Clin North Am 1996;29(5):795–805.

80. Driscoll PV, Ramachandrula A, Drezner DA, et al. Characteristics of cerumen in diabetic patients: a key to understanding malignant external otitis? Otolaryngol Head Neck Surg 1993;109(4):676–9.

81. Kwon BJ, Han MH, Oh SH, et al. MRI findings and spreading patterns of necrotizing external otitis: is a poor outcome predictable? Clin Radiol 2006;61: 495–504.

82. Chang CH, Shu MT, Lee JC, et al. Treatments and outcome of malignant tumors of external auditory canal. Am J Otolaryngol 2009;30:44–8.

83. Hermans R. External ear imaging. In: Lemmerling M, Kolias S, editors. Radiology of the petrous bone. New York, Berlin, Heidelberg: Springer-Verlag; 2004. p. 15–30.

84. Kenning TJ, Willcox TO, Artz GJ, et al. Surgical management of temporal meningoencephaloceles, cerebrospinal fluid leaks, and intracranial hypertension: treatment paradigm and outcomes. Neurosurg Focus 2012;32(6):E6.

Magnetic Resonance Imaging of the Pediatric Neck: An Overview

Karuna V. Shekdar, MD[a],*, David M. Mirsky, MD[a],
Ken Kazahaya, MD, MBA[b], Larissa T. Bilaniuk, MD[a]

KEYWORDS

- Pediatric neck MR imaging • Anomalies of the branchial apparatus • Cystic neck lesions in a child
- Solid neck lesions in a child • Rhabdomyosarcoma • Fibromatosis colli

KEY POINTS

- Magnetic resonance imaging does not involve ionizing radiation, and is ideally suited for characterization of pediatric neck lesions located in anatomically complex areas such as the floor of the mouth and deep neck spaces.
- The leading differential considerations for a cystic lesion on the floor of the mouth include a thyroglossal duct cyst, a dermoid/congenital inclusion cyst, a ranula, and a foregut duplication cyst.
- Anomalies of the second branchial cleft are the most common of the branchial-apparatus anomalies. These lesions typically displace the submandibular gland anteriorly and the sternocleidomastoid muscle posterolaterally.
- A nontender fusiform mass involving unilateral sternocleidomastoid muscle in a young infant is often pathognomonic of fibromatosis colli.
- Lymphatic malformations are large transspatial, multiloculated masses with heterogeneous signal intensity that may demonstrate fluid levels secondary to hemorrhage.
- An enhancing solid mass, associated with the carotid sheath and unilateral Horner syndrome, should raise concern for neuroblastoma.
- Aggressive soft-tissue masses in the pediatric head and neck with transspatial involvement, especially when accompanied by osseous destruction, are most commonly associated with rhabdomyosarcomas.

INTRODUCTION

Evaluation of neck lesions in the pediatric age group can be a diagnostic challenge. The evaluation begins with clinical history and thorough physical examination. Imaging, either ultrasonography (US), computed tomography (CT), or magnetic resonance (MR) imaging, is used to further characterize these lesions. US is a quick imaging modality, which does not involve ionizing radiation and is helpful in characterizing or in confirming cystic nature of lesion and, to a certain extent, in defining the relationship of lesions with surrounding normal structures. However, US is limited in evaluating lesions that are deep seated or very small. CT is superior to US regarding cross-sectional evaluation of masses

Funding sources: None.
Conflict of interest: None.
[a] Division of Neuroradiology, Department of Radiology, The Children's Hospital of Philadelphia, Perelman School of Medicine at the University of Pennsylvania, 324 South 34th Street, Philadelphia, PA 19104, USA;
[b] Division of Pediatric Otolaryngology, The Children's Hospital of Philadelphia, Perelman School of Medicine at the University of Pennsylvania, 324 South 34th Street, Philadelphia, PA 19104, USA
* Corresponding author.
E-mail address: shekdar@email.chop.edu

mri.theclinics.com

that are deep seated. CT is also superior for detection of calcification, and with the new ultrafast scanners CT is the investigation of choice in the setting of an emergency involving trauma, acute infection, or airway compromise. However, CT involves ionizing radiation, which can be potentially harmful in the pediatric age group to sensitive organs such as the thyroid gland.[1,2] MR imaging does not involve ionizing radiation, has superior contrast resolution, and has an inherently high signal-to-noise ratio, making it ideal for evaluating various neck lesions. MR is ideally suited for evaluation of masses located in anatomically complex areas such as the floor of the mouth and deep neck spaces. MR can characterize a lesion better, can accurately demonstrate the full extent of the mass along with its relationship with the surrounding structures, and provides important information for presurgical planning.

This article provides an overview of the utility of MR imaging in the evaluation of various neck lesions in the pediatric population.

TECHNICAL ASPECTS

A typical neck MR study includes multiplanar T1-weighted and T2-weighted images. It is recommended that T2-weighted images be done with fat saturation. Depending on the clinical indication for the study, the slice thickness needs to be tailored according to the lesion being evaluated. For example, for evaluation of subcentimeter lesions and small tracts and fistulae, the slice thickness may have to be as thin as 2 mm. Addition of HASTE (Half-Fourier Single short Turbo Echo) sequences is particularly valuable for identifying cystic lesions and fluid-filled sinus tracts, shown in **Figs. 1** and **2**. Contrast-enhanced MR imaging is essential for the evaluation of most lesions that are congenital, inflammatory/infectious, or of neoplastic etiology. Postcontrast T1 imaging with fat suppression is helpful in correctly identifying subtle enhancement. Addition of diffusion-weighted (DW) imaging is particularly useful in the evaluation of suspected dermal inclusion cysts (see **Fig. 1**), abscesses, or neoplastic lesions, for better characterization of these lesions and help in arriving at a specific diagnosis. At their institution the authors routinely use DW imaging and obtain apparent diffusion coefficient (ADC) maps in MR evaluation of the neck. The average duration of a neck MR imaging study is approximately 30 to 40 minutes. The older children are able to hold still for the duration of the MR study without the use of sedation. However, infants and young children often require preprocedural sedation to maintain a motionless state, thus ensuring high-quality MR imaging.

A discussion of the detailed anatomy of the neck spaces is beyond the scope of this article. The reader is referred to further excellent literature for this information.[3,4] The distribution of the different neck lesions according to their location is summarized in **Table 1**.

Knowledge of the embryologic origin of neck structures is helpful in the understanding and detection of pediatric neck lesions. Relevant embryology is discussed here, along with thyroglossal duct cysts (TGDCs), anomalies of the branchial apparatus, and thymic cysts.

THYROGLOSSAL DUCT CYST

During the fourth week of gestation, the thyroid primordium originates as a diverticulum from the floor of the pharynx (tuberculum impar) at the site of the future foramen cecum at the base of the tongue.[5] The gland migrates inferiorly through the peripharyngeal connective tissue just anterior to the hyoid bone and laryngeal cartilages and descends in the neck anterior to the thyrohyoid membrane and deep to the strap muscles, reaching its final position in the lower midline of the neck by the seventh week of gestation. The anlage of the gland is connected to the tongue by the thyroglossal duct during its migration. The thyroglossal duct obliterates between the fifth and tenth week of gestation, leaving behind a proximal remnant at the foramen cecum and a distal remnant: the pyramidal lobe of the thyroid gland. The duct is intimately associated with the developing hyoid bone.[6] Failure of obliteration of the thyroglossal duct before the formation of the mesodermal anlage of the hyoid bone results in its persistence during development and after birth. The line defined by the embryologic descent of the thyroid gland is the site where the anomalies of the thyroglossal duct can occur.

Anomalies of the thyroglossal duct constitute the majority of the congenital midline cervical masses seen in children. It has been estimated that they account for about 70% of congenital neck anomalies, and are the second most common benign neck mass in pediatric patients behind benign cervical lymphadenopathy.[6] TGDCs are approximately 3 times more common than anomalies of the branchial apparatus.[7]

TGDCs arise as cystic expansion of the remnant of the thyroglossal duct tract.[6] TGDCs are located adjacent to the hyoid bone (60%), between the hyoid bone and the base of the tongue (24%), and infrahyoid (13%). Three percent of TGDCs may be intralingual in location.[6,8] TGDCs are intimately related to the hyoid bone, either juxtahyoid

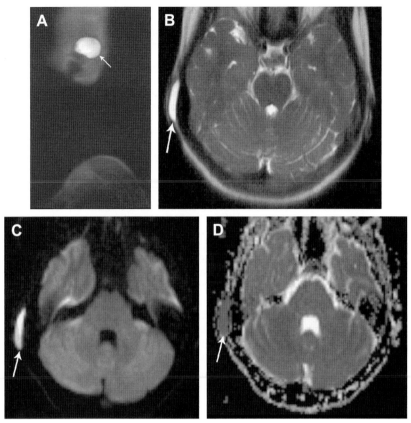

Fig. 1. Congenital inclusion cyst/epidermoid, posterior to the right auricle (*arrows*). (*A, B*) Sagittal and axial half-Fourier single short turbo echo (HASTE) showing bright fluid signal consistent with a cyst. (*C*) Axial diffusion and (*D*) Apparent diffusion coefficient (ADC) map showing restricted diffusion.

or infrahyoid. Most of these (75%) are in or slightly off the midline (25%) but within 2 cm of the midline (**Fig. 3**A).[8] The paramedian location is usually seen with the infrahyoid TGDCs (**Fig. 3**B).

On MR imaging, a noncomplicated TGDC is hypointense on T1, hyperintense on T2, and bright on HASTE sequences, reflecting fluid content. Sagittal MR images are particularly useful in determining the extent of the lesion before resection. Such lesions may be unilocular or multiloculated

and occasionally have septations. There is no peripheral rim enhancement unless there has been prior inflammation. This classic appearance is seen in fewer than half of cases.[6] A peripheral rim of enhancement is seen if there has been prior infection or inflammation (**Fig. 4**).[6] In the case of infection or hemorrhage a thick irregular rim may be demonstrated, and the signal intensity of the contents may vary according to the presence of proteinaceous or hemorrhagic debris within the

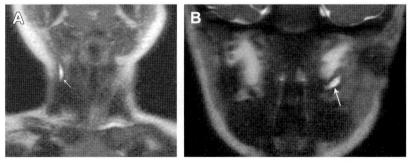

Fig. 2. (*A, B*) Utility of thin-section HASTE coronal images showing fluid-filled, tiny, bilateral branchial sinus tracks (*arrows*).

Table 1
Differential diagnosis of pediatric neck masses based on their location

Location	Lesions
Floor of the mouth	Thyroglossal duct cyst (midline) Foregut duplication cyst Dermoid, epidermoid Ranula Lymphatic malformation Teratoma Vascular lesions (ie, hemangioma, venous vascular lesions)
Periauricular	Lymphadenitis Anomalies of first branchial cleft Atypical mycobacterial infection Lymphatic malformation
Submandibular	Lymphadenitis Anomalies of second branchial cleft Atypical mycobacterial infection Lymphatic malformation Vascular lesions (ie, hemangioma, venous vascular lesions)
Carotid	Lymphadenitis Branchial-cleft anomalies Lymphatic malformation Neurogenic tumors: neuroblastoma, neurofibroma Vascular lesions (ie, hemangioma, venous vascular lesions)
Neck anterior	Thyroglossal duct cyst (midline or within 2 cm of midline) Thymic cyst/ectopic thymus Lymphatic malformation Lymphadenitis Teratoma
Supraclavicular	Lymphoma Metastatic disease Lymphadenitis Lymphatic malformation
Posterior neck occipital	Lymphadenitis Lymphoma Lymphatic malformation Vascular lesions (ie, hemangioma, venous vascular lesions)

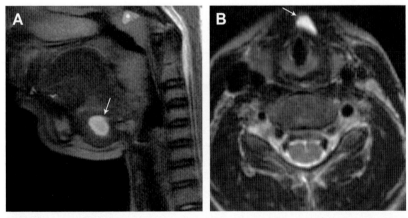

Fig. 3. Thyroglossal duct cyst (TGDC). (*A*) Sagittal T2-weighted image shows TGDC in most common location at base of the tongue (*arrow*). Incidentally noted is a small retention cyst in the adenoids (*asterisk*). In another patient (*B*), Axial T2-weighted image shows an infrahyoid TGDC slightly to left of midline subjacent to strap muscles (*arrow*).

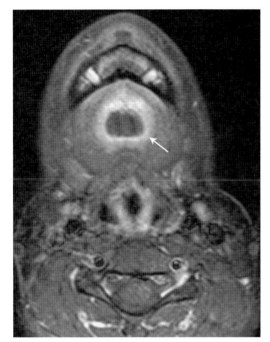

Fig. 4. Infected TGDC. Contrast-enhanced axial T1-weighted fat-saturated image demonstrates a thick rim of enhancement (*arrow*).

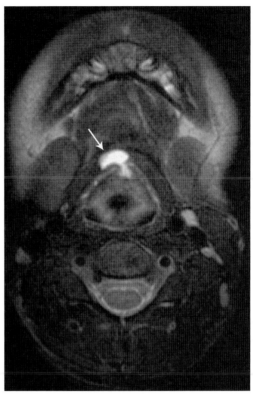

Fig. 5. Recurrent TGDC. Axial T2-weighted image with fat saturation demonstrates a lobulated cystic mass (*arrow*) traversing the anterior aspect of the hyoid bone via a defect created from prior TGDC resection.

cyst. Thickening of the surrounding strap muscles and cutaneous induration of the subcutaneous fat can be related to TGDC inflammation. Association of a solid mass with a TGDC usually represents ectopic thyroid tissue. Coexisting malignancy may be found within 1% of TGDCs. Malignancy usually arises from ectopic thyroid tissue and is typically a papillary carcinoma.[9,10] Papillary carcinoma may be seen on MR imaging as a soft-tissue mass, which enhances with contrast and usually contains foci of mineralization/calcification.

Thyroglossal duct cysts are treated by surgical excision. Typically a Sistrunk procedure is used, which involves complete resection of the entire TGDC along with excision of the midportion of the hyoid bone and any associated tract. Occasionally, following simple cyst excision or even the Sistrunk procedure, the TGDC may recur. MR imaging is again valuable in evaluation of recurrent cysts.[11] **Fig. 5** illustrates a case of recurrence of a TGDC following the Sistrunk procedure.

What the Ear/Nose/Throat (ENT) Surgeon Wants to Know

1. Whether the TGDC is a single cyst or if it is multifocal; location with regard to the surrounding anatomy: foramen cecum, base of tongue musculature, and hyoid bone.
2. Whether the thyroid gland is present in a normal location in the lower neck. Is there evidence of lingual thyroid?
3. If there is a recurrence the location and size of the recurrent TGDC, and if there are more than one foci of recurrence.

LINGUAL THYROID

Arrest of the migration of the thyroid anlage between 3 and 7 weeks of gestation results in an ectopic location of the thyroid gland at the tongue base, usually at foramen cecum. The imaging features of the lingual thyroid resemble that of thyroid gland tissue, that is, iso- to hyperintense on T1-weighted images and mild to strikingly hyperintense on T2-weighted images, with more enhancement than for the tongue (**Fig. 6**). Once a lingual thyroid is identified, it is important to assess by imaging whether an orthotopic thyroid tissue is present and if there are additional sites of ectopic thyroid tissue in the neck. A radioisotope scan is usually performed to help assess or confirm such findings.[12]

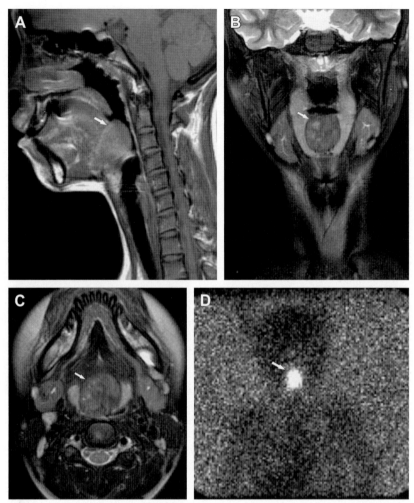

Fig. 6. Lingual thyroid. (*A*) Sagittal T1-weighted, (*B*) coronal T2-weighted, and (*C*) axial T2-weighted images demonstrate a well-circumscribed mass (*arrow*) at the base of the tongue. (*D*) Planar image from an iodine-123 uptake scan demonstrates a single focus of radiotracer activity in the lingual region without any focal activity in the normal thyroid bed.

CONGENITAL INCLUSION CYSTS/DERMOIDS AND EPIDERMOIDS

The term congenital inclusion cyst is commonly used in reference to both dermoid and epidermoid cysts. These cysts arise from elements of the ectoderm and are lined by squamous epithelium. Dermoid cysts include components of all 3 layers of the ectoderm and may include adnexal structures such as teeth, hair, and sebaceous glands. Dermoid cysts may also contain lipid material derived from sebaceous secretions. Epidermoid cysts include debris from the desquamated epithelium from 2 layers of the ectoderm containing keratin and cholesterol derived from the breakdown of cell membranes.

The oral cavity is the second most common location of dermoid cysts in the head and neck regions, the most common location being the orbital area.[13]

Dermoid cysts in the oral cavity are in the region of the floor of the mouth and are typically found in the midline.[13] These cysts may be located on the dorsum of the tongue and the hard or soft palate. Sublingual dermoid cysts are centered above the mylohyoid muscle and present as submucosal lesions in the floor of the mouth. Submental dermoid cysts are centered below the mylohyoid muscle.

On MR imaging dermoid cysts are usually well-demarcated, unilocular midline masses located within the submandibular or the sublingual space. Presence of fat within the lesion is a characteristic feature of a dermoid cyst. Dermoid cysts are most commonly moderately hyperintense on T1-weighted images because of the presence of lipids; however, the signal characteristics on T1 images may be variable and can be isointense relative to muscle. On T2-weighted images they are usually hyperintense. Heterogeneity, fluid-fluid levels, and calcification may be present (**Fig. 7**). Many dermoid cysts show restricted diffusion.

Epidermal inclusion cysts have fluid-signal characteristics that are T1-hypointense and T2-hyperintense. Diffusion restriction is a characteristic feature of epidermal inclusion cysts or epidermoids (see **Fig. 1**).[14]

ENT Surgeon Comment

MR imaging is valuable in demonstrating the exact location of the dermoid cyst with respect to the mylohyoid muscle using the multiplanar imaging capability, which is most helpful for planning surgical resection and approach. Dermoid cysts located superior to the mylohyoid muscle typically require a transoral surgical approach, whereas those cysts located inferior or superficial to the mylohyoid muscle require an external submandibular approach.[15]

RANULA

A ranula is a pseudocyst containing extravasated mucus from the sublingual salivary glands. Ranulas are considered pseudocysts, as they lack a true epithelial lining. A simple ranula is a cystic collection confined to the sublingual space in the floor of the mouth. A diving or plunging ranula typically presents with a swelling in the submandibular region or upper neck as the result of mucus extravasating inferior to the mylohyoid muscle.

On MR imaging, a ranula typically demonstrates signal consistent with fluid that is hypointense on T1-weighted images and hyperintense on T2-weighted images (**Fig. 8**). Thin linear enhancement of the wall may be seen following contrast. If there has been recent infection or inflammation, the wall may be thick with irregular enhancement. A simple ranula has either an oval or lenticular shape, and if bilateral may assume a horseshoe shape. On imaging a plunging ranula has a comet shape and may have a tail in the sublingual space (**Fig. 9**). The presence of the tail is a characteristic

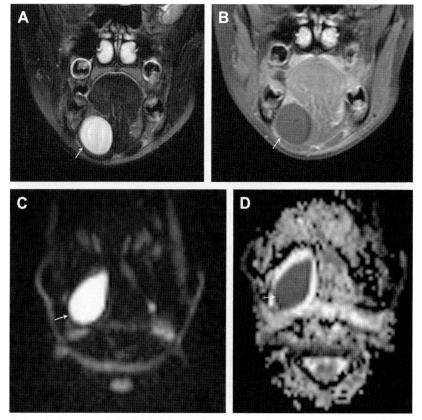

Fig. 7. Congenital inclusion cyst/epidermoid, (*A*) Coronal T2-weighted and (*B*) fat-saturated postcontrast coronal T1-weighted images reveal an ovoid mass involving the floor of the mouth, eccentric to the right (*arrow*). (*C*) Diffusion-weighted image and (*D*) corresponding ADC map showing restricted diffusion (*arrow*).

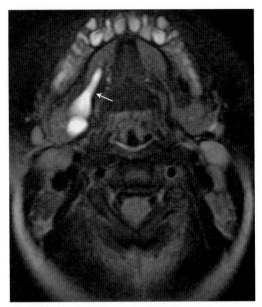

Fig. 8. Simple ranula. Axial T2-weighted fat-saturated image demonstrates a multiloculated cystic mass within the right sublingual space (*arrow*).

feature of a plunging ranula, and when they are large enough they may extend into the upper neck and parapharyngeal space.[16]

ENT Surgeon Comment

Management of a ranula typically requires resection of the ipsilateral sublingual gland and intraoral drainage of the mucus collection. Simple transoral drainage and/or marsupialization of a ranula may be performed, but has a high recurrence rate. Therefore, transoral resection of the sublingual gland with drainage of the mucus collection is a recommended technique. The submandibular duct and lingual nerve should be carefully preserved, as they typically run along the medial

aspect of the dissection. Complete resection of the pseudocyst is unnecessary, as there is no epithelial lining of the collection and the origin of the fluid is the sublingual gland, which is completely excised. Confirmation of the diagnosis of a ranula can be made by analyzing the fluid composition, as it typically will have lower sodium, chloride, and glucose levels, and higher amylase levels, than a similar-appearing collection from a cystic hygroma. A biopsy of the wall of the pseudocyst may also be sent for confirmation.

ANOMALIES OF THE BRANCHIAL APPARATUS

Anomalies of the branchial apparatus account for 17% of all pediatric neck masses, and are the second most common developmental neck abnormality after the TGDC.

To understand the different anomalies arising from the branchial apparatus, it is crucial to have knowledge about their embryologic origin. All the structures of the neck are derived from the branchial apparatus, which consists of paired pharyngeal arches, clefts, pouches, and membranes.[5] During the fourth to seventh weeks of the human embryonic development 6 paired branchial arches are initially formed. The first branchial arch is either not formed or quickly degenerates in the body. Five ectodermal-lined branchial clefts and 5 endodermal-lined pharyngeal pouches separate the 6 arches. A closing membrane is present at the interface of the pharyngeal pouches and the branchial clefts. The external auditory canal forms from the first cleft, and the tympanic cavity, mastoid air cells, and Eustachian tube develop from the first pouch. The palatine tonsil is a derivative of the second pouch. The second cleft disappears completely. Incomplete obliteration of the branchial apparatus results in the formation of branchial cysts, sinuses, or fistulae. Regardless of the different theories about the origin of these

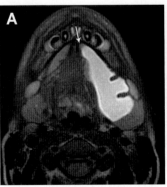
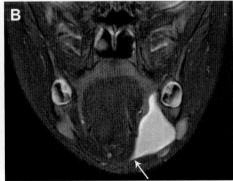

Fig. 9. Diving ranula. Axial (*A*) and coronal (*B*) T2-weighted fat-saturated images showing a diving ranula with characteristic tail (*arrow*).

congenital cervical anomalies, the most popular accepted hypothesis concerns the branchial remnants that lead to anomalies of the branchial apparatus, of which anomalies of the second branchial cleft are the most common.[17] With continued development of the neck, the second branchial arch overgrows the third and the fourth branchial clefts and fuses with the lateral branchial wall. An ectodermal-lined cavity known as the cervical sinus of His is formed. Incomplete obliteration of the cervical sinus plays an important role in the development of anomalies of the second branchial cleft. A line drawn from the oropharyngeal tonsillar fossa to the supraclavicular region of the neck represents the site of anomalies of the second branchial cleft.[17]

Based on their location, anomalies of the branchial apparatus are classified according to the proposed pouch or cleft of origin. The majority are anomalies of the second branchial apparatus, followed by those of the first branchial cleft.[18] Anomalies of the third and particularly the fourth branchial apparatus are extremely rare. **Table 2** summarizes the location and common clinical presentation of anomalies of the branchial apparatus.

MR imaging is particularly useful in the evaluation of anomalies of the branchial apparatus and in understanding their relationship to the surrounding structures.[18,19]

Anomalies of the First Branchial Apparatus

Anomalies of the first branchial cleft can occur anywhere along the embryologic tract extending from the submandibular triangle and terminating at the cartilaginous-bony junction of the external auditory canal, coursing through the parotid gland, with a variable relationship with the facial nerve.[17]

The majority of first-branchial anomalies are unilocular cysts, within the parotid gland or around the external auditory canal. Fistulae typically extend from the floor of the external auditory canal through the parotid gland, to an opening located between the sternocleidomastoid muscle, hyoid bone, and angle of the mandible.[17] The appearance of the cyst on MR imaging depends on the contents of the cyst. Simple cystic lesions demonstrate fluid-signal characteristics with hypointense signal on T1-weighted images and hyperintense signal on T2-weighted images (**Fig. 10**). With increasing protein content or infections there is a higher signal on T1-weighted images. There may be enhancement and a thick wall if the cyst has been infected.[18] A first-branchial anomaly has a variable relation to the facial nerve. The location of the branchial anomaly and its relationship to the facial nerve should be specifically determined before surgery if possible. MR imaging is especially useful in determining these important factors prior to surgery.[18] Care must be taken during surgery, as the nerve may be displaced laterally if the anomaly runs medial to the nerve, putting the nerve at risk during the approach to the anomaly.

Anomalies of the Second Branchial Cleft

The typical location of these lesions is in the submandibular space along the anterior border of the sternocleidomastoid muscle, but can be anywhere along the developmental path of the second branchial arch.

On MR imaging these lesions typically demonstrate a cystic nature, with low signal on T1-weighted images and high signal on T2-weighted images. Signal characteristics may vary according

Table 2		
Location and clinical features of anomalies of the branchial apparatus		
Type	**Location**	**Clinical Presentation**
First	External auditory canal, parotid region	Mass around external auditory canal, chronic unexplained otorrhea, or recurrent parotid gland abscess
Second	Submandibular region, lateral to carotid vessels	Painless mass at mandibular angle or lateral neck in a child or young adult
Third	Posterior triangle of neck, usually left side	Unexplained recurrent deep or lateral neck infection/abscesses Draining cervical sinus Mass in posterolateral neck expanding after respiratory tract infection
Fourth	Sinus tract opening at pyriform sinus usually on the left	Mass on lower third of neck usually on the left side Recurrent neck abscesses Recurrent suppurative thyroiditis

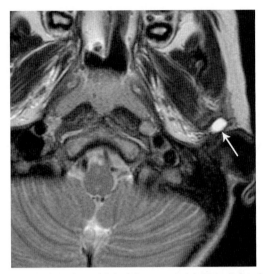

Fig. 10. First branchial cleft cyst. Axial T2-weighted image demonstrates a small well-circumscribed cystic lesion (*arrow*) anterior to the left external auditory canal, posterior to the left mandibular condylar head.

to the protein content within the cyst. With high proteinaceous fluid content there may be increased signal on T1, and decreased or intermediate T2 signal intensity. The most common of the cysts of the second branchial cleft is the Bailey type 2. Such cysts displace the submandibular gland anteriorly, push the carotid space vessels medially or posteromedially, and displace the sternocleidomastoid muscle posterolaterally (**Fig. 11**).[18] The typical path of an anomaly of the

second branchial cleft is over the glossopharyngeal nerve and hypoglossal nerves, between the internal and external carotid arteries, penetrating through the pharyngeal musculature to communicate with the oropharynx in the region of the tonsillar fossa. Occasionally a beak sign may be seen as a small soft tissue pointing medially between the internal and external carotid arteries, and is considered a pathognomonic imaging feature of a cyst of the second branchial cleft.[18]

Anomalies of the Third and Fourth Branchial Clefts

Developmental anomalies of the third and the fourth branchial clefts are extremely rare, and are almost always formed on the left side. Cysts of the third branchial cleft usually present as a mass in the posterior cervical triangle,[18] and are considered the most common congenital lesion of the posterior cervical space after lymphangiomas. A characteristic fistula of third-branchial origin communicates externally along the anterior border of the sternocleidomastoid muscle, similar to a second-branchial anomaly, only more caudally. A third-branchial anomaly follows the predicted embryologic course extending from the supraclavicular fossa to the lateral aspect of the piriform sinus. The tract descends within the carotid sheath posterior to the common and internal carotid arteries and anterior to the vagus nerve, between the hypoglossal and glossopharyngeal nerves, and penetrates the thyrohyoid membrane to communicate with the upper

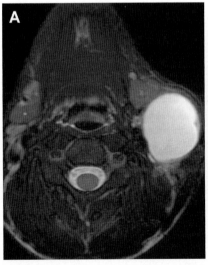
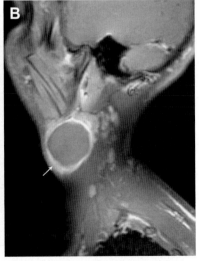

Fig. 11. Infected type 2 branchial cleft cyst. (*A*) Axial T2-weighted image with fat saturation demonstrates a well-circumscribed cystic mass within the left neck, lateral to the left common carotid artery bifurcation and anterior to the left sternocleidomastoid muscle. (*B*) Contrast-enhanced sagittal T1-weighted fat-saturated image reveals thick rim of enhancement (*arrow*) about the mass.

part of the piriform sinus, anterior to the superior laryngeal nerve. The possibility of a cyst of the third branchial cleft can be suggested on MR imaging when the lesion is situated in the lateral compartment of the neck, posterior to the common carotid artery and jugular vein, and is in the posterior triangle of the neck. These lesions may extend inferiorly to the level of the thyroid gland.

Differentiating anomalies of the third branchial cleft from those of the fourth may be difficult because both have a relationship with the piriform sinus. The difference between these two lesions is in their relationship to the superior laryngeal nerve (nerve of the fourth arch).[18] The lesions above this structure originate from the third branchial cleft and those below are derived from the fourth branchial cleft. The fourth-branchial anomaly typically opens into the apex of the piriform sinus.

Cysts of the third branchial cleft are mostly seen as a unilocular cystic mass on MR imaging. The signal depends on the contents and the wall thickness, and enhancement and surrounding changes vary according to the associated inflammatory changes. An internal fistula arising from the apex of the piriform sinus would be a remnant of the fourth pouch. When the sinus tracts are fluid-filled or inflamed they may be seen on MR imaging with the help of HASTE sequences and fat-suppressed, contrast-enhanced T1-weighted sequences. However, the gold standard for evaluation of these sinuses and fistulae is direct visualization by fluoroscopy following injection of contrast material (Figs. 12 and 13).[18,19]

What the ENT Surgeon Wants to Know

Anatomic location of the cyst and associated track along with the relationship to the parotid gland, carotid sheath, internal and external carotid arteries, and piriform sinus, as defined herein.

THYMIC CYSTS AND RESTS

The embryologic development of the thymus is from ventral sacculation of the third pharyngeal pouch at approximately 6 weeks of development of the human embryo.[20] The thymopharyngeal tract elongates and descends into the mediastinum, with obliteration of the lumen by approximately 7 to 8 weeks and there is fusion of the tract in the mediastinum by the ninth week of development. The most common theory postulated for the formation of thymic cysts is that they probably arise from the embryologic remnants of the thymopharyngeal duct.[20]

The rests of the thymic tissue in the neck can be present anywhere along the embryologic path of descent from the angle of the mandible to the mediastinum (Fig. 14). It has been estimated that residual thymic tissue in the neck is found in 1.8% to 21% of individuals.[20] It usually presents as an asymptomatic neck mass and is one of the differential diagnoses of neck masses in children. It is important to identify the thymic rests for what they are, and avoid unnecessary anxiety or intervention (Fig. 15).[21]

Thymic cysts are either unilocular or multilocular cysts. These masses extend almost parallel to the sternocleidomastoid muscle in the lower neck and are more commonly on the left. The MR appearance is hypointensity on T1-weighted images and hyperintensity on T2-weighted images.[19,22]

LYMPHATIC MALFORMATIONS

Lymphatic anomalies constitute about 5% of benign tumors of infancy and childhood.[23] These tumors most commonly present in newborn infants, and most of these (up to 90%) are diagnosed by 2 years of age.[23] The most common

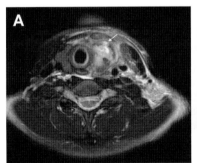
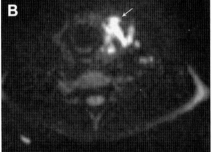

Fig. 12. Type 4 branchial cleft cyst. (A) Axial T2-weighted image with fat saturation and (B) axial diffusion image reveal a lobulated collection centered within the left lobe of the thyroid gland with restricted diffusion and surrounding inflammation (arrow). This patient had a history of recurrent suppurative thyroiditis.

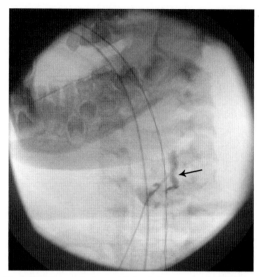

Fig. 13. Type 4 branchial cleft cyst. Fistulogram demonstrating a thin linear tract directed superiorly toward the expected location of the left piriform sinus (*arrow*).

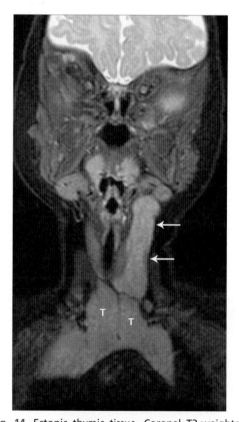

Fig. 14. Ectopic thymic tissue. Coronal T2-weighted fat-saturated image demonstrates cervical extension of thymic tissue (T) with an elongated soft-tissue mass (*arrows*) extending cephalad within the left neck, which follows thymic signal intensity on all pulse sequences.

location of lymphatic malformations is the extra-cranial head and neck.[7]

Lymphatic malformations are thought to arise from an early sequestration of embryonic lymphatic channels, which prevents normal drainage into the venous system and results in progressive enlargement of the isolated lymphatic spaces. Another popular hypothesis is congenital obstruction of lymphatic drainage, resulting in formation of these large lymphatic spaces.[7]

Within the neck the most common location is the posterior cervical triangle, followed by the submandibular region. These masses are usually large and therefore render themselves to antenatal detection by either US or MR. Such lesions are known to enlarge commensurate with the growth of the child. A sudden increase in their size is known to occur with spontaneous hemorrhage, trauma, or infection. These masses often extend transspatially, and when large are at risk for critical compromise of the airway.

MR imaging is the preferred cross-sectional modality for evaluation of lymphatic anomalies, as it can completely demonstrate the extent and morphology of the lesion and its relationship to the adjacent soft tissues and vital structures. Signal within the lesions on T1-weighted images is variable from hypointense to hyperintense, depending on the contents. Hemorrhage within the cystic locules can give rise to fluid-fluid levels as well as extensive T1 shortening. On T2-weighted images these lymphatic malformations are characteristically hyperintense. Heterogeneous hypointensity within these lesions on T2-weighted images is most often due to blood products. Postcontrast T1-weighted images may demonstrate enhancement of internal septations and on the wall of the lesion.[24] Typically their MR appearance is of a large multiloculated mass without a clearly defined wall. Lymphatic malformations are large transspatial masses, without respect for fascial boundaries, and may extend into multiple spaces of the neck. These lesions commonly arise in the posterior triangle of the neck, but may also extend into the retropharyngeal space as well as into the mediastinum. Lymphatic malformations are commonly divided into macrocystic or microcystic lesions. When they become infected or occur after sclerotharapy, lesions demonstrate enhancing walls and thick internal septations (**Fig. 16**). Lack of feeding arteries or draining veins and absence of phleboliths allow for differentiation of lymphatic anomalies from primary vascular malformations.

ENT Surgeon Comment

An increasing number of lymphatic malformations are treated with sclerotherapy with injection of

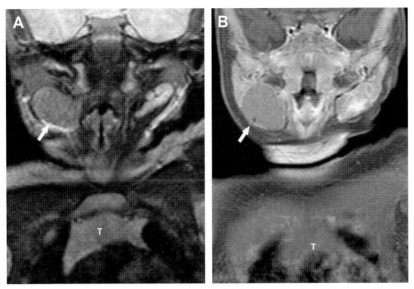

Fig. 15. Ectopic thymic tissue. (*A*) Coronal T2-weighted and (*B*) contrast-enhanced coronal T1-weighted images demonstrate a mass within the right neck posterior to the submandibular gland and lateral to the carotid space (*arrow*), which follows signal intensity of the orthotopic thymus gland (T) on all pulse sequences.

doxycycline or other sclerosing agent.[25,26] Macrocystic lesions are noted to be more amenable to sclerotherapy than are microcystic lesions. Sclerotherapy has been shown to cause significant shrinkage in the size of macrocystic lymphatic malformations. MR imaging is very useful in monitoring response to treatment in these lymphatic malformations (**Fig. 17**).[26]

VASCULAR LESIONS
Hemangioma

Hemangiomas, the most common tumors of the head and neck in infancy and childhood, typically present in early infancy, demonstrate rapid growth in the first year of life, and undergo fatty replacement and subsequent involution by adolescence.[27]

Most of the hemangiomas are superficial, and imaging studies are not required. Deep or large hemangiomas are typically single and are located in the parotid space, submandibular space, or sublingual space. These tumors do not respect fascial boundaries, and multiple masses may be commonly encountered.

MR is the imaging modality of choice. MR demonstrates these masses as typically isointense to muscle on T1-weighted images and hyperintense on T2-weighted images, with some heterogeneity. Avid enhancement is a hallmark of these lesions, which can be optimally evaluated

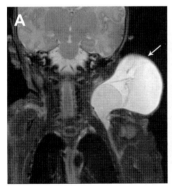
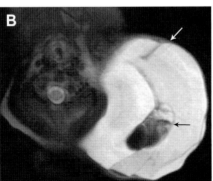
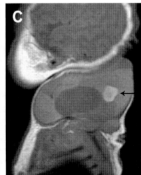

Fig. 16. Lymphatic malformation. (*A*) Coronal T2-weighted, (*B*) axial T2-weighted, and (*C*) sagittal T1-weighted images illustrate a transspatial multiloculated cystic mass arising from the left neck (*white arrow*). Note T1 and T2 shortening from blood products within the mass (*black arrow*).

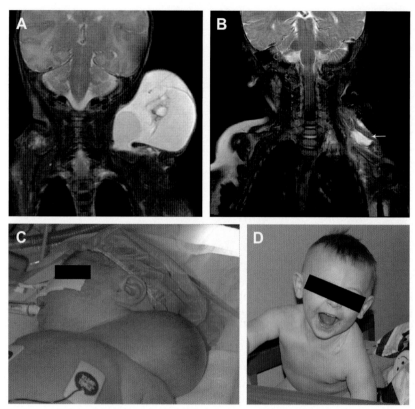

Fig. 17. Treatment response in a lymphatic malformation treated with sclerotherapy. Coronal T2-weighted image with fat saturation, presclerotherapy (*A*) and postsclerotherapy (*B*). Clinical photographs pretreatment (*C*) and posttreatment (*D*) show an excellent response with significant decrease in the lesion size (*arrow in B*).

with fat-suppressed T1-weighted imaging (**Fig. 18**). A search should always be made for similar lesions or satellite lesions. When imaged during the proliferative phase in infancy these hemangiomas contain prominent vascular structures, and can be seen as large-flow voids on spin-echo sequences and flow-related enhancement on gradient-echo sequences. MR angiography can demonstrate large feeding vessels. The involuting hemangiomas become low-flow lesions and may show areas of high T1 signal intensity attributable to fatty replacement, and may not enhance as avidly.

Large infiltrative hemangiomas are seen with Kasabach-Meritt syndrome. Multiple hemangiomas may be seen in the setting of PHACE syndrome (Posterior fossa, Hemangioma, Arterial lesions, Cardiac abnormality, Eye abnormality) (**Fig. 19**).

Venous Vascular Malformations

Venous vascular malformations are low-flow anomalies. Unlike hemangiomas, venous vascular malformations do not involute. Their growth is commensurate with the growth of the patient, and can be distinguished from hemangiomas by the

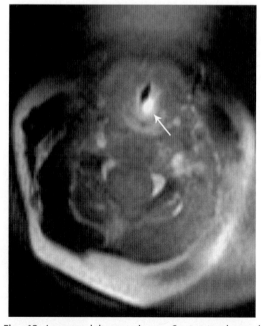

Fig. 18. Laryngeal hemangioma. Contrast-enhanced axial T1-weighted fat-saturated image demonstrates an avidly enhancing hemangioma of the left vocal cord (*arrow*).

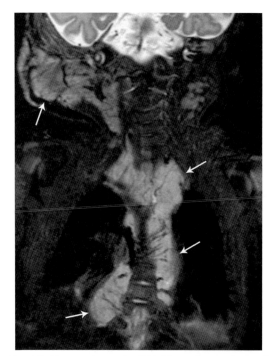

Fig. 19. Hemangiomas in PHACE syndrome. Coronal T2-weighted fat-saturated image demonstrates numerous hyperintense, bilateral paraspinal hemangiomas (*arrows*) with additional involvement of the right neck.

presence of venous lakes and phleboliths. Venous lakes are prominent dilated veins of homogeneously high signal intensity on T2-weighted images. Phleboliths are small foci of low signal intensity on all pulse sequences within these venous lakes, and can be identified with gradient-echo or susceptibility-weighted imaging (**Fig. 20**).[24]

What the ENT Surgeon Wants to Know

Anatomic boundaries and information on critical structures adjacent to the lesion.

THROMBOSIS OF THE INTERNAL JUGULAR VEIN

Acute or subacute thrombosis of the internal jugular vein may be associated with adjacent tissue inflammation or infection. Jugular vein thrombosis may become chronic if the clot persists even after soft-tissue inflammation has subsided.

Thrombosis of the internal jugular vein (IJV) may appear as lack of normal flow void. Signal changes on MR imaging of the thrombus depend on the age of the thrombus. Acute thrombus in the IJV is usually hyperintense, whereas subacute thrombus may have an isointense to hypointense signal. Fat-suppressed sequences may demonstrate acute

thrombus as isointense on T1-weighted images, and a subacute clot may demonstrate high signal due to presence of methemoglobin on fat-suppressed T1-weighted images. Enhancement may also depend on the age of the clot, with an acute clot showing avid diffuse enhancement or peripheral enhancement, whereas there is lack of enhancement in a more chronic clot. There may be presence of surrounding flow voids and enhancement within the developing collaterals. MR venography demonstrates lack of flow-related signal in the involved jugular vein. Chronic jugular vein thrombosis may result in complete obliteration of the vascular lumen of the affected vessel. Adjacent venous collaterals are usually present in the more chronic stages.[28]

Lemierre syndrome is a rare postoropharyngitis complication characterized by septic thrombophlebitis of the ipsilateral IJV.[24,28] An anaerobe, *Fusobacterium necrophorum*, is commonly the causal microorganism (**Fig. 21**). This process can progress to septicemia, septic embolization, and formation of metastatic abscess. An uncommon dangerous complication of Lemierre syndrome is pulmonary embolism.

NEOPLASMS
Teratoma

Teratomas are tumors arising from ectopic, totipotent, embryonic germ cells. Teratomas that arise in the head and neck are usually large masses, many of which are evident at birth or detected antenatally. Teratomas comprise all 3 germ layers, and commonly neuroepithelial and thyroid elements.[13] The most common sites of involvement are the upper cervical region and the nasopharynx. Although the vast majority of teratomas in children are benign lesions, malignant teratomas can occur occasionally.[13]

On MR imaging, teratomas are typically bulky, multiloculated masses with heterogeneous signal depending on the composition. Presence of fat and calcification and areas of hemorrhage are typical. Because of their large size, they may be associated with considerable morbidity. Affected infants have symptoms of respiratory obstruction from deviation and compression of the airway.[13] Maternal polyhydramnios is a known complication in fetuses with teratomas, owing to the inability of the infant to swallow amniotic fluid (**Fig. 22**).

What the ENT Surgeon Wants to Know

Extent of lesion and its relationship to critical structures, namely vessels, nerves, airway deviation, and distortion of normal anatomy. Correct delineation of distorted anatomy is critical because

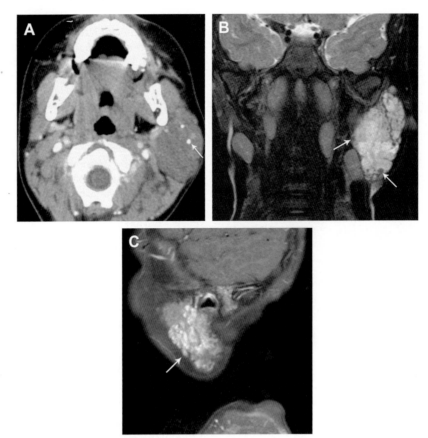

Fig. 20. Venous vascular malformation. (*A*) Contrast-enhanced axial CT image demonstrates punctate calcifications/phleboliths (*arrow*) within the left parotid mass. (*B*) Coronal T2-weighted and (*C*) contrast-enhanced sagittal T1-weighted fat-saturated images reveal a well-circumscribed multiloculated hyperintense enhancing mass within the superficial lobe of the left parotid gland, with focal round hypointensities/phleboliths (*arrows*).

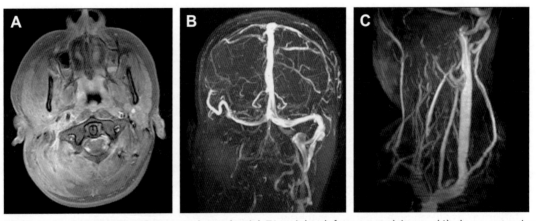

Fig. 21. Lemierre syndrome. Contrast-enhanced axial T1-weighted fat-saturated image (*A*) shows extensive inflammation in the right neck with diffuse enhancement secondary to infective/inflammatory changes and lack of right IJV flow void. Coronal maximum-intensity projection images from MR venography of head (*B*) and neck (*C*) show lack of flow-related enhancement, consistent with thrombosis of the right IJV, and right sigmoid sinus but normal flow-related enhancement in the left IJV and sigmoid sinus.

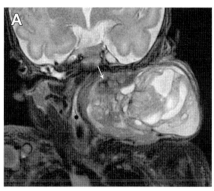
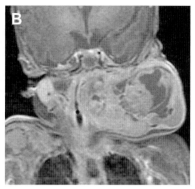

Fig. 22. Cervical teratoma. (*A*) Coronal T2-weighted image and (*B*) contrast-enhanced coronal T1-weighted image with fat saturation show a huge, soft-tissue mass with several solid and cystic components, which involves almost entire left neck, and with areas of T2 shortening (*arrow*) and heterogeneous enhancement, in a 2-day-old infant diagnosed prenatally with neck teratoma, and delivered via the EXIT (ex utero intrapartum treatment) procedure. Note that the oropharynx (*asterisk*) is deviated to the right.

teratomatous tissue left behind has a propensity to become malignant.

FIBROMATOSIS COLLI

Fibromatosis colli is a nonneoplastic condition characterized by benign enlargement of the sternocleidomastoid muscle (SCM). It is also known as sternocleidomastoid pseudotumor of infancy. The enlargement may be diffuse or focal. When focal it is seen to more commonly involve the middle to the lower third of the SCM. It has been noted more commonly on the right side than the left. There is no discrete mass or lymphadenopathy. This presentation is typically seen within the first week of life and has been associated with birth trauma. The head is typically tilted up and away from the affected SCM because of the foreshortening of the muscle. Pathologically there is a fibrocollagenous infiltration of the sternocleidomastoid.[28]

The diagnosis of fibromatosis colli is based on clinical history and physical examination, often confirmed by US. On MR imaging there is fusiform enlargement of the involved SCM. The enlarged SCM is sharply defined. The signal intensity can vary, usually iso- to hypointense to muscle on T1-weighted images and heterogeneous signal on T2-weighted images, with scattered hypointense areas interspersed with hyperintensity (**Fig. 23**). It has been postulated that hypointense zones within may be caused by areas of fibrosis.[29] Surrounding inflammatory changes and lymphadenopathy are conspicuously absent.

Teaching Point

Nontender fusiform mass involving unilateral sternocleidomastoid muscle in a young infant is almost always pathognomonic of fibromatosis colli.[30]

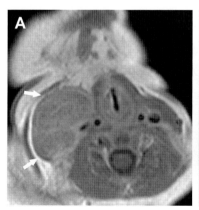
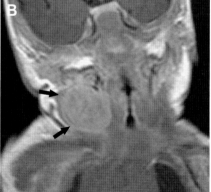

Fig. 23. Fibromatosis colli. (*A*) Contrast-enhanced axial T1-weighted (*white arrows*) and (*B*) contrast-enhanced coronal T1-weighted (*black arrows*) images demonstrate fusiform enlargement and enhancement of the right sternocleidomastoid muscle.

AGGRESSIVE FIBROMATOSIS

Aggressive fibromatosis is a benign but locally aggressive fibrous tumor with a tendency to infiltrate adjacent tissues. It belongs to the group of extra-abdominal desmoid tumors, and commonly affects the muscles of the head and neck. Compared with fibromatosis colli, aggressive fibromatosis can present as a swelling at any time, commonly during the first 2 years of life. It usually does not produce metastatic disease. Aggressive fibromatosis is known to recur following treatment.

MR imaging studies demonstrate a poorly circumscribed isointense to slightly hyperintense signal compared with muscle on both T1- and T2-weighted images, with intense enhancement after contrast administration.[31] The areas of low signal on the T2-weighted images are again thought to indicate fibrous tissue. There is usually absence of metastatic disease. Invasion of the surrounding fat planes and muscles may be present.

Teaching Point

Poorly circumscribed, enhancing lesion involving muscles of the head and neck with predominant low signal intensity relative to muscle, without any lymphadenopathy, points toward aggressive fibromatosis.

What the ENT Surgeon Wants to Know

Once again, key items are extent and anatomic boundaries. With this tumor the best management is gross resection but with the need to try to preserve function, as it is a benign disease.[32,33] One needs to know the precise anatomic location and what structures are nearby or involved.

NEUROGENIC TUMORS
Neurofibroma

Neurofibromas can occur in the neck in patients with neurofibromatosis type 1 (NF1). These lesions may be a single large plexiform neurofibroma or multiple small neurofibromas. Neurofibromas may be present along with other stigmata of NF1. MR imaging is ideally suited for assessing the extent of these lesions; they are isointense to muscle on T1-weighted images and hyperintense on T2-weighted images, with variable enhancement.[34] When imaged in cross section neurofibromas demonstrate the characteristic central T2 hypointensity that is pathognomonic of a neurofibroma (**Fig. 24**).

Imaging pearl

Using multiplanar short-tau inversion recovery fat-suppression sequences can be a quick method of assessing the extent of large lesions. Surveillance imaging of large plexiform neurofibromas can evaluate the relationship of the large mass to vital

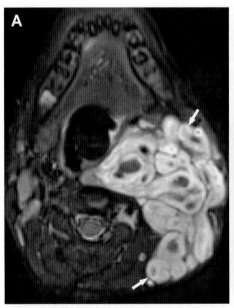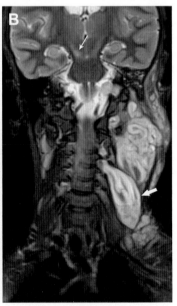

Fig. 24. Plexiform neurofibromas in neurofibromatosis type 1. (*A*) Axial and (*B*) coronal T2-weighted fat-saturated images demonstrate large, lobulated infiltrative masses involving the deep spaces of the left neck (*thick arrows*). Note is made of patchy hyperintense foci (*thin arrow*) within the midbrain, in keeping with spongiform changes of neurofibromatosis type 1.

structures such as the airway, neural structures, neck vessels, and the spinal cord.

Schwannoma

Schwannomas may originate in the neck and are most commonly found in the carotid space, and may be single or multiple. Multiple schwannomas can be associated with neurofibromatosis type 2.

On MR imaging schwannomas are typically well-defined ovoid structures, with intermediate signal intensity on T1-weighted and T2-weighted images, and demonstrate intense contrast enhancement. Central cystic areas may be found within the mass, and these do not enhance following contrast administration (**Fig. 25**).[34] Images of an isolated left vagal schwannoma are shown in **Fig. 26**.

Teaching point

Well-defined, intensely enhancing mass typically in the carotid space with central areas of necrosis is likely to represent a schwannoma. Multiple schwannomas may be present in the setting of neurofibromatosis type 2.

ENT surgeon comment

To help differentiate between schwannomas and paragangliomas/carotid-body tumors, the location and orientation to the great vessels is critical, that is, displacement versus splaying of vessels. The amount of encasement of the carotid is also important (90°, 180°, >180°, total encasement): this will make a surgical difference. Also, distance of the lesion from the skull base is important because if the lesion is too close to the skull base there may be increased risk in getting around the lesion, requiring consideration for a carotid balloon occlusion and carotid bypass.

Neuroblastoma

Neuroblastomas are malignant tumors of primitive neural crest cells. The majority of neuroblastomas involving the head and neck are metastatic lesions from primary abdominal tumors. About 1% to 5% may present as primary cervical neuroblastomas. Cervical involvement usually occurs along the course of the sympathetic chain, with the most common location being in the posterior carotid space.[34]

The signal characteristics on MR imaging are typically intermediate signal on T1-weighted images and moderately hyperintense signal on T2-weighted images. The lesion may be heterogeneous if intralesional calcification, hemorrhage, or necrosis is present (**Fig. 27**).[24] Unlike the neuroblastomas found in the abdomen, the primary cervical neuroblastoma often displaces the carotid sheath vessels rather than encasing them. MR imaging is useful in identifying any mediastinal or intraspinal extension of the neuroblastoma. Meta-iodobenzylguanidine scanning may be needed as a more specific method of staging and evaluating the response to therapy in neuroblastoma.

Teaching point

Enhancing solid masses associated with the carotid sheath in the neck with clinical presentation of a child with unilateral Horner syndrome, with or without palpable neck mass, should make one consider a neuroblastoma.

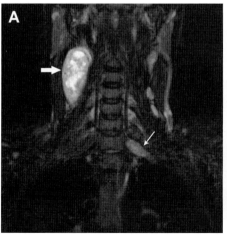
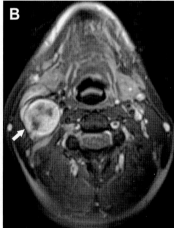

Fig. 25. Schwannomas in neurofibromatosis type 2. (*A*) Coronal T2-weighted and (*B*) contrast-enhanced axial T1-weighted fat-saturated images demonstrate a well-circumscribed elongated enhancing mass in the right carotid space, with areas of cystic change/necrosis within (*thick arrow*). Note is made of an additional schwannoma involving a lower cervical exiting nerve root in *A* (*thin arrow*).

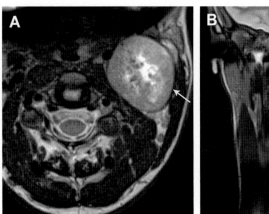
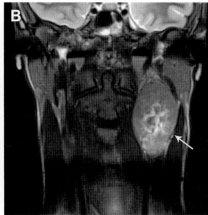

Fig. 26. Isolated vagal schwannoma. (*A*) Axial and (*B*) coronal T2-weighted fat-saturated images demonstrate a well-circumscribed mass in the left carotid space (*arrow*). Note the characteristic areas of cystic change/necrosis within the schwannoma.

LYMPHOMAS

Hodgkin Disease

Hodgkin disease is a lymphoproliferative malignancy predominantly affecting adolescents and young adults. Hodgkin disease is rarely extranodal, with 90% of lesions arising in lymph nodes. It is uncommon to see Hodgkin disease in children younger than 5 years.[35]

Non-Hodgkin Lymphoma

Unlike Hodgkin disease, non-Hodgkin lymphoma is seen in children between 2 and 12 years of age. Non-Hodgkin lymphoma may develop in various congenital and acquired immune deficiency states. In contrast to Hodgkin disease, extranodal sites are commonly involved in children with non-Hodgkin lymphoma.[35] The primary extranodal sites in the head and neck include the nasopharynx, parotid, skin, and bone. Most patients

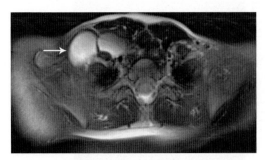

Fig. 27. Neuroblastoma. Axial T2-weighted image with fat saturation shows hyperintense lobulated solid masses around the carotid sheath (*arrow*) in this 11-month-old infant presenting with right Horner syndrome.

with non-Hodgkin lymphoma have advanced disease at the time of presentation.

Burkitt Lymphoma

Burkitt lymphoma is a rapidly proliferative form of non-Hodgkin lymphoma and has been divided into two separate forms, African and American. The disease is almost exclusively seen in children. The African form is considered endemic and is characterized by a distinctive distribution. The face and jaw are the most commonly affected sites. However, other sites may be involved. Almost all patients have high antibody titers to Epstein-Barr virus. By contrast, the American Burkitt lymphoma does not have a strong association with Epstein-Barr virus. The cervical nodes may be affected, and facial and mandibular masses are rare in the American type.[35]

For imaging of the lymphomas CT is the preferred technique; however, MR imaging is performed for lesions that arise within the soft tissues of the head and neck because it allows for better delineation. Involvement of the soft tissues by lymphoma is characterized by a mass that is almost isointense in signal characteristics to the surrounding musculature on T1-weighted images and slightly hyperintense on T2-weighted images, and with variable enhancement characteristics. The margins of the lesion are usually well defined (**Figs. 28** and **29**). Typically the adjacent bone is remodeled rather than infiltrated, although rarely bony destruction may be seen. Lymph nodes involved by lymphoma are usually discretely enlarged, or may form a conglomerate and present as a large solid mass. Necrosis and calcification are uncommon in the enlarged nodes but may occasionally be present after treatment.[28]

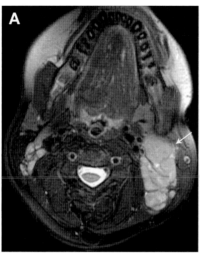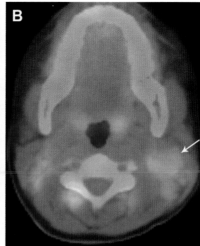

Fig. 28. Hodgkin lymphoma. (*A*) Axial T2-weighted image shows conglomerate lymphadenopathy within the left neck (*arrow*), which demonstrates avid fluorodeoxyglucose uptake on (*B*) positron emission tomography/CT.

It may not be possible by imaging to distinguish Hodgkin disease from non-Hodgkin lymphoma. ¹⁸F-Fluorodeoxyglucose positron emission tomography (FDG-PET) is increasingly used for Hodgkin disease to assess the complete extent of the disease and to monitor response to treatment.

Teaching Point

A young patient with painless neck and mediastinal lymphadenopathy and with a clinical history of fever, night sweats, and weight loss should lead to consideration of lymphoma, likely Hodgkin disease.

Posttransplant Lymphoproliferative Disorder

Posttransplant lymphoproliferative disorder (PTLD) is defined as uncontrolled lymphoid overgrowth in a transplant recipient or in a patient on immunosuppressive therapy, and represents a spectrum of disease varying from lymphoid hyperplasia to malignancy. This condition is more common in pediatric transplant patients, and is seen to occur in up to 80% of cases within the first year following transplant. MR imaging is the best imaging tool for evaluation of these patients. On MR imaging PTLD is seen as markedly increased lymph nodal tissue, or as clusters of lymph nodes, or as a solid mass. Isointense to hypointense signal may be seen on T1-weighted imaging, and an intermediate signal on T2-weighted images may demonstrate necrotic areas (**Fig. 30**).[36] Following contrast administration there is intense enhancement, and if there are necrotic areas they are seen to lack enhancement. PTLDs are known to demonstrate increased uptake on

FDG-PET. FDG-PET may be used for staging and to assess response to treatment.

Teaching point

Intensely enhancing, aggressive-looking solid mass in the neck region of a patient with a history of transplant or immunosuppression should warrant consideration of PTLD.

ENT surgeon comment

Typically the history and description will be adequate. The position of the nodes are usually noted; if they are palpable and there is a surface marker, this is useful information, especially if there are nodes that look involved and may be easy to access for biopsy without significant morbidity.

SARCOMAS AND CARCINOMAS
Rhabdomyosarcoma

Rhabdomyosarcoma is the second most common malignancy following lymphoma and the most common soft-tissue malignancy to involve the pediatric extracranial head and neck. It is a malignant neoplasm of striated muscle. Histologically rhabdomyosarcoma is classified into 4 separate types: the embryonal and botryoid forms are more common in infants and children, whereas the alveolar form is seen predominantly in adolescents and has a worse prognosis. The last variety is the well-differentiated pleomorphic form, which is most commonly seen in adults.[37]

The most common location of rhabdomyosarcoma within the head and neck in children is the orbit, followed by the nasopharynx, paranasal sinuses, temporal bone, paravertebral soft tissues,

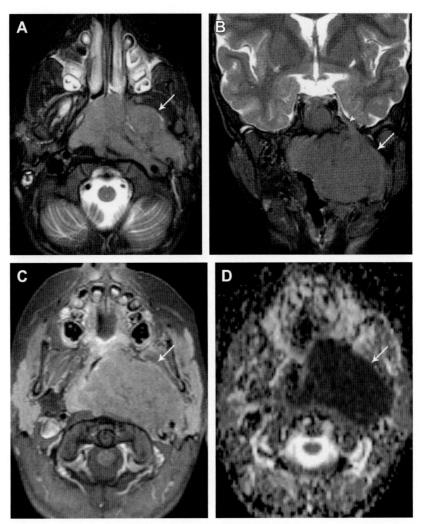

Fig. 29. Burkitt lymphoma. (*A*) Axial and (*B*) coronal T2-weighted, and (*C*) contrast-enhanced axial T1-weighted fat-saturated images demonstrate a large enhancing nasopharyngeal mass (*arrow*), extending into the left parapharyngeal and left carotid spaces and with skull base involvement via the left foramen ovale (*arrowhead in B*). (*D*) ADC map reveals marked restricted diffusion intrinsic to the mass (*arrow*).

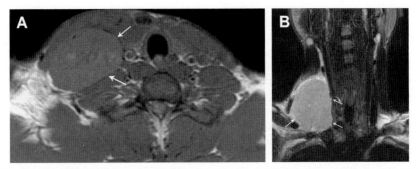

Fig. 30. Posttransplant lymphoproliferative disorder in a liver-transplant patient. (*A*) Axial T1-weighted and (*B*) coronal T2-weighted images illustrate a large well-circumscribed mass within the right supraclavicular region (*arrows*).

and lungs. Rhabdomyosarcomas present as soft-tissue mass with iso- to hypointense T1-weighted signal and hyperintense T2-weighted signal related to the muscle. The tumor mass may show variable contrast enhancement. Aggressive local destruction, and transspatial extension and intracranial extension with parameningeal spread may be noted.[38] Osseous destruction and erosion is common but may not be present in all cases. Prognosis of the tumors with intracranial spread and parameningeal involvement is poor, and hence it is very important that such characteristics are detected and noted before therapy and preoperatively (**Fig. 31**).[39]

Teaching point

Aggressive soft-tissue masses of the head and neck with transspatial extension accompanied by osseous destruction in a pediatric patient indicates a rhabdomyosarcoma. It is very important by imaging to delineate the complete extent of the tumor, demonstrate its relationship to important structures, and detect intracranial extension.

What the ENT Surgeon Wants to Know

1. As noted, it is important to delineate the extent of the malignancy, as the greater the tumor mass that can be resected, the better the prognosis. Ideally complete excision is preferred, but not at the risk of significant functional or cosmetic morbidity. If complete resection is possible, this will reduce the amount of adjuvant therapy required.

2. If gross resection is not feasible, a biopsy of the lesion must be obtained, and imaging can reveal the best access to the lesion.

Nasopharyngeal Carcinoma

This tumor accounts for almost 80% of head and neck malignancies in adults, but in the pediatric age group it accounts for only about 4% of the lesions involving the upper aerodigestive tract. Similar to Burkitt lymphoma, nasopharyngeal carcinoma (NPC) has a strong association with Epstein-Barr virus. There are 3 types of NPC classified by the World Health Organization: Type 1 is squamous cell carcinoma; Type 2a is keratinizing undifferentiated carcinoma; and Type 2b is non-keratinizing undifferentiated carcinoma. Type 2b, the nonkeratinizing undifferentiated form, is the most common, and is most strongly associated with Epstein-Barr virus infection of cancerous cells. In children, the nasopharynx is the most common site of the squamous cell malignancy. Sometimes histologic differentiation between squamous cell carcinoma, neuroblastoma, and non-Hodgkin lymphoma in a nasopharyngeal mass may be difficult. However, the age of the patient, location of the mass, and imaging characteristics help in the differential diagnosis. The most common presentation is cervical lymphadenopathy, in particular an enlarged posterior cervical lymph node. Most patients have cervical lymph node metastases at the time of presentation. Nasopharyngeal carcinoma can demonstrate intracranial spread by direct invasion of the skull

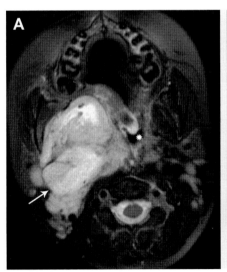
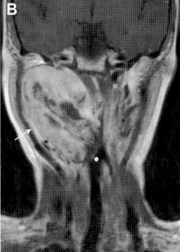

Fig. 31. Rhabdomyosarcoma. (*A*) Axial T2-weighted and (*B*) contrast-enhanced coronal T1-weighted images reveal a large right parapharyngeal space mass (*arrow*), resulting in moderate mass effect on the adjacent airway (*asterisk*).

base, extension along the vessels, or perineural spread along the cranial nerves (**Fig. 32**).[40]

Teaching point

Although it is difficult by imaging to differentiate squamous cell carcinoma from rhabdomyosarcoma, location in the nasopharynx, intracranial extension, and perineural spread may indicate a squamous cell carcinoma, although an older pediatric patient, male gender, and Asian descent would favor a carcinoma.

ENT surgeon comment

Staging for NPC is by clinical and radiologic findings.

> Stage I: small tumor confined to nasopharynx
> Stage II: tumor extending locally or any evidence of limited neck (nodal) disease
> Stage III: larger tumor with or without neck disease, or tumor with bilateral neck disease
> Stage IV: intracranial or infratemporal involvement of tumor, extensive neck disease, or any distant metastasis

Fibrosarcoma

Fibrosarcoma is the second most common sarcoma involving the extracranial head and neck in children. The areas involved include the sinonasal region, face, larynx, and hypopharynx. Metastatic spread is infrequent (**Fig. 33**).[28]

A variety of other sarcomas have been described to occur in the head and neck in children, such as Ewing sarcoma, chondrosarcoma, and certain varieties of osteosarcoma particularly involving the face and jaw. Some advanced cases of neurofibromatosis are at increased risk for developing neurofibrosarcoma. Another type of sarcoma very unique to young pediatric patients is an atypical teratoid rhabdoid tumor, a highly malignant tumor of primitive variety that usually is seen intracranially, but may rarely be present at the skull base and the neck. Such tumors carry a uniformly dismal prognosis (**Fig. 34**).[28]

What the ENT surgeon wants to know

Again, precise delineation of extent of lesion and its related anatomy.

The differential imaging characteristics of common transspatial masses in the pediatric age group are summarized in **Table 3**.

PEDIATRIC THYROID CANCER

The incidence of head and neck malignancies including thyroid cancer has increased by almost 25% during the last 20 years. Thyroid carcinoma is the second most common malignancy in adolescent, Caucasian females. Most pediatric thyroid cancers are of the papillary type. Pediatric thyroid cancers usually present at an advanced stage. A painless, noninflammatory metastatic cervical mass is usually the presenting symptom in about 40% to 60% of patients.[28]

Ultrasound and nuclear medicine studies are the mainstay in the imaging evaluation of thyroid cancer. MR is also useful in that it does not use iodinated contrast, as CT does, for contrast studies. The use of iodinated contrast can

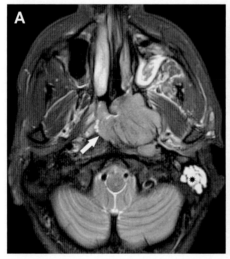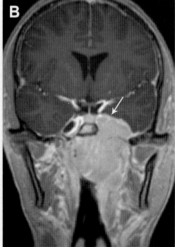

Fig. 32. Nasopharyngeal carcinoma. (*A*) Axial T2-weighted and (*B*) contrast-enhanced coronal T1-weighted images reveal a left nasopharyngeal mass (*arrow*) with skull-base invasion and involvement of the left cavernous sinus (*thin arrow in B*). Note is made of postobstructive-fluid opacification of the left mastoid air cells (*asterisk*).

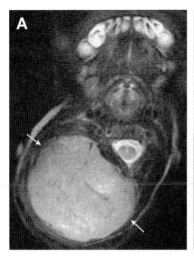

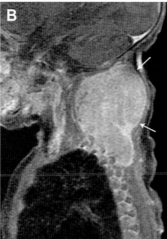

Fig. 33. Fibrosarcoma. (A) Axial T2-weighted and (B) contrast-enhanced sagittal T1-weighted fat-saturated images illustrate a large, hyperintense enhancing mass within the right posterior neck (arrows) with no intraspinal involvement.

significantly delay postsurgical radioactive-iodine treatment of thyroid malignancies.

The role of MR imaging in the evaluation of thyroid cancer is predominantly to characterize the disease and assess the extent of nodal metastatic disease or invasive disease, if there is concern for invasion of the trachea or if there is involvement of the recurrent laryngeal nerve. It is also useful in assessment of complications related to treatment and in evaluation of recurrent thyroid malignancy (Fig. 35).[41]

What the ENT Surgeon Wants to Know

Any suspicious lymphadenopathy, nodal loss of hilum, calcifications, and invasion of trachea/esophagus.

INFECTIOUS AND INFLAMMATORY CONDITIONS
Infectious Lymphadenitis

Cervical lymphadenopathy is a common occurrence in children. The condition most commonly presents as a transient response to a benign local or generalized infection. The infectious agents drain into the afferent lymphatic channels of lymph nodes, leading to activation of lymphocytes and enlargement of lymph nodes. The enlarged nodes are referred to as reactive nodes.

Suppurative lymphadenitis refers to infected nodes that have undergone liquefaction necrosis, with pus within them. Acute bilateral cervical lymphadenopathy usually is caused by a viral upper respiratory tract infection or streptococcal

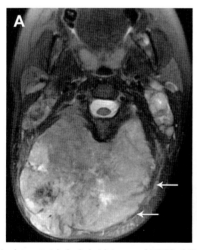

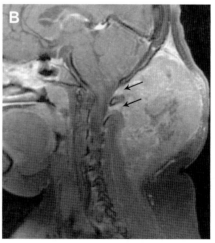

Fig. 34. Atypical teratoid rhabdoid tumor (ATRT). (A) Axial T2-weighted and (B) contrast-enhanced sagittal T1-weighted fat-saturated images reveal a large partially necrotic enhancing mass (white arrows) within the posterior neck extending into the bilateral C0-C1 and C1-C2 neural foramina (black arrows) without spinal canal compromise.

Table 3
MR imaging characteristics of common transspatial neck masses in children

Type	MR Imaging Features
Lymphatic malformation	Large multiloculated mass. T1 signal variable or hypo-, iso-, or hyperintense. T2 signal heterogeneously hyperintense Fluid levels if hemorrhage present Enhancement present along septae or walls if infected or treated
Venous vascular lesion	Heterogeneous signal on T1 and T2, with presence of venous lakes (prominent dilated veins), which are of homogeneously high signal intensity on T2-weighted images, and phleboliths (small foci of low signal intensity) on all pulse sequences best seen on gradient-echo or susceptibility-weighted imaging
Rhabdomyosarcoma	Soft-tissue mass with iso- to hypointense T1 signal and hyperintense T2 signal relative to muscle, with variable contrast enhancement Aggressive local destruction Intracranial extension with parameningeal spread and osseous destruction often present
Teratoma	Large multiloculated masses with heterogeneous signal depending on the composition Presence of fat and calcification and areas of hemorrhage are typical Enhancement common and patchy
Neurogenic tumors	Usually large plexiform neurofibromas Isointense to muscle on T1-weighted images and hyperintense on T2-weighted images, with variable enhancement Characteristic central T2 hypointensity when imaged in cross section

pharyngitis. Acute unilateral cervical lymphadenitis can be caused by streptococcal or staphylococcal infections in about 40% to 80% of cases[28] Some of the most common causes of subacute or chronic

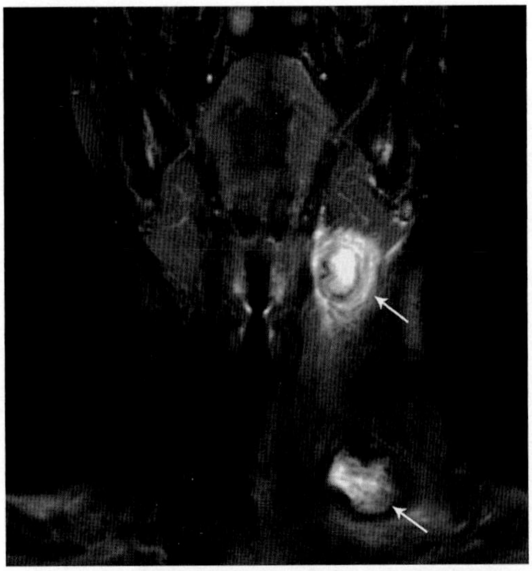

Fig. 35. Thyroid cancer lymph node metastases. Coronal T2-weighted fat-saturated image shows multiple necrotic lymph nodes in the left neck in this patient with papillary thyroid cancer, status postthyroidectomy and modified left radical neck dissection.

infectious lymphadenitis are cat-scratch disease, mycobacterial infection, and toxoplasmosis.

Contrast-enhanced CT is the preferred imaging modality for evaluation of suspected suppurative lymphadenitis in the neck. Occasionally MR imaging may be used to evaluate the complications of suppurative cervical lymphadenitis. The mainstay of imaging includes T2-weighted sequences and postcontrast T1-weighted images with fat saturation. DW imaging is increasingly useful in assessing collections and abscess formation.[28]

It should be noted that the size criteria for normal lymph nodes in children is larger than that for adults. Lymph nodes up to 2.5 cm in diameter in the internal jugular chain may still be normal in the pediatric age group. Also, the presence of Rouviere or retropharyngeal lymph nodes is not necessarily considered pathologic in the pediatric population (**Fig. 36**).

Infected lymph nodes on MR imaging are characterized by homogeneous enlargement, loss of internal architecture and the fatty hilum, and increased enhancement of the involved lymph nodes. Necrotic centers have an appearance more like fluid, with hypointense T1 and hyperintense T2 signal. With pus formation or complete liquefaction, these areas may demonstrate restricted diffusion with low ADC values (**Fig. 37**).[24] Associated findings in suppurative lymphadenopathy include

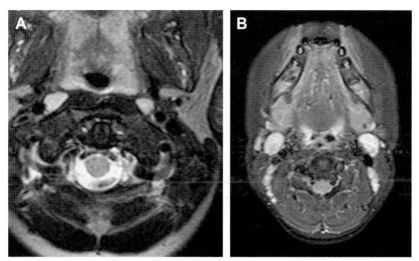

Fig. 36. Nonpathologic lymph node enlargement. Axial T2-weighted (*A*) and axial post-contrast T1-weighted (*B*) images with fat saturation show prominent Rouviere nodes and prominent cervical chain lymph nodes, which are not considered pathologic.

surrounding cellulitis as well as adjacent muscle thickening. Often there is associated nonsuppurative or reactive lymphadenopathy in the adjacent lymph node stations.

What the ENT surgeon wants to know

1. Size of necrotic or liquefied node if present.
2. Location in neck (height): toward skull base, above the palate, level of oropharnyx, or hypopharynx.
3. Location with respect to great vessels (medial or lateral), as this can determine method of

surgical approach if the nodal collection needs to be drained. If medial to the great vessels, a transoral route is necessary; if lateral to the great vessels, an external approach is better suited.
4. Patency of the jugular vein: narrowing or occlusion/thrombosis.
5. Deviation of airway or impingement on airway.

Tuberculous Lymphadenopathy

Cervical lymphadenitis caused by *Mycobacterium tuberculosis* infection is the most common site of

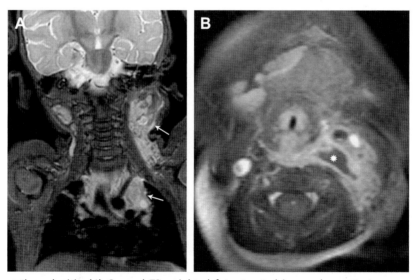

Fig. 37. Suppurative adenitis. (*A*) Coronal T2-weighted fat-saturated image demonstrates a conglomerate of multiple enlarged left cervical and few mediastinal lymph nodes with surrounding inflammation (*arrows*). (*B*) Contrast-enhanced axial T1-weighted fat-saturated image demonstrates frank abscess formation (*asterisk*) within the left paravertebral space.

extrapulmonary tuberculous adenopathy. It typically involves the internal jugular and posterior cervical nodes and is more commonly unilateral. On MR imaging, centrally necrotic lymph nodes or conglomerate lymph node mass with thick irregular peripheral enhancement may be noted (**Fig. 38**). Characteristically on MR spectroscopy, choline and creatinine is not found in the affected lymph nodes in *M tuberculosis*, but is seen in malignant lymph nodes.[28]

On CT scanning, nodal calcifications may be evident. Additional associated findings in the lungs and mediastinal adenopathy is common. There is increased FDG uptake on PET imaging, indicating active disease. The PET tracer ^{11}C-choline has low uptake in *M tuberculosis*.

Nontuberculous Mycobacterial Lymphadenopathy (Atypical Mycobacterial Infection)

Cervical adenopathy can also be caused by infections from *Mycobacterium avium intracellulare*, which is most common, or by other strains of mycobacteria such as *Mycobacterium scrofulaceum* and *Mycobacterium kansasii*. These infections are considered nontuberculous or of atypical mycobacterial type. Cervical adenopathy is commonly characterized by large nontender lymphadenopathy with disproportionately mild or absent clinical symptoms. On imaging, necrotic lymphadenopathy is common, with the lack of surrounding cellulitis (**Fig. 39**).[28] Persistent preauricular or submandibular lymphadenopathy in a child who appears to be systemically well should raise concern for nontuberculous mycobacterial lymphadenopathy. Associated violaceous pigmentation of the overlying skin has also been reportedly associated with nontuberculous bacterial lymphadenitis.[28] Imaging is useful in determining the extent of lymph node involvement.

Teaching point
Consider nontuberculous mycobacterial infection in pediatric cervical lymph node mass that does not respond to standard treatment, or necrotic nodes with minimal surrounding inflammation.[42,43]

Treatment is mainly surgical, with curettage of the affected node(s). Adjuvant antimicrobial therapy is also often included in the management of this disorder. Infectious disease specialists should be included in the management. Recurrent disease may require more extensive debridement; however, often these nodes may be in close proximity to the facial nerve.

Although most of the lymphadenopathies are of infectious etiology, occasionally they may be due to a more serious disorder of neoplastic origin such as lymphoma or neuroblastoma. Supraclavicular or posterior cervical lymphadenopathy is at much higher risk for being malignant than is anterior cervical lymphadenopathy.[28]

Deep Neck Infections

Typical locations of pediatric deep neck infections involve the retropharyngeal or parapharyngeal spaces. Knowledge of these is important, as infection spreading into these spaces can be potentially life threatening. These infections may be secondary to suppurative lymphadenitis, abscess formation, or traumatic inoculation of infection. Usually the presenting symptoms are fever,

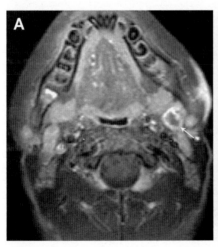 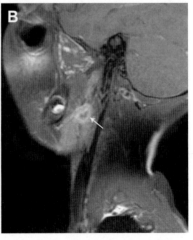

Fig. 38. Tuberculous adenitis. Contrast-enhanced (*A*) axial and (*B*) sagittal T1-weighted fat-saturated images demonstrate left cervical necrotic adenopathy with thick enhancing rim (*arrow*). Note the relative lack of surrounding inflammation compared with that seen in **Fig. 37**.

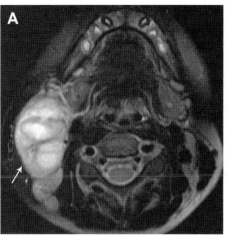
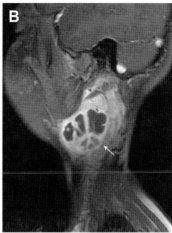

Fig. 39. Nontuberculous mycobacterial adenitis. (A) Axial T2-weighted and (B) contrast-enhanced sagittal T1-weighted fat-saturated images demonstrate a conglomerate nodal mass (arrow) within the right level-2 region, with nonenhancing necrotic areas within.

dysphagia, limited range of motion, neck mass, and a high leukocyte count.

The role of imaging is to identify the location of infection, and to characterize it as a cellulitis versus phlegmon formation versus a well-formed abscess. Although contrast-enhanced CT preceded by a lateral neck radiograph are traditional modalities for imaging, MR imaging is sometimes used to determine the complete extent of the process and to assess for vascular complications. Differentiation of a phlegmon from an abscess may sometimes not be completely reliable on CT. On MR imaging, the involved area of cellulitis is characterized by poorly marginated, diffuse T1 hypointense and T2 hyperintense signal, and nonspecific enhancement. An abscess in formation or fully formed would demonstrate focal low T1 hypointense signal and higher T2 hyperintense signal, with peripheral enhancement. DW imaging

reveals restriction of diffusion in areas of abscess formation (Fig. 40).[24]

While characterizing deep neck infections it is critical to identify their effect on vital structures, for example, the airway and the neck vessels. Large infective collections and retropharyngeal abscesses can cause a mass effect, displacement, or partial effacement of the airway. There may be narrowing of the cervical internal carotid artery caused by spasm. The IJV can be displaced and flattened. A complication of infection of the deep neck space in children can result in inflammatory thrombophlebitis and occlusion of the IJV (Lemierre disease) (see Fig. 21).[24]

A potential space posterior to the retropharyngeal space between the cervical fascial layers is known as the danger space. This space is continuous inferiorly with the posterior mediastinum. Infections in the retropharyngeal space may enter

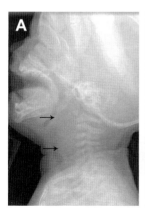
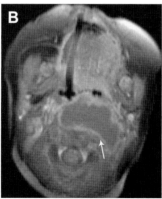
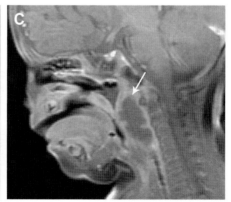

Fig. 40. Retropharyngeal abscess. (A) Lateral radiograph illustrates widening of the prevertebral soft tissues (black arrows). Contrast-enhanced (B) axial and (C) sagittal T1-weighted fat-saturated images reveal a lobulated, rim-enhancing collection (white arrow) within the retropharyngeal space.

the danger space because of the close proximity, and then dissect down to the mediastinum.[24] Hence, it is important to determine the inferior extent of all infections involving the retropharynx, which is better delineated by MR imaging.[28]

What the ENT surgeon wants to know

Location, size, and characterization of deep neck infections: size of phlegmon and/or collection if present. Location relative to great vessels, medial or lateral, and effect on airway may be important if the patient requires surgical treatment, so the anesthesiologist would want to be aware of any deviation or impingement on the airway.

NECK TRAUMA AND ITS COMPLICATIONS

The most common cause of external injuries in the neck region in children is motor vehicle accidents, foreign bodies, or penetrating objects. Penetrating oropharyngeal injury usually occurs when a child falls with a foreign body such as a pencil or a stick inside the mouth.

CT is the imaging modality of choice to quickly demonstrate the extent of the injury, identify any foreign body, and assess the degree of airway compromise and integrity of the laryngeal cartilages. In the setting of a stable patient with severe penetrating oropharyngeal injury or neck trauma, MR imaging with MR angiography and MR venography are used for the detection of possible dissection of the internal carotid artery or IJV injury.[28] Late posttraumatic vascular complications such as pseudoaneurysm formation can also be optimally assessed with MR angiography.

SUMMARY

MR imaging is an established diagnostic tool in the evaluation of pediatric neck lesions. The specific advantages of using MR imaging in the pediatric neck lie in MR imaging not involving ionizing radiation and providing superior resolution on images. MR imaging can provide better characterization of lesions and anatomic delineation of various pediatric neck abnormalities, and provide important information for presurgical planning when surgery is indicated.

REFERENCES

1. Shore RE. Issues and epidemiological evidence regarding radiation-induced thyroid cancer. Radiat Res 1992;131(1):98–111.
2. Ron E, Lubin JH, Shore RE, et al. Thyroid cancer after exposure to external radiation: a pooled analysis of seven studies. Radiat Res 1995;141(3):259–77.
3. Langman J, editor. Medical embryology. 3rd edition. Baltimore (MD): Williams & Wilkins; 1975.
4. Moore K, editor. The developing human. Philadelphia: Saunders; 1988.
5. Sadler T, editor. Langman's medical embryology. 6th edition. Baltimore (MD): Williams and Wilkins; 1990.
6. Allard RH. The thyroglossal cyst. Head Neck Surg 1982;5(2):134–46.
7. Koeller KK, Alamo L, Adair CF, et al. Congenital cystic masses of the neck: radiologic-pathologic correlation. Radiographics 1999;19(1):121–46 [quiz: 152–3].
8. el-Silimy OE, Bradley PJ. Thyroglossal tract anomalies. Clin Otolaryngol Allied Sci 1985;10(6):329–34.
9. Heshmati HM, Fatourechi V, van Heerden JA, et al. Thyroglossal duct carcinoma: report of 12 cases. Mayo Clin Proc 1997;72(4):315–9.
10. Doshi SV, Cruz RM, Hilsinger RL Jr. Thyroglossal duct carcinoma: a large case series. Ann Otol Rhinol Laryngol 2001;110(8):734–8.
11. Ostlie DJ, Burjonrappa SC, Snyder CL, et al. Thyroglossal duct infections and surgical outcomes. J Pediatr Surg 2004;39(3):396–9 [discussion: 396–9].
12. Arekapudi SR, Varma DR. Lingual thyroid. Pediatr Radiol 2007;37(9):940.
13. Smirniotopoulos JG, Chiechi MV. Teratomas, dermoids, and epidermoids of the head and neck. Radiographics 1995;15(6):1437–55.
14. Al-Khateeb TH, Al-Masri NM, Al-Zoubi F. Cutaneous cysts of the head and neck. J Oral Maxillofac Surg 2009;67(1):52–7.
15. Lee SS, Persing JA. Refinement in technique for pediatric dermoid cyst excision: technical note. Plast Reconstr Surg 2008;122(4):1059–61.
16. Harrison JD. Modern management and pathophysiology of ranula: literature review. Head Neck 2010;32(10):1310–20.
17. Benson MT, Dalen K, Mancuso AA, et al. Congenital anomalies of the branchial apparatus: embryology and pathologic anatomy. Radiographics 1992;12(5):943–60.
18. Mukherji SK, Fatterpekar G, Castillo M, et al. Imaging of congenital anomalies of the branchial apparatus. Neuroimaging Clin N Am 2000;10(1):75–93, viii.
19. Ibrahim M, Hammoud K, Maheshwari M, et al. Congenital cystic lesions of the head and neck. Neuroimaging Clin N Am 2011;21(3):621–39, viii.
20. Tovi F, Mares AJ. The aberrant cervical thymus. Embryology, pathology, and clinical implications. Am J Surg 1978;136(5):631–7.
21. Zielke AM, Swischuk LE, Hernandez JA. Ectopic cervical thymic tissue: can imaging obviate biopsy and surgical removal? Pediatr Radiol 2007;37(11):1174–7.
22. Molina PL, Siegel MJ, Glazer HS. Thymic masses on MR imaging. AJR Am J Roentgenol 1990;155(3):495–500.

23. Zadvinskis DP, Benson MT, Kerr HH, et al. Congenital malformations of the cervicothoracic lymphatic system: embryology and pathogenesis. Radiographics 1992;12(6):1175–89.

24. Harnsberger H, editor. Diagnostic imaging: head and neck. Salt Lake city, UT: Amirsys; Elsevier Saunders; 2004.

25. Nehra D, Jacobson L, Barnes P, et al. Doxycycline sclerotherapy as primary treatment of head and neck lymphatic malformations in children. J Pediatr Surg 2008;43(3):451–60.

26. Cahill AM, Nijs E, Ballah D, et al. Percutaneous sclerotherapy in neonatal and infant head and neck lymphatic malformations: a single center experience. J Pediatr Surg 2011;46(11): 2083–95.

27. Marler JJ, Mulliken JB. Vascular anomalies: classification, diagnosis, and natural history. Facial Plast Surg Clin North Am 2001;9(4):495–504.

28. Tortori-Donati P, editor. Pediatric neuroradiology: brain, head, neck and spine. Berlin, Heidelberg (Germany), New York: Springer; 2005.

29. Ablin DS, Jain K, Howell L, et al. Ultrasound and MR imaging of fibromatosis colli (sternomastoid tumor of infancy). Pediatr Radiol 1998;28(4):230–3.

30. Lowry KC, Estroff JA, Rahbar R. The presentation and management of fibromatosis colli. Ear Nose Throat J 2010;89(9):E4–8.

31. Ahn JM, Yoon HK, Suh YL, et al. Infantile fibromatosis in childhood: findings on MR imaging and pathologic correlation. Clin Radiol 2000;55(1): 19–24.

32. Abdelkader M, Riad M, Williams A. Aggressive fibromatosis of the head and neck (desmoid tumours). J Laryngol Otol 2001;115(10):772–6.

33. Sharma A, Ngan BY, Sandor GK, et al. Pediatric aggressive fibromatosis of the head and neck: a 20-year retrospective review. J Pediatr Surg 2008; 43(9):1596–604.

34. Weber AL, Montandon C, Robson CD. Neurogenic tumors of the neck. Radiol Clin North Am 2000;38(5): 1077–90.

35. Weber AL, Rahemtullah A, Ferry JA. Hodgkin and non-Hodgkin lymphoma of the head and neck: clinical, pathologic, and imaging evaluation. Neuroimaging Clin N Am 2003;13(3):371–92.

36. Borhani AA, Hosseinzadeh K, Almusa O, et al. Imaging of posttransplantation lymphoproliferative disorder after solid organ transplantation. Radiographics 2009;29(4):981–1000 [discussion: 1000–2].

37. McCarville MB, Spunt SL, Pappo AS. Rhabdomyosarcoma in pediatric patients: the good, the bad, and the unusual. AJR Am J Roentgenol 2001; 176(6):1563–9.

38. Yousem DM, Lexa FJ, Bilaniuk LT, et al. Rhabdomyosarcomas in the head and neck: MR imaging evaluation. Radiology 1990;177(3):683–6.

39. Breneman JC, Lyden E, Pappo AS, et al. Prognostic factors and clinical outcomes in children and adolescents with metastatic rhabdomyosarcoma—a report from the Intergroup Rhabdomyosarcoma Study IV. J Clin Oncol 2003;21(1):78–84.

40. Stambuk HE, Patel SG, Mosier KM, et al. Nasopharyngeal carcinoma: recognizing the radiographic features in children. AJNR Am J Neuroradiol 2005; 26(6):1575–9.

41. Kaplan SL, Mandel SJ, Muller R, et al. The role of MR imaging in detecting nodal disease in thyroidectomy patients with rising thyroglobulin levels. AJNR Am J Neuroradiol 2009;30(3):608–12.

42. Hanck C, Fleisch F, Katz G. Imaging appearance of nontuberculous mycobacterial infection of the neck. AJNR Am J Neuroradiol 2004;25(2):349 [author reply: 349–50].

43. Robson CD, Hazra R, Barnes PD, et al. Nontuberculous mycobacterial infection of the head and neck in immunocompetent children: CT and MR findings. AJNR Am J Neuroradiol 1999;20(10):1829–35.

Fetal MRI: Head and Neck

David M. Mirsky, MD*, Karuna V. Shekdar, MD,
Larissa T. Bilaniuk, MD

KEYWORDS

- Fetal head and neck magnetic resonance imaging • Craniosynostosis • Cleft lip and palate
- Micrognathia • Lymphatic malformation • Teratoma • Goiter

KEY POINTS

- Magnetic resonance imaging (MRI) is an useful adjunct to ultrasound in the work-up of fetal head and neck pathology. It is a safe and effective imaging modality for which there have been no proven harmful effects to the developing human fetus from limited exposure.
- Common indications for fetal head and neck imaging include: lymphatic malformation, teratoma, hemangioma, facial cleft, and goiter.
- MRI can be helpful in assessing airway obstruction, which may impact prenatal management and delivery planning.
- Cleft lip/palate represents the most common anomaly of the fetal face. A midline defect should prompt one to carefully scrutinize the intracranial contents, as there is an increased association with holoprosencephaly.
- Micrognathia is rarely an isolated finding and when detected on fetal MRI, it may serve as the initial clue that the fetus has an underlying syndrome or genetic abnormality.

INTRODUCTION

Over the last 3 decades, magnetic resonance imaging (MRI) has become an useful adjunct to ultrasound in the work-up of fetal head and neck pathology.[1,2] MRI is particularly important in cases where there is concern for airway compromise, as clear delineation of fetal anatomy is crucial, particularly if fetal or perinatal interventional procedures are being considered and for scheduling and deciding on type of delivery.[3,4] Additionally, given the high association of fetal head and neck pathology and concomitant central nervous system (CNS) abnormalities, MRI allows for detailed structural evaluation of the brain for detecting coexisting pathology and to assess for any intracranial extension of extracranial disease processes. MRI is not limited by the ossified calvarium and skull base, as is the case with ultrasound, particularly later in gestation.[2,5] Lastly MRI, with its multiplanar imaging ability and high signal-to-noise ratio, provides superior delineation of the anatomically complex areas such as the floor of the mouth and deep neck spaces.[5]

The focus of this article is on the evaluation of fetal head and neck pathology using MRI.

SAFETY OF FETAL MRI

Since the inception of fetal MR imaging in the early 1980s there have been no proven harmful effects to the developing human fetus from limited exposure to the changing electromagnetic fields occurring during MRI.[6,7] Several studies have failed to demonstrate any adverse long-term effects on children who were imaged as fetuses.[8] MRI is a safe and effective imaging modality for further

Funding sources: None.
Conflict of interest: None.
Division of Neuroradiology, Department of Radiology, The Children's Hospital of Philadelphia, Perelman School of Medicine at the University of Pennsylvania, 324 South 34th Street, Philadelphia, PA 19104, USA
* Corresponding author.
E-mail address: mirsky@gmail.com

mri.theclinics.com

characterizing fetal anomalies that are limited in their assessment by sonography alone.[9]

Given the lack of conclusive data documenting deleterious effects of MRI at 1.5 T, the current guidelines by the American College of Radiology do not stipulate any special consideration regarding MRI of the fetus at any stage of pregnancy.[10] However, in the United States, fetal MRI is generally not performed in the first trimester of gestation given the theoretical concern for teratogenesis. Furthermore, it is difficult to acquire high-quality images in very young fetuses by MRI.

Use of intravenous contrast in MRI in pregnancy is a relative contraindication. Gadolinium crosses the placenta and is considered a pregnancy class C drug (ie, gadolinium administration during pregnancy has not been proven to be completely safe in people).[11]

TECHNICAL ASPECTS

Various types of coils can be used for fetal MRI. A body coil alone or a body phased-array coil in combination with a surface coil situated on the mother's abdomen is commonly used. Images are acquired in the sagittal, axial, and coronal planes relative to the fetal facial profile. At the authors' institution, the half-Fourier single-shot turbo spin-echo (HASTE) sequence serves as the mainstay of MRI of the fetus. HASTE sequences provide heavily T2-weighted (T2W) images with low susceptibility weighting in a very short time, enabling good discrimination of fetal facial features.[9] Sequential slice capability and interleaving allows for high-quality imaging despite fetal movement. Susceptibility weighted sequences such as extremely rapid gradient echo, echo planar imaging (EPI) are very useful in the detection of hemorrhage and mineralization, and thus help in characterizing and in distinguishing head and neck masses such as lymphatic malformations, teratomas, and congenital hemangiomas/vascular malformations. T1-weighted (T1W) images have limited utility in the evaluation of fetal head and neck pathology apart from certain specific scenarios such as fetal goiter and in cases of large hemorrhages. Cine imaging is routinely acquired in fetal head and neck imaging, as it is useful in assessing the swallowing mechanism and patency of the aerodigestive tract.

As stated previously, images are acquired in 3 orthogonal planes with respect to the fetal face. Similar to postnatal life, the sagittal view provides a good evaluation of the fetal profile, including the frontal and nasal bones, hard palate, tongue, and mandible. Coronal images are useful in assessing the integrity of the fetal lips and palate as well as providing delineation of the eyes, nose, and ears. Axial images help assess the different compartments of the neck and are also valuable in evaluating the fetal facial structures and variations in cranial morphology.

Many congenital anomalies of the head and neck are associated with concomitant abnormalities of the fetal spine, heart, kidneys, or limbs and digits. Careful inspection of the visualized portions of the fetal body during a head and neck examination may provide additional information to suspect an underlying syndrome, sequence, or association.

On average, a routine fetal neuroimaging examination takes approximately 30 to 40 minutes. At the authors' institution, no sedation is provided to the mother of the fetus.[12]

INDICATIONS FOR FETAL HEAD AND NECK IMAGING

MRI of the fetal head and neck is primarily used as a problem-solving technique when fetal anomalies cannot be completely assessed with sonography. MRI is not used as a screening tool. Common indications for fetal head and neck imaging include: lymphatic malformation, teratoma, hemangioma, facial cleft, and goiter. Other less common indications include abnormal shape of cranium, scalp, jaw, and orbital anomalies. As described previously, MRI can be helpful in assessing airway obstruction, which may impact prenatal management and delivery planning.

ABNORMAL CALVARIUM

Abnormalities of the fetal skull can be related to calvarial size, shape, and mineralization. There are many causes for an abnormal fetal skull size and shape. Macrocephaly is a common presentation on fetal MRI, often related to an underlying abnormality such as hydrocephalus, abnormal development (Fig. 1A), intracranial tumor (see Fig. 1B), or megalencephaly. Microcephaly can be seen with various syndromes and malformations (Fig. 2A, B) and can also be caused by volume loss or brain destruction secondary to infection, ischemia, and hemorrhage. An abnormal fetal skull shape may be related to a variety of causes, many of which have an underlying genetic mutation. Loss of subarachnoid space and collapse of the calvarial bones around the brain produce a characteristic lemon shape that is seen with neural tube defects. A triangular strawberry-shaped configuration to the head is associated with trisomy 18. Spalding's sign (Fig. 3A, B) refers to overlapping of calvarial bones as the brain collapses following fetal demise. The fetal head may also become

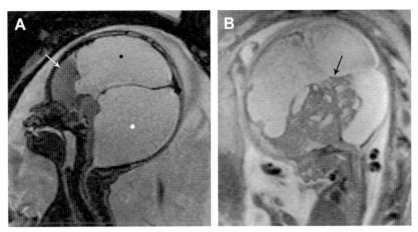

Fig. 1. Macrocephaly. (*A*) Midline sagittal image reveals an enlarged head in a fetus with alobar holoprosencephaly. A thin band of cerebral mantle (*white arrow*) is seen anteriorly, and a midline interhemispheric cyst is present (*black asterisk*). Note the large posterior fossa cyst (*white asterisk*). (*B*) Massively enlarged head seen in a different fetus secondary to a large intracranial teratoma (*black arrow*) containing both cystic and solid components.

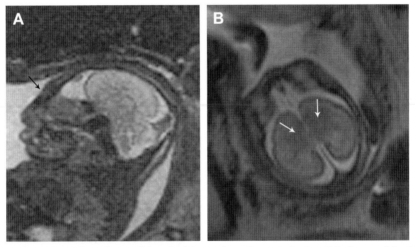

Fig. 2. Microcephaly. (*A*) Profoundly small head with resultant frontal sloping (*black arrow*) in this fetus with semilobar holoprosencephaly. (*B*) Axial image demonstrates absence of the frontal horns (*white arrows*) with only portions of the posterior lateral ventricles present.

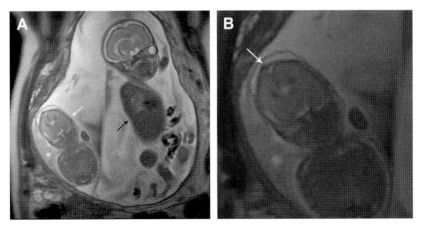

Fig. 3. Spalding sign. (*A*) Fetal demise in a twin gestation with significant size discrepancy between the small dead fetus (*white arrow*) and the normal-appearing live fetus (*black arrow*). (*B*) Overlapping of the cranial bones (*white arrow*) and subcutaneous edema are seen at the vertex of the demised twin.

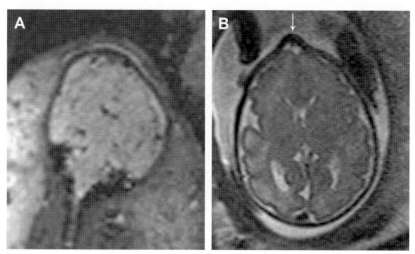

Fig. 4. Craniosynostoses. (*A*) Coronal image demonstrates abnormal asymmetric calvarial flattening secondary to unilateral coronal synostosis. (*B*) Trigonocephalic deformity of the calvarium (*white arrow*) noted in a different fetus is related to abnormal early fusion of the metopic suture. (*From* Shekdar K, Feygin T. Fetal neuroimaging. Neuroimaging Clin N Am 2011;21(3):697; with permission.)

deformed in cases of severe oligohydramnios or anhydramnios.

The craniosynostoses refer to a collection of disorders all characterized by premature fusion of 1 or more cranial sutures resulting in inhibition of calvarial growth at right angles to the fused suture (**Fig. 4**A, B). This leads to characteristic morphology of both the calvarium and the face. Both syndromal and nonsyndromal forms of craniosynostosis exist. In the context of syndromal craniosynostoses, often times other skeletal findings may help make the prenatal diagnosis.

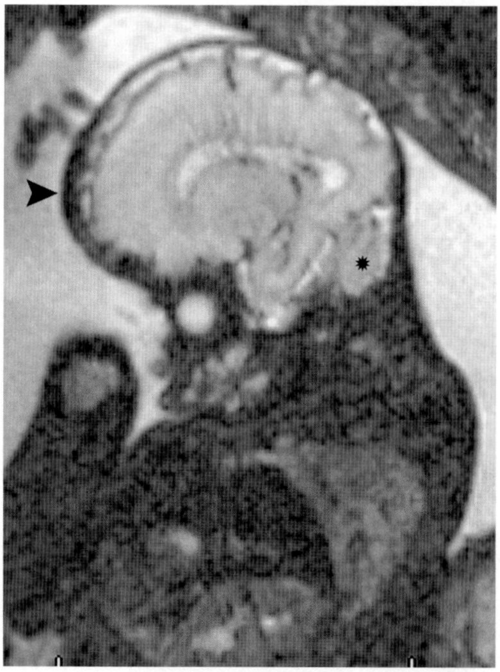

Fig. 5. Apert syndrome. Sagittal EPI image illustrates a dysmorphic skull with frontal bossing (*black arrowhead*) and a small posterior fossa (*black asterisk*). (*From* Shekdar K, Feygin T. Fetal neuroimaging. Neuroimaging Clin N Am 2011;21(3):697; with permission.)

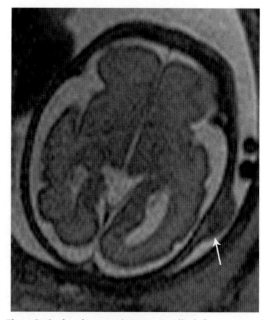

Fig. 6. Scalp hemangioma. Small left temporal scalp mass (*white arrow*) causing minimal flattening of the underlying cranium however no intracranial extension.

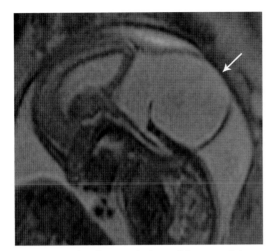

Fig. 7. Cephalocele. Herniation of intracranial contents (*white arrow*) noted through a large defect within the occipital bone.

Apert syndrome (**Fig. 5**) is a craniofacial dysostosis characterized by coronal craniosynostosis plus or minus other sutures, midface hypoplasia, and syndactyly of the hands and feet (mitten hands).[13]

SCALP MASSES

Causes of fetal scalp masses are many and varied. The most common causes include hemangioma (**Fig. 6**), lymphatic malformation, and congenital inclusion cysts. Fetal MRI plays an important role in cases where there is concern for a cephalocele both in the confirmation of the calvarial defect, which sometimes may be falsely detected on sonography due to scanning angle, as well as to define the intracranial anatomy in cases of true calvarial defects (**Fig. 7**).[14] A clue to the fact that one may be dealing with a cephalocele or an atretic cephalocele is to look for abnormalities of the venous sinus anatomy.

ABNORMAL ORBITS
Hypotelorism

Hypotelorism refers to the eyes being abnormally close together, resulting in a decreased interocular diameter (IOD: inner-to-inner margin between orbits) and binocular diameter (BOD: outer-to-outer margin of both orbits). While there are standardized measurements of interocular and binocular diameters, an easy approach to recognizing hypotelorism is that a normal IOD should roughly equal a single orbit width. Findings need to be correlated with ultrasound, which has established standardized measurements. Hypotelorism is rarely seen in isolation and is often associated with midline malformations of the brain, such as holoprosencephaly (**Fig. 8A, B**). Identifying hypotelorism on a fetal MRI should prompt one to scrutinize the intracranial contents for associated brain anomalies. Hypotelorism can also occur with other chromosomal abnormalities, syndromes, and abnormal calvarial development as described previously.[15]

Hypertelorism

Hypertelorism, or abnormally wide-set eyes, should be recognized when the IOD is larger than a single orbit width (**Fig 9**). As with hypotelorism, isolated primary hypertelorism is rare. Hypertelorism has many associations including

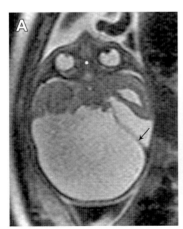

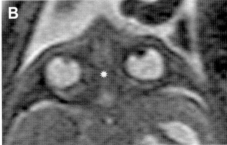

Fig. 8. Hypotelorism. (*A, B*) Decreased interocular diameter (*white asterisks*) is noted in this fetus with a large posterior fossa cyst (*black arrow*).

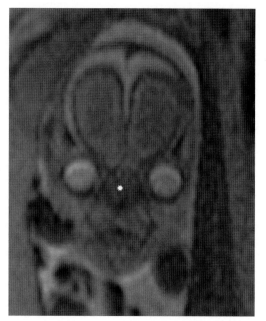

Fig. 9. Hypertelorism. Increased interocular diameter (*white asterisk*) was present in this fetus noted to have an underlying chromosomal anomaly.

craniosynostoses, anterior encephalocele, midline facial masses, and chromosomal aberrations.[15] Maternal intake of antiepileptic drugs has even been associated as a cause of hypertelorism.

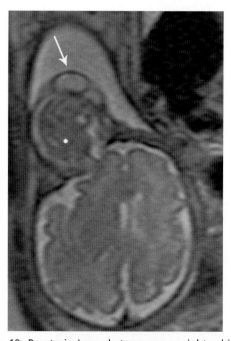

Fig. 10. Proptosis. Large heterogeneous right orbital teratoma (*white asterisk*) causing marked expansion and deformity of the right orbit as well as significant proptosis of the right globe (*white arrow*).

Proptosis

Proptosis refers to the forward displacement of the globes. The appearance of proptosis may be due to shallow orbits in association with a craniosynostosis. Rarely, proptosis may be the presenting feature of an orbital mass (**Fig. 10**) or orbital encephalocele.

Microphthalmia/Anophthalmia

Mircophthalmia is a globe that measures below the fifth percentile for gestational age. It is a feature of many conditions and is frequently seen with triploidy, trisomy 13, Aicardi syndrome, and CHARGE (coloboma, heart defects, choanal atresia, retarded growth and development, genital anomalies, and ear anomalies) association, and Walker-Warburg syndrome.[16] Anophthalmia, or an absent globe, may occur when the optic vesicle fails to form appropriately. This can be unilateral or bilateral (**Fig. 11**).

CLEFT LIP AND PALATE

Cleft lip and palate refers to failure of fusion (majority of cases) of the lip and palate segments during embryogenesis. Eighty percent of patients with a cleft lip will also have a cleft palate. Cleft lip and cleft palate represent the most common anomalies of the fetal face. There are 4 types of clefts consisting of unilateral (**Fig. 12**A–C), bilateral (**Fig. 13**), and midline (**Fig. 14**A–C), with the rate

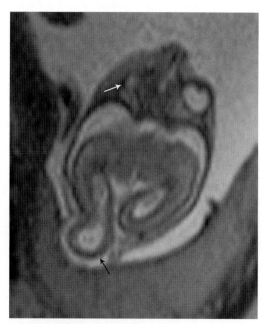

Fig. 11. Anophthalmia. Absent right optic globe (*white arrow*) in this fetus that also has an occipital cephalocele (*black arrow*).

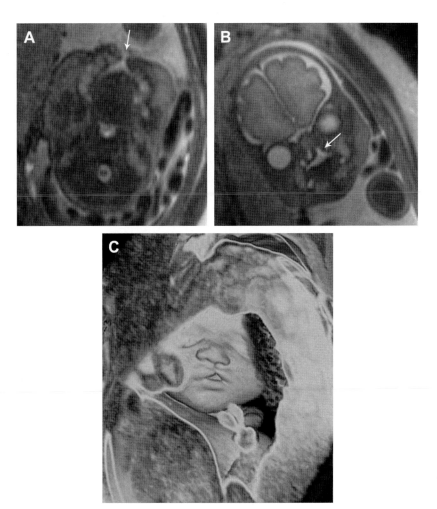

Fig. 12. Unilateral cleft lip and palate. (*A*) Axial and (*B*) coronal images reveal a unilateral left-sided defect (*white arrows*). (*C*) 3-dimensional reformatted image illustrates the deformed fetal face. (*From* Shekdar K, Feygin T. Fetal neuroimaging. Neuroimaging Clin N Am 2011;21(3):696; with permission.)

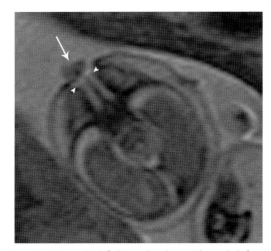

Fig. 13. Bilateral cleft lip and palate. Bilateral defects (*white arrowheads*) are present with a characteristic midline triangular tissue seen between the 2 clefts (*white arrow*).

of underlying aneuploidy increasing from types 1 through 4. The most common associated chromosomal abnormality is trisomy 13 and trisomy 18, and in these settings cleft lip/cleft palate is rarely an isolated finding.[17] Various infections and teratogens have also been implicated as the underlying etiology of this deformity.

Fetal MRI is very good at defining an amniotic fluid-filled cleft.[18] When complete, the cleft extends through the upper lip to involve the hard palate (see **Fig. 12**A, B). With its multiplanar capability, MRI is particularly useful in visualizing the posterior soft palate.[19] Unilateral cleft lip without cleft palate, as well as closely apposed cleft lip/cleft palate, can be difficult to visualize on fetal MRI. Bilateral cleft lip/cleft palate has a characteristic premaxillary protrusion on profile view resulting from elevation of the median nasal prominence. In the axial plane, a midline triangular

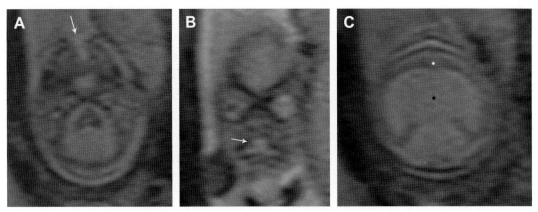

Fig. 14. Midline cleft lip and palate. (*A*) Axial and (*B*) coronal images demonstrate a wide midline defect (*white arrows*). (*C*) Note the horseshoe-shaped mantle of brain parenchyma anteriorly (*white asterisk*) and large monoventricle (*black asterisk*) in this fetus with alobar holoprosencephaly.

tissue is seen between the 2 clefts (see **Fig. 13**). Midline cleft lip/cleft palate results from medial maxillary agenesis and is often associated with midface hypoplasia. A midline defect should prompt one to carefully scrutinize the intracranial contents, as there is an increased association with holoprosencephaly (see **Fig. 14A–C**).

ABNORMAL MANDIBLE
Micrognathia

Micrognathia, a small mandible, is often seen in association with retrognathia, an abnormal position of the mandible (receding chin) (**Fig. 15**). It can be an isolated finding or may occur in a variety of conditions, such as hemifacial microsomia

(Goldenhar syndrome), Pierre Robin sequence (**Fig. 16**), and Treacher Collins syndrome.[20] Chromosomal abnormalities have been reported in as many as 66% of fetuses with micrognathia, commonly trisomy 13 and trisomy 18. Micrognathia is rarely an isolated finding and when detected on fetal MRI, it may serve as the initial clue that the fetus has an underlying syndrome or genetic abnormality. A detailed assessment for additional anomalies will help with genetic counseling for the parents. Of note, a normal-appearing mandible at 20 weeks of gestation does not exclude micrognathia, as significant mandibular growth

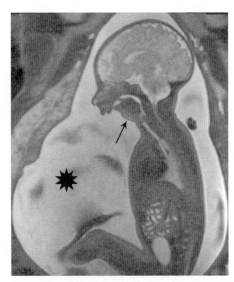

Fig. 16. Pierre-Robin sequence. Severe micrognathia (*black arrow*) impairs normal swallowing in this fetus with polyhydramnios (*black asterisk*). (*From* Shekdar K, Feygin T. Fetal neuroimaging. Neuroimaging Clin N Am 2011;21(3):696; with permission.)

Fig. 15. Micrognathia. Small and retruded mandible (*white arrow*) present with the tongue filling the small oral cavity.

occurs in the third trimester. Therefore, in younger fetuses, the mandible often appears small. In addition, asymmetrically angulated sections can give the wrong impression of a small mandible.

Micrognathia is related to a defect in the first and second branchial arches. Mandibular hypoplasia results in a small oral cavity with superior and posterior displacement of the tongue and failure of palate fusion. These children often have impaired swallowing and can present with polyhydramnios. Given the risk of airway compromise in these children, many require a scheduled delivery using the ex utero intrapartum treatment (EXIT) procedure at tertiary care centers.

Agnathia is an extremely rare malformation. It is commonly associated with microstomia (small mouth) and absent tongue.

CYSTIC LESIONS OF THE ORAL CAVITY

Cystic lesions of the fetal oral cavity are rare (**Fig. 17**A, B). They include congenital epithelial inclusion cysts, such as dermoid and epidermoid, enteric duplication cysts, and lymphatic malformations. Because of the potential airway obstruction and respiratory distress at delivery, many of these patients require the EXIT procedure.

INCREASED NUCHAL TRANSLUCENCY

The nuchal translucency (NT) reflects a sonographic measurement of the nuchal skin and subcutaneous tissue. It should be obtained in a standardized imaging plane. Nuchal thickness increases with gestational age in the normal fetus. Causes of abnormally increased NT are varied and include redundant nuchal skin, edema, lymphedema, and sometimes lymphatic malformations. An NT greater than or equal to 3 mm at 11

to 14 weeks of gestation is always abnormal and is associated with an increased risk of fetal aneuploidy, such as trisomies 21, 18, and 13, and Turner syndrome (XO).[21] It is for this reason that increased NT detected within the first trimester should warrant offering fetal karyotyping. At such early gestational age, fetal evaluations are performed with ultrasound.

MASSES OF THE FACE AND NECK
Lymphatic Malformation

Significant accumulation of lymphatic fluid within the subcutaneous spaces of the posterior neck results in a multiseptated nuchal collection. This is the most common fetal posterior cystic neck mass and is the result of failed/delayed jugular venous–lymphatic connection,[22] most appropriately termed a lymphatic malformation (**Fig. 18**A, B). In the old nomenclature, it was referred to as a cystic hygroma. Lymphatic malformations are typically located within the posterior subcutaneous tissues, although they frequently wrap around laterally and may involve only 1 side of the neck, causing postural abnormality. They can be massive, trans-spatial masses insinuating between vessels and other normal structures (**Fig. 19**A–C). Internal fluid–fluid levels containing blood products are not uncommon and are well identified on MRI.[9] Lymphatic malformations are frequently associated with fetal hydrops and as with increased NT associated with chromosomal abnormalities (**Fig. 20**A, B).

Teratomas

Teratomas are germ cell tumors, and most are composed of tissues derived from all 3 germ layers. The head and neck are the most common sites for

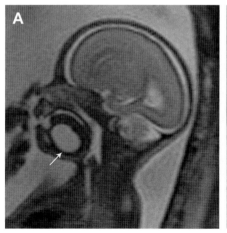
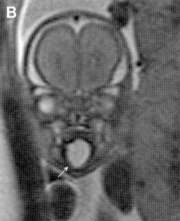

Fig. 17. Cystic lesion of the oral cavity. (*A*) Sagittal and (*B*) coronal images reveal a well-circumscribed cystic mass (*white arrows*) within the oral cavity at the floor of the mouth.

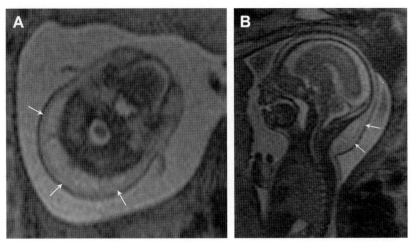

Fig. 18. Lymphatic malformation. (*A*) Axial and (*B*) sagittal images illustrate a multiseptated nuchal collection (*white arrows*) extending caudally into the lower neck.

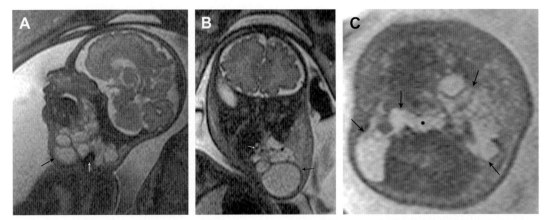

Fig. 19. Large lymphatic malformation. (*A*) Sagittal, (*B*) coronal, and (*C*) axial images demonstrate a large transspatial multicystic mass (*black arrows*) involving superficial and deep aspects of the left neck. There is involvement of the contralateral side via extension across the retropharynx (*black asterisk*). The mass encompasses and displaces major cervical vasculature, which remains patent (*white arrows*).

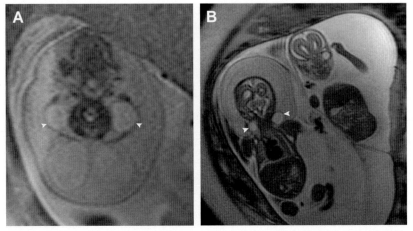

Fig. 20. Lymphatic malformation and hydrops. (*A*) Axial and (*B*) coronal images illustrate a large multicystic neck mass (*white arrowheads*) in a fetus that is part of a twin gestation. Note the associated hydrops in the fetus with the neck mass.

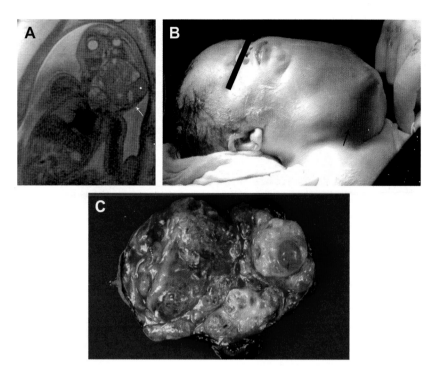

Fig. 21. Cervical teratoma. (*A*) Large, heterogeneous anterior neck mass (*white arrow*) containing solid (*white asterisk*) and cystic components. (*B*) Clinical picture (*printed with parental permission*) obtained following delivery reveals the marked neck deformity (*black arrow*). (*C*) Pathologic specimen provided following resection.

teratomas after the sacrococcygeal region. Fetal MRI is excellent in determining anatomic extent. Teratomas typically demonstrate mixed signal intensity due to their complex composition, often containing cystic and solid components as well as calcifications and hemorrhage. Calcifications are virtually pathognomonic of teratomas, and they can be recognized as areas of susceptibility on EPI.[9]

Cervical teratomas present as anterior neck masses that infiltrate the surrounding structures (**Fig. 21**A–C). They often cause hyperextension of the neck, resulting in malpresentation and dystocia precluding vaginal delivery. The EXIT procedure provides a controlled environment to secure an airway.[23]

Teratomas arising within the oral/nasal cavity or pharynx most commonly arise from the hard or soft palate. They can be large, fungating oral masses causing the jaw to be held in a fixed open position (**Fig. 22**). Polyhdramnios secondary to pharyngeal obstruction is not uncommon. Hydrops may develop with large masses. Important in the evaluation of oral teratomas is to carefully look for intracranial extension.

The orbit represents a rare location for primary teratoma development; more often it is affected secondarily by inferior growth from an intracranial teratoma. Teratomas can be particularly vascular and can parasitize blood from the brain. Orbital teratomas are characteristically massive tumors that cause severe facial deformity (**Fig. 23**A, B). In postnatal life, they present as extreme unilateral proptosis with marked stretching of the eyelids (see **Fig. 23**B).

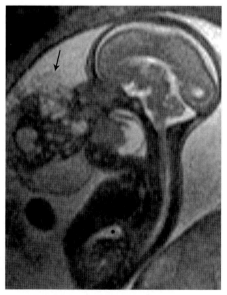

Fig. 22. Oral teratoma. Large, fungating oral mass (*black arrow*) causing the jaw to be held in a fixed open position. Note the patent aerodigestive tract with fluid in the fetal stomach (*black asterisk*).

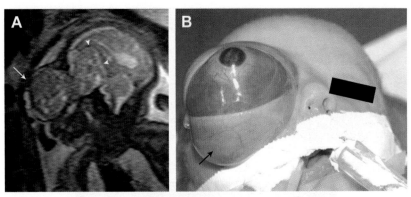

Fig. 23. Orbital teratoma. (*A*) Large, dumbbell-shaped right orbital mass (*white arrow*) with intracranial extension (*white arrowheads*). (*B*) Clinical picture (*printed with parental permission*) obtained following delivery demonstrates significant proptosis (*black arrow*).

Congenital Hemangiomas

Congenital hemangiomas (CHs) are rare vascular tumors that grow in utero, in contradistinction to infantile hemangiomas, which typically appear postnatally around 2 weeks of age.[24] Two subtypes of CH exist, the rapidly involuting CH (RICH), which usually involutes by 8 to 14 months of postnatal life, and the noninvoluting CH (NICH), which may persist into late childhood.[25,26] CHs can grow gradually or rapidly during pregnancy and on rare occasion may cause fetal heart failure, polyhydramnios, and hydrops. MRI is useful for assessing size, location, and internal characteristics. CHs are usually large, well-circumscribed solid masses with prominent arterial and venous flow (**Fig. 24**A, B). Heterogeneous flow voids may be noted on T2W imaging or EPI.[27] It is because of their heterogeneity that they may appear similar to teratomas.

GOITER

Fetal goiter may be due to maternal hyper- or hypothyroidism. In the hyperthyroid state, maternal thyroid-stimulating antibodies cross the placenta and stimulate the fetal thyroid. In the hypothyroid state, fetal thyroid enlargement is most commonly due to maternal antithyroid medication or endemic iodine deficiency.[28] Rarely, fetal thyromegaly may be the result of inborn errors of thyroid metabolism. On MRI, fetal goiter presents as an anterior neck mass that is characteristically homogeneously hyperintense on T1W imaging due to the intrinsic iodine content (**Fig. 25**).[29] Fetal goiter may obstruct swallowing or compress the trachea, resulting in polyhydramnios and airway compromise at birth, necessitating the EXIT procedure. Intrauterine growth restriction is common. Skeletal maturation may be accelerated or delayed depending on the underlying etiology for thyroid enlargement,

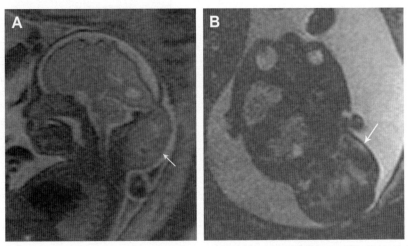

Fig. 24. Hemangioma. (*A*) Sagittal and (*B*) axial images reveal a large, well-circumscribed, posterior neck mass (*white arrows*) with mild distortion and flattening of the underlying calvarium.

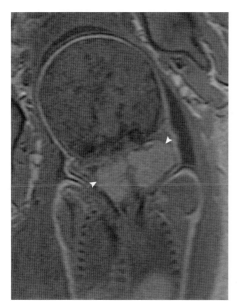

Fig. 25. Goiter. Coronal T1-weighted image demonstrates an enlarged, homogeneously hyperintense thyroid gland (*white arrowheads*).

maternal hyperthyroidism, or hypothyroidism, respectively. It should be noted that fetal goiter can occur even in the maternal euthyroid state.

SUMMARY

MRI has become a standard tool in the armamentarium of radiologists in working up suspected fetal head and neck pathology, providing a supplement to sonography in helping to guide diagnosis and management. Advances in fetal medicine and surgery have further solidified MRI's role in the field of prenatal imaging.

REFERENCES

1. Dinh D, Wright R, Hanigan W. The use of magnetic resonance imaging for the diagnosis of fetal intracranial anomalies. Childs Nerv Syst 1990;6(4): 212–5.
2. Levine D, Barnes PD, Madsen JR, et al. Fetal central nervous system anomalies: MR imaging augments sonographic diagnosis. Radiology 1997; 204(3):635–42.
3. Kathary N, Bulas DI, Newman KD, et al. MRI imaging of fetal neck masses with airway compromise: utility in delivery planning. Pediatr Radiol 2001;31(10):727–31.
4. Stevens GH, Schoot BC, Smets MJ, et al. The ex utero intrapartum treatment (EXIT) procedure in fetal neck masses: a case report and review of the literature. Eur J Obstet Gynecol Reprod Biol 2002;100(2): 246–50.
5. Poutamo J, Vanninen R, Partanen K, et al. Magnetic resonance imaging supplements ultrasonographic imaging of the posterior fossa, pharynx and neck in malformed fetuses. Ultrasound Obstet Gynecol 1999;13(5):327–34.
6. Schwartz JL, Crooks LE. NMR imaging produces no observable mutations or cytotoxicity in mammalian cells. AJR Am J Roentgenol 1982;139(3):583–5.
7. Thomas A, Morris PG. The effects of NMR exposure on living organisms. I. A microbial assay. Br J Radiol 1981;54(643):615–21.
8. Baker PN, Johnson IR, Harvey PR, et al. A three-year follow-up of children imaged in utero with echo-planar magnetic resonance. Am J Obstet Gynecol 1994;170(1 Pt 1):32–3.
9. Simon EM, Goldstein RB, Coakley FV, et al. Fast MR imaging of fetal CNS anomalies in utero. AJNR Am J Neuroradiol 2000;21(9):1688–98.
10. American College of Radiology (ACR), Society for Pediatric Radiology (SPR). ACR-SPR practice guideline for the safe and optimal performance of fetal magnetic resonance imaging (MRI). Reston (VA): American College of Radiology (ACR); 2010. Available at: http://www.acr.org/SecondaryMainMenu Categories/quality_safety/guidelines/pediatric/Fetal-MRI.aspx. Accessed May 15, 2012.
11. Runge VM. Safety of approved MR contrast media for intravenous injection. J Magn Reson Imaging 2000;12(2):205–13.
12. Shekdar K, Feygin T. Fetal neuroimaging. Neuroimaging Clin N Am 2011;21(3):677–703.
13. Hansen WF, Rijsinghani A, Grant S, et al. Prenatal diagnosis of Apert syndrome. Fetal Diagn Ther 2004;19(2):127–30.
14. Lau TK, Leung TN, Leung TY, et al. Fetal scalp cysts: challenge in diagnosis and counseling. J Ultrasound Med 2001;20(2):175–7.
15. Trout T, Budorick NE, Pretorius DH, et al. Significance of orbital measurements in the fetus. J Ultrasound Med 1994;13(12):937–43.
16. Babcook C. The fetal face and neck. Philadelphia: W.B. Saunders; 2000.
17. Merritt L. Part 1. Understanding the embryology and genetics of cleft lip and palate. Adv Neonatal Care 2005;5(2):64–71.
18. Stroustrup Smith A, Estroff JA, Barnewolt CE, et al. Prenatal diagnosis of cleft lip and cleft palate using MRI. AJR Am J Roentgenol 2004;183(1):229–35.
19. Ghi T, Tani G, Savelli L, et al. Prenatal imaging of facial clefts by magnetic resonance imaging with emphasis on the posterior palate. Prenat Diagn 2003;23(12):970–5.
20. Bromley B, Benacerraf BR. Fetal micrognathia: associated anomalies and outcome. J Ultrasound Med 1994;13(7):529–33.
21. Pandya PP, Kondylios A, Hilbert L, et al. Chromosomal defects and outcome in 1015 fetuses with

increased nuchal translucency. Ultrasound Obstet Gynecol 1995;5(1):15–9.

22. von Kaisenberg CS, Nicolaides KH, Brand-Saberi B. Lymphatic vessel hypoplasia in fetuses with Turner syndrome. Humanit Rep 1999;14(3):823–6.

23. Bouchard S, Johnson MP, Flake AW, et al. The EXIT procedure: experience and outcome in 31 cases. J Pediatr Surg 2002;37(3):418–26.

24. Marler JJ, Fishman SJ, Upton J, et al. Prenatal diagnosis of vascular anomalies. J Pediatr Surg 2002; 37(3):318–26.

25. Boon LM, Enjolras O, Mulliken JB. Congenital hemangioma: evidence of accelerated involution. J Pediatr 1996;128(3):329–35.

26. Enjolras O, Mulliken JB, Boon LM, et al. Noninvoluting congenital hemangioma: a rare cutaneous vascular anomaly. Plast Reconstr Surg 2001;107(7): 1647–54.

27. Robson CD, Barnewolt CE. MR imaging of fetal head and neck anomalies. Neuroimaging Clin N Am 2004; 14(2):273–91.

28. Radetti G, Zavallone A, Gentili L, et al. Foetal and neonatal thyroid disorders. Minerva Pediatr 2002; 54(5):383–400.

29. Karabulut N, Martin DR, Yang M, et al. MR imaging findings in fetal goiter caused by maternal graves disease. J Comput Assist Tomogr 2002;26(4): 538–40.

Index

Note: Page numbers of article titles are in **boldface** type.

Moving?

Make sure your subscription moves with you!

To notify us of your new address, find your **Clinics Account Number** (located on your mailing label above your name), and contact customer service at:

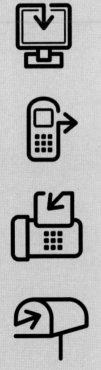

Email: journalscustomerservice-usa@elsevier.com

800-654-2452 (subscribers in the U.S. & Canada)
314-447-8871 (subscribers outside of the U.S. & Canada)

Fax number: 314-447-8029

Elsevier Health Sciences Division
Subscription Customer Service
3251 Riverport Lane
Maryland Heights, MO 63043

*To ensure uninterrupted delivery of your subscription, please notify us at least 4 weeks in advance of move.

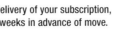